W9-CIR-675

CHILDBIRTH WITHOUT FEAR

*the text of this book is printed
on 100% recycled paper*

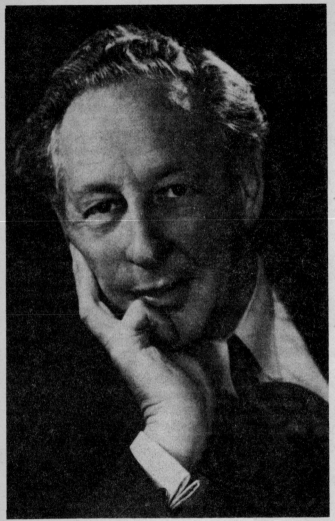

Grantly Dick-Read, M.D.

Prager

CHILDBIRTH WITHOUT FEAR

*The Original Approach to
Natural Childbirth*

GRANTLY DICK-READ, M.D.

NEW FOURTH EDITION

Revised and Edited by

Helen Wessel and Harlan F. Ellis, M.D.

PERENNIAL LIBRARY
Harper & Row, Publishers
New York, Hagerstown, San Francisco, London

CHILDBIRTH WITHOUT FEAR: THE ORIGINAL APPROACH TO NATURAL CHILD-
BIRTH. New Fourth Edition. Copyright 1944, 1953 by Grantly Dick-Read.
Renewed 1972 by Jessica Dick-Read Bennett. Copyright © 1959, 1972 by
Jessica Dick-Read. All rights reserved. Printed in the United States of
America. No part of this book may be used or reproduced in any manner
whatsoever without written permission except in the case of brief quotations
embodied in critical articles and reviews. For information address Harper &
Row, Publishers, Inc., 10 East 53d Street, New York, N.Y. 10022. Published
simultaneously in Canada by Fitzhenry & Whiteside Limited, Toronto.

First PERENNIAL LIBRARY edition published 1979.

ISBN: 0-06-080490-4

79 80 81 82 83 10 9 8 7 6 5 4 3 2

Contents

Acknowledgments xiii

Foreword xv

Preface xix

Part I

THE PRINCIPLES OF NATURAL CHILDBIRTH

1. Childbirth as a Natural Process 3

2. Mental Imagery 13
   Sources of Imagery
   Historical and Religious Influences
   Ancient Practices and Pagan Religions
   The Middle Ages
   The Sixteenth and Seventeenth Centuries
   The Last Hundred Years
   Natural Law
   A New Look

3. Education in Pregnancy 37

4. The Conduct of Labor 52
   Onset of Labor (Elation)
   To the Maternity Nurse
   First Stage of Labor (Relaxation)
   The Transition
   Anesthetics and Analgesics

Second Stage of Labor (Amnesia)
Crowning
Third Stage of Labor (Exaltation)

5. Childbirth and the Family   81
The Husband
Mother-Baby
The Home

6. Childbirth in Perspective, Harlan Ellis, M.D.   103
What is Natural Childbirth?
Natural Childbirth and Pain
Natural Childbirth and Relaxation
Natural Childbirth and the Husband
Natural Childbirth and the Hospital
Natural Childbirth: A Team Effort
Natural Childbirth: A Continuum
Natural Childbirth: The Problems
Natural Childbirth: Special Benefits
Natural Childbirth: A Challenge
    To Make Childbirth an Emotionally Positive Event
    To Discourage Separation of Mother and Newborn
    To Update Standard Orthodox Prenatal Care
The Newborn Potential
    Physical Potential
    Mental Potential
    Emotional Potential
Natural Childbirth: An Ideal Program
    Personnel
        The Obstetrician and His Prenatal Office Staff
        *The Hospital and the Staff of the Hospital
            Maternity Ward*
    *The Natural Childbirth and Family-Centered
        Maternity Care Program*
    Classes in Early Pregnancy
    Classes in Late Pregnancy
    Postpartum Hospital Classes
Natural Childbirth: An Ideal Example

Conclusion
Bibliographical References for Chapter 6

     Part II

THE PRACTICE OF NATURAL CHILDBIRTH

7. Prenatal Health   147
   Diet
   Clothing
   Personal Hygiene

8. Education   152
   Fertilization
   Development of the Human Baby
   The Uterus During Pregnancy
   The Muscle Layers of the Uterus
   Fear-Tension-Pain
   Hospital Tour

9. Breathing   162
   Full Deep Breathing
   "Work" Breathing
   "Sleep" Breathing
   Breath-holding
   Rapid Breathing

10. Relaxation   168
   Preparation for Relaxation
   Recognizing Tension
   Practicing Relaxation
   Breathing
   Positions for Relaxation
   Residual Tension

11. Physical Fitness   184
   Posture
   Exercises
     Pelvic Rock
     Squatting, with variations

Firming the Breasts
Labor Position
Firming Pelvic Floor Muscles

12. Labor (First-Stage Labor)   196
   Onset of Labor
   Early First-Stage Labor
   Late First-Stage Labor
      Position
      Breathing
      Relaxation
      Discomfort
   Transition
   Summary of First-Stage Labor

13. Birth (Second-Stage Labor)   211
   Early Second-Stage Labor
      The Husband
      Position
   Well-Established Second-Stage Labor
      Breathing
      Relaxation
      Anesthesia
   Birth
   Summary of Second-Stage Labor

14. Immediate Newborn Period (Third-Stage Labor)   225
   Addendum: Instructions on the Immediate Routine
            Care of the Newborn

15. Natural Childbirth in Emergency   234

16. Care of the Newborn   240
   Body Contact
   Colostrum
   Feeding on Demand
   Baby's Perfect Food
   Rooming-In
   Addendum: Infant Care in the Nursery
              Suggested Rooming In Procedures

17. The New Mother   251
    Afterpains
    Lochia
    Care of the Nipples
    Breastfeeding
    Rooming-In
    Diet
    Postnatal Exercises
        Breathing
        Firming Pelvic Floor
        Firming Abdominal Muscles
        Firming the Breasts
        Pelvic Rock
        Conclusion

        Part III

THE PIONEER OF NATURAL CHILDBIRTH

18. Early Impressions   263

19. Prophet Without Honor   282

20. Man Without a Country   300

21. The Women of Africa   313

22. Some Misunderstandings   324

23. American Tour   333

24. In Conclusion   354

        Part IV

THE PHYSIOLOGY OF CHILDBIRTH

25. The Physiology of Childbirth   362
    Structure of the Uterus and Birth Canal
        The Uterus
        The Cervix Uteri
        The Vaginal Canal

x   CONTENTS

    The Vulva
   Automatic Contraction of the Uterus
    Nerve Supply of Uterus, Vagina and Vulva
    Factors Relevant to Nerve Supply
    Pain
   Influences of Emotion Upon Labor
    The Mechanics of Fear
    Mechanics of Dilatation
   Bibliographical References for Chapter 25

Epilogue: Pioneers Pass On, Jessica Dick-Read   392

APPENDIX

Glossary of Terms for Lay Readers   397

Sources of Information   401

Sources of Supplies   403

Bibliography   404
   Pregnancy and Childbirth
   Related Subjects
   Films

Index   409

Illustrations

GRANTLY DICK-READ FRONTISPIECE

1. Position for early second stage   109
2–5. Husband massaging back   110–111
6–7. Husband giving emotional support   115
8. Husband and newborn   115
9–10. Inverted chair as backrest   119
Infant warmer in background   119
11–12. Giving birth on birth table without stirrups   120
13. Baby kept horizontal after birth   121
14. Maternal newborn closeness   121
15. Walking to room after giving birth   122
16. Full-term infant in uterus   156
17–19. Muscle layers of the uterus   159
20–21. Quiet diaphragmatic breathing   165
22–23. Learning relaxation   174
24–25. Husband checking relaxation   175
26. Reclining chair position   180
27–28. Relaxing in left lateral position   180, 181
29. Husband checking relaxation   181
30–31. Relaxation in pregnancy and labor   182
32–33. Pelvic rocking   188
34. Squatting   189
35–36. Squatting, variation a   189
37–38. Squatting, variations b, c   190
39. Sitting Indian style   191

40. Firming the breasts   191
41–42. Second-stage pushing, practice and real   192
43–44. Second-stage resting, practice and real   193
45–46. Arrival at hospital in labor   198
47–49. First-stage labor   201
50–53. In labor with twins   203
54–56. Early second-stage in labor room   213
57. Husband scrubbing before accompanying wife
        to birth room   215
58. Accompanying wife to birth room   215
59. Resting against backrest in birth room
        (in labor with twins)   215
60. Bearing down in second-stage labor   217
61. Resting between contractions   217
62. Baby's head born   223
63. Baby's body emerges   223
64. Physician showing baby to mother   227
65. Proud parents admiring newborn   227
66. Physician showing placenta   229
67. Physician showing membranes   229
68. Twins!   231
69. Walking to room after giving birth to twins   231
70–72. Skin-to-skin contact   242, 243

Acknowledgments

Our special thanks are given to the following persons
for their cooperation in the preparation of this edition:

Jessica Dick-Read Bennett for her encouragement,
and for her help in obtaining copies of Dr. Dick-Read's
other books and manuscripts;

Harold E. Grove for his confidence, advice, and
patience in helping work out the many details involved
in such a project as this;

Gary Davis, Fireside Portraits, for the long hours he
spent taking photographs to demonstrate the various
points that were needed to amplify the text;

The central California couples who so willingly
served as models for the pictures, both while in training for their own natural childbirth babies and at the
time of birth;

The Sierra Community Hospital, for its full cooperation in developing a natural childbirth program, and for
their patience with all the extra photography needed
for this book.

Our long-suffering children and spouses, who patiently accepted the many intrusions of camera and
typewriter into the normal household routines.

H. W., H. E.

Foreword

It has been over fifty years since Grantly Dick-Read (1890–1959) first prepared a monograph on his carefully developed philosophy of childbirth. At that time, the concept of childbirth as a positive experience, free from suffering, was a shocking and revolutionary idea, unacceptable to many, for almost all women in labor were delivered under deep anesthesia.

But he was not to be deterred from the truth he had discovered, and the intervening years have proven the validity of his teaching. In the 1920s he not only defied tradition by educating his women patients for labor and birth, but even set up classes for their husbands as well. Today the concept of prenatal education for both husbands and wives, no longer controversial, is widely adopted.

But Grantly Dick-Read was a man out of step with his time in many other important ways, in addition to his approach to childbearing. He was one of those who set the pace for succeeding generations, and in the years since his death social changes in the world have brought to public attention the importance of many of the things he was advocating during his lifetime.

Among his "heretical" ideas were his outspokenness against environmental pollution, as well as against the "pollution" of people's minds by false fears and their bodies by drugs. His approach to obstetrics was fastidiously scientific, but he also brought to bear upon it an interdisciplinary interest, relating psychology, sociology, and anthropology to his studies in physiology and the natural sciences. He continually emphasized the importance of treating the patient as a whole person, and not just concentrating upon a physical mechanism within her body.

In order to limit his practice to obstetrics, he entered group practice at a time when it was such a new concept that it created an outcry. He shocked many people with his proposals that teen-agers should be taught such important matters as sex, reproduction, and family life in the schools.

He was a man "against the establishment," not opposing it arbitrarily, but continually questioning the maintenance of the status quo at the expense of creativity and truth. He spoke out against the futility of cold scientism, materialism, and social prestige at the expense of an awareness of human relationships and metaphysical realities.

He was vocal in expressing the equality of the black man as a human being, and the need the white man has to learn from the lore of black history and wisdom.

None of these views made him popular with many of his contemporaries!

Then, at the height of his successful obstetric practice, at forty years of age, Grantly Dick-Read wrote a book that was to change the course of obstetric history. He had proven from his own experiences as a physician his belief that childbirth is a natural physiological process not meant to be painful, and because he had built his teaching around a study of the "laws of nature," he chose for his book the title *Natural Childbirth*. He had not the faintest notion that this book title would be taken as a "name" for this kind of childbirth experience! Indeed, though often misunderstood, the term became a household word everywhere, for when the book was published, in 1933, Grantly Dick-Read rose from the relative obscurity of a local medical practice into a target for the ire or praise of people all over the world. The rest of his life followed the course of such great medical pioneers as Simpson, Semmelweis, Lister, Pasteur, and many others who were rejected by their contemporaries but whose teachings nevertheless became the foundation stones for future medical progress.

Grantly Dick-Read did not envision his teaching on childbirth as an "end" to discovery, but as a true foundation from which many further discoveries could be made. He was not afraid to challenge tradition by asking the disturbing question, "Why?" If he were here today, he would encourage the young people of the 1970s to keep on asking questions, to keep on challenging tradition, to keep on testing current medical practices and theories, including his own, for validity. All those who share his faith in the consistency and orderliness of natural law, which we disregard at our own peril, will continue in the search for truth.

Helen Wessel
Harlan Ellis, M.D.

1972

Preface

There has been no subject during recent years that has claimed so much attention as obstetrics. Learned societies have invited lectures and discussions upon its practice and teaching, and committees have been set up by the government for the purpose of investigating maternal and infant mortality. Medical journals have published a vast amount of literature concerning the abnormalities and complications of childbirth, while the lay press rarely misses an opportunity to bring before the public any information upon the subject that can be gleaned from the transactions of the societies and associations of the medical profession. Vast improvement has resulted in both knowledge and technique, but, unhappily, statistics have not shown a relatively pronounced advance upon those of ten or fifteen years ago.

An effort has been made in the following pages to regard childbirth from a different angle. A large percentage of the dangers and complications can be avoided by careful prenatal observation and instruction. An exact knowledge of the shape and size of the pelvis, and of the position and development of the fetus, prevents problems because such knowledge leads to the application of correct treatment.

But it is generally agreed that one of the most important

This Preface first appeared in the original edition of *Natural Childbirth* in 1933 (London: Heinemann, Publishers). The editors include it here because its accuracy and relevancy after forty years is most remarkable.

factors in the production of complicated labor, and therefore of maternal and infant mortality, is the inability of obstetricians to stand by and allow the natural and uninterrupted course of labor. It may be an excess of zeal, or anxiety born of ignorance, but it is an unquestionable fact that interference is still one of the greatest dangers with which both mother and child have to contend.

But there is another aspect of interference, and it should not be attributed, without careful consideration, to any motives other than those of misdirected kindness. Forceps are frequently applied at the beginning of the second stage under the misapprehension that it is neither modern nor moral to allow the woman to continue in her suffering. To the same end, anesthetics of various sorts are given without an accurate knowledge of their effect upon the mechanism—muscular, nervous, and circulatory.

It is not fully realized that the majority of "pelvic" invalids suffer from the mistaken application of human sympathy. But it is equally obvious that *if there is suffering, it should be allayed.***** Therefore the problem arises: how can prolonged suffering be prevented or stopped without the risk of injury to the mother or child? For which is the greater immorality, to allow an agonizing labor or to injure mother, child, or both?†

It becomes clear that the solution to this problem lies in an investigation of pain. In certain chapters that follow, the various influences to which cultured women are subjected have been considered, and the whole question of pain reviewed from the point of view of both the phylogeny and ontogeny of the species.

A new attitude toward childbirth has been evolved, and deductions upon which treatment is based made from the premises of experience, and the results have been gratifying.

It must not be presumed that a full understanding is obtained by simply recognizing the principles; their application will require greater patience from the scientist and the aca-

---

* Italics added.
† Correction of one does not necessarily correct the other!—Ed.

demically minded physician than from those whose conception of this doctoring is unhampered by the ever-present bugbear of abnormality.

Had it not been for the enthusiasm of those who have accepted this teaching, these pages would not have appeared in print. It must not be presumed that any claim is made to invariable success: where there are anatomical abnormalities, the operative procedure of modern obstetrics is unhesitatingly resorted to; and again, abnormal conditions of the mother's mind may impair its sensibility and receptivity.

The first and most obvious benefit that results from the care of the mother psychical as well as the mother physical is the natural perfection of labor, and the almost complete absence of many of the complications of the second and third stages.

Perhaps a feature that is even more pleasing is the happiness of motherhood, and the manner in which both mother and baby thrive following the birth.

If, in spite of all, there is pain, it should be immediately overcome. Painless labor is the greatest gift that our profession can make to humanity, but if painless labor is obtained at the cost of the integrity of the function, it becomes a choice between two evils.

Childbirth is the perfection of womanhood, and the beautifying of the maternal conscience is one of its most acceptable rewards, not only for the mother herself, but for her home, the community, and the nation. Thousands of women today have their babies born under what are known as modern humanitarian conditions—they are the first to disclaim any knowledge of the beauties of childbirth, they are the first to tell the doctor how easy it is for a man to be enthusiastic—but those who have known all and suffered little are not slow to sympathize with mere man in that he can never know the joy that is the reward of natural reproduction.

Grantly Dick-Read, M.D.

1933

THE PRINCIPLES OF NATURAL CHILDBIRTH

Grantly Dick-Read first published *Childbirth Without Fear* in the United States with the subtitle "The Principles and Practice of Natural Childbirth." For this current edition, in an attempt to bring to the reader the best of his teaching in a comprehensive overview, we have gathered all his writings on the subject over the years and extracted the most vital parts.

Part I presents the basic philosophical principles upon which his teaching is best carried out. For a contemporary evaluation of this subject, readers are invited to turn first to Chapter 6, "Childbirth in Perspective."

Grantly Dick-Read's principles of prophylactic or physiological childbirth, as he named his teaching in the 1920s and 1930s, have a carefully thought-out scientific base. The physiological and functional facts that form the basis for these preventive principles are outlined in Chapter 25, "The Physiology of Childbirth," the material for which is compiled from his earlier, more medically oriented writings, never before published in the United States. Readers interested in a more detailed scientific study of the physiology of natural childbirth are invited to examine this chapter.

1

Childbirth as a Natural Process

We cannot think of motherhood only in terms of its satisfactory completion. We must look back into the life of a young woman and consider the thoughts and experiences that eventually lead her to become a mother. We need not delve into that experimental playground of psychologists popularly known as the "sex life." We have only to recall the normal sequence of events every healthy-minded girl and young woman of our time goes through. At an early age she learns all the happiness of love; it is an emotional development that radiates from a young girl. It will often be found that in her untrained and undifferentiated affection life holds some joys too deep and too unfathomable for her to understand. This irresistible urge to love is so mysterious that my daughter, when fifteen years of age, wrote to me from school:

I wish you could explain to me why I feel as I do this term; it has never been like it before. I am so deliriously happy. There is no reason that I know of, but I am fond of everybody. I seem to see the good in them, and want to *think* lovely things, as if I were possessed of a heavenly spirit making me so much better than my real self.

And so, with every girl in varying degrees this power which will rule her life begins to develop at an early age, until in due course she finds herself in love, and here her emotional life becomes concentrated, with all its thrills, its joys, and its anxieties, upon one semi-divine individual. It is the spiritual refinement of her own ideal, and in the normal course of events she becomes engaged, but unwilling to believe that there are others who are equally fortunate, and blissfully ignorant of the fact that she is but an instrument in the design of nature. Eventually she marries, and if all goes well she conceives and prepares to bear her child.

The average woman associates all that is beautiful in her life with this series of events. It is the implementation of the power of life by the universal forces that govern all things to the end that the human race shall survive. From earliest girlhood, each forward step in this progression is made because of a desire to bring her joy or a fuller realization of her dreams. The law of life does not beat a woman on by either fear or physical necessity, but attracts her to develop by the presentation of increasingly beautiful experiences, which she is not slow to grasp. Love may be beset by anxieties and doubts, but of itself it stimulates all the noblest and greatest qualities by which human nature is characterized at its best. It is the greatest power in the world, and without it the races of mankind would be finished in a few generations.

When the time comes for giving birth, each woman must be treated according to her understanding. Childbirth is divided into three definite stages by signs and symptoms. The first stage is not just the opening of the outlet of the uterus; it presents certain features of the process of labor, all of which can be shown to be purposeful. Where education has been satisfactory and the beginning of labor can be seen as a joyful prelude to her child's arrival, a woman is conscious of each uterine contraction as a promise of her highest ambition. Elation, rejoicing, and a strong sense of contentment and relief are the natural emotional reactions to the onset of labor.

I use the term "elation" in its strict meaning. It is not a simple happiness, but an exaltation of the mind resulting from the feeling of success and pride in the confident approach of the reward of pregnancy. Many women become conscious of their own importance at this time, and the strong instinct of self-assertion may be observed. Such women will telephone their friends, and many will advertise widely to the world the fact that at last the great moment has come. This is a time when doctors are not often with their patients, but a doctor may detect this elation when a woman who does not fear labor calls on the telephone when she thinks she has begun labor. She will say, with a cheerful spirit, "I think I have started. Isn't that great?" or, "Things are happening—I am so thankful." This emotional state was described to me by a vivacious, intelligent girl in simple yet dramatic words.

"I have never known such a sense of joy," she said. "I walked out into the garden; I felt an irresistible desire to parade myself. I made a point of going to speak to the gardener. I told the chauffeur to be ready to go out in the car at any moment. I have no idea why, but it seemed as near as I could reasonably go to telling him that my baby was coming. I walked down the drive and up and down the road for five or ten minutes, feeling in the back of my mind a hope that I should meet some of my friends. My time had come, my baby was on its way—after all it was true. I believe now that I actually exaggerated my shape."

This is only one example of many instances that have been told to me. Although few women will volunteer, without questioning or an inquiry being made, to describe the profoundly stimulating emotions that accompany the onset of labor when complete confidence in its outcome dispels all fear, most women do not hesitate to say they are glad when their baby is coming at last.

To all nurses, mothers, doctors, and husbands, I say: Do nothing to destroy the cheerful courage and confidence of the woman who has begun labor with her mind in that state; bury your own anxiety and fear and share with her the spirit of victory about to be achieved. You will thereby assist in paving the way for her progress to uncomplicated motherhood and ward off the greatest enemy to her neuromuscular perfection.

There are few greater obstetric crimes than to become a serious busybody who demands compliance with illogical and baseless conservative principles, requesting silence, speaking in whispers, parading a mass of so-called essentials ready to deal with all emergencies. The kindly sympathy and word of warning advice are disturbing to a happy woman who sees only the impending joy of her child's arrival, and believes it will come quickly and easily. Elation is an emotional state, but it has profound physical manifestations; it is not only a part of the reward of childbirth, it is a phenomenon of which nature, to facilitate the safe reproduction of her species, takes most subtle advantage.

The first stage of labor demands peaceful relaxation, quiet assurance, and the ignoring mentally of what is going on in the womb, or *uterus*. Any effort actively to assist first-stage contractions will defeat its own ends. The secret of rapid opening of the outlet (the *cervix*) of the uterus is to allow the skeletal muscles to become limp and thus let the uterus work by itself. The more relaxed and unresisting both the abdominal muscles and the muscles of the pelvic floor below the uterus are, so much more easily can each uterine contraction pull the cervix over the baby's head and press the head gently down into the birth canal. If the woman's muscles outside the uterus are tensed and rigid—as they will be if, for example she grabs something tightly with her hands, resisting the contraction—this will tighten the circular muscles of the cervix. This creates in the uterus the need to work harder to push the baby out, and causes pain.

Relaxation must be recognized as a necessary phenomenon of natural labor, and it should be accompanied by an alienation of the mind from any active interest in the uterine function. How often have I said, "You can do nothing to help yet—allow your uterus to get on with its work undisturbed by your inquisitive interest. If you interfere it will resent it, and hurt you." Almost invariably that advice, when acted upon, results in the relief of pain and discomfort caused unwittingly by efforts to assist.

But even if efficient relaxation is practiced, there is always the possibility of a few relatively painful contractions at the end of the first stage—the final dilation of the cervical canal. On many occasions I have formed the opinion that the only true pains of normal labor, if present at all, are the last few contractions that completely dilate the cervix. When this discomfort is recognized and its significance appreciated, a woman may confidently be asked to put up with about six or eight such contractions. The reaction to such a request is almost invariably an easy compliance. "If it is only six or eight, I don't mind, but I thought it might be going on and getting worse all the time now." And so it proves true; this short phase passes into the more definite but completely different second stage. The discomfort of the end of the first stage lifts, either gradually or suddenly, depending upon the mode of onset of the bearing-down reflex.

I have in mind a nurse who attended cases with me until she herself was seven months pregnant. About two weeks after her baby boy was born I had an opportunity to ask her in detail what she thought about the whole process. We discussed at length everything that had happened during her pregnancy and labor. She had closely followed my teaching, which she had seen practiced in the maternity home, and her final judgment was that she could not understand why some women made such a fuss about having a baby. At one point only— and then for a very few contractions—was she in discomfort, but other than that the whole thing, as she put it, was an exciting and marvelous experience.

As the second stage becomes fully established, acquired social habits and manners are thrown off. The woman becomes aware of the conscious effort demanded of her to help, so far as possible, in the expulsion of her child. She is engrossed in her task, concentrating upon the all-important occupation of the moment. When the muscular effort ceases, her mind and body relax and she passes into a restful, sleepy state, sometimes into a deep, snoring slumber. This condition of complete alienation from other thoughts and associations either causes or passes into a state of amnesia and partial anesthesia; the perception is dulled and the interpretation of stimuli through the normal channels is clouded. She rests peacefully, arousing only to work with each contraction.

I cannot lay too much stress upon the necessity for recognizing this *amnesiac state,* and the changes in perception, interpretation, and reaction that accompany it. If control is removed from a mind that is undisturbed and confident, a quiet peace remains, a fact best demonstrated by the relative absence of discomfort when a woman retains both confidence and courage. "Hard work, yes—the hardest work I have ever known," was the comment of a fearless woman. The physical reactions to the emotional state in the second stage must be more clearly understood if interference is to be avoided in normal labor.

Take, for another example, the grunting moans during a second-stage contraction. In a natural, uncomplicated labor they vary, not only according to the strength of the woman's muscular activity, but according to her emotional state, and they have no association with physical pain. The large majority of undrugged and fully informed women have very little if any discomfort with second-stage contractions, but a deal of hard work. Their grunts and moans are like those of a man who pulls successfully upon a rope, the physical strain at the utmost. His determination adds to the violence of his effort; when he relaxes, it is with a groan of satisfaction and relief that he may rest in preparation for the next pull, and having rested he is ready for a renewal of his exertion. So he struggles in the sure confidence of victory until at last his objective is attained, and according to his valuation of the prize, so is the joy with which he hails success. His contortions have not been accompanied by physical agony, though his facial expression may well have represented it. His groans have been physiological, for our bodies abhor a sudden change of tension and most of all a sudden drop of intra-abdominal pressure. The diaphragm must be gradually released and the muscles of the chest slowly relaxed from the strain of their rigidity. There is nothing to cause purely physical pain, but the partial closure of the larynx, which produces the grunt, groan, or long-drawn-out moan, is a part of the design for safety after effort.

There is yet one more observation upon the natural anesthesia and analgesia of the second stage. The stretching of the *vulva* (external genitals) just before the baby is born is felt as a burning sensation. But this is temporary, and the actual passage of the baby through the vulva is often accomplished with so little sensation that the woman is with difficulty persuaded her baby has arrived; until she sees or hears it she is unwilling to believe it is born. In a natural labor the *perineum,* the area between the vulva and the anus, is practically insensitive.

It is my custom to lift up the crying child, even before the cord is cut, so that the mother may see "with her own eyes" the reality of her dreams (fig. 64, p. 227). I have been told that no woman should see her baby until it has been bathed and dressed; my patients, however, are the first to grasp the small fingers and touch gingerly the soft skin of the infant's cheek. They are the first to marvel at the miracle of their own performance; to them indeed is due the inspiring reward of full and conscious realization. That there is anything unsightly in the appearance of a newborn babe is nonsense; that a mother might be shocked at her own baby is fantastic. Its first cry remains an indelible memory on the mind of a mother; this is the song that carried her upon its wings to an ecstasy mere man seems quite unable to comprehend. But like all other natural emotional states, it is part of a great design; its magnitude is significant of its important purpose. No mother and no child should be denied that great mystical association. It is not only advantageous for the immediate present, to perfect the restoration of the muscles and tissues involved in the birth to their nonpregnant state, as we shall see in a moment, but it lays a foundation of unity of both body and spirit upon which the whole edifice of mother love will stand.

Many times I have called attention to the wonderful picture of happiness that we see at a natural birth. Women of all ages and types have testified to this "greatest happiness in their lives." It is a moment when, in the full consciousness of their achievement, they experience the most intense emotional joy. "I have never felt anything so marvelous—it cannot be compared to ordinary pleasure." If this is intended, and is one of the series of physical and emotional states in the natural law of parturition, what reason can we assign to it? Why should the serious hard work of the second stage, with its dulled senses, lowered receptivity to certain stimuli, and sleepy relaxation between the contractions, suddenly disappear? It is not just an accident that the brilliant sunlight of motherhood breaks through and dispels for all time the clouds of her labor. No change in human emotions is more dramatic. The quick temper that flashes from calm to rage, with all its disturbing variations of sound and appearance, is dull and crude when compared with this amazing transformation. I have sometimes been constrained to desert my established custom of observing with impersonal interest the phenomena of childbirth. Such an aura of beauty has filled the whole atmosphere of the room, and such superhuman loveliness has swept over the features of the woman whose baby is crying in her hands, that I wonder if I am right in my stolid abstinence from spiritual participation. "Strange talk," my reader may remark, "from a two-hundred-pound athlete!" But with all sincerity I repeat that I myself have experienced a sense of happiness much more akin to reverence and awe than to the simple satisfaction of just another natural birth.

This phenomenon is so definite and so inevitable, if preceded by the uncomplicated events of a relaxed and relatively painless labor, that it is not unreasonable to ascribe to it some result. All emotional states have a definite purpose, and the more closely we examine the physiological changes consequent upon emotional activity, the more apparent does the functional advantage of such states become. The overwhelming delight activates the sympathetic nervous system, and all the forces of that great protective mechanism are brought into play. The inhibitory fibers no longer lie relaxed and passive in the birth canal; the circular bands bind firmly the muscles of expulsion, and the uterus, as if in answer to the cry of the newborn child, becomes hard and remains contracted. Let every obstetrician feel once the brisk contraction of the uterus when the mother hears her child; it is the natural stimulus to close the great blood sinuses, rendering the placental site anemic and so hastening the separation of the useless afterbirth. "No bleeding at all" is frequently recorded, except the ounce or two of placental blood that comes away at the end of the third stage. Thus the physical reaction to this natural emotional state protects the mother from delayed expulsion of the afterbirth, excessive loss of blood, and postpartum shock.

But this is not all. When exhilaration and intense joy are experienced, physical changes occur that are readily diagnosable at sight and strangely infectious. The ecstasy of love that floods the whole personality when the earliest call of a new life awakens a woman to the realization of motherhood is a transport akin to mysticism. It is the spiritual perfection of physical achievement. Many women have written to me of this highest plane of human happiness: "Something of which no woman should be deprived," "a moment no words can describe," and so on. What does it mean? I do not know what inference should be drawn from such spontaneous and superlative expressions. The thoughts and words of women who watch their babies being born are so constant that in spite of the different terms in which they are couched they must be included in the purposeful phenomena of labor. Excitement, emotionalism, or sentimentality may be offered as an explanation, but it does not account for the uniformity of these manifestations in that most variable and unpredictable field, the mind of woman. Young mothers with no pretensions to piety have unhesitatingly told me that at the birth of their child they felt nearness to God, or the presence of a superhuman being—"a heavenly feeling that they have never known before"—and that it was difficult for them to believe in the reality of the present. They spoke with awe and respect for the unpremeditated wonder of their experience.

And so, when a child is born unhampered by the limitations we moderns put upon the natural laws, I am humbled before the miracle of birth and all the host of wonders that awaken its mechanism. It lives, we do not know why; indeed, we do not know the source of life itself. But here, from the indestructible forces of the universe, arrives a new human form. It is unlike any other we have ever seen, different in a thousand ways from its most similar brother. It has, however, the great common denominator of all humanity, life, that inestimable gift which from the first moment is our responsibility—life, which arrives, is marred or magnified, and passes on. Is it surprising that, at a moment of such stupendous significance, the woman who has been chosen to be the perfected instrument in the natural law of survival should be rewarded by a sense of exaltation? A new life, which of its very potential power is greater than death, should be logically heralded with pride and joy. In every newborn child there is new hope—to every mother the people should give thanks.

2

Mental Imagery

Francis Galton wrote much on the importance of mental imagery that has been overlooked in the modern teaching of medicine.* His investigations emphasize the vividness with which images, based upon thought and association, can be reproduced in the mind. Sights, sounds, and associations, real and imaginary, imprint themselves upon the human mind to mold and influence its reactions.

Is it unreasonable that we should pause to consider the mental image of labor within the mind of a woman? Is it not essential that we should create by education and instruction the true and natural happiness of motherhood within the vision of her mind? The mental picture of her anticipated experience should be the image of all that is beautiful in the fulfillment of her love. For the body is only a vehicle in which and from which a child is miraculously made and produced. It is the *mind* of woman that knows passion and desires the fulfillment of her biological purpose. It is the mind—its receptivity and its ability to integrate the fund of new thoughts and feeling that are the physiological visitations of love and pregnancy—that molds and fashions the child. It is the mind that bears the spiritual imprint of the newborn child and around it writes indelibly the mysterious circumscription of love.

But as Pavlov points out in his important work on condi-

* Sir Francis Galton, *Inquiries Into Human Faculty and Its Development* (London: Macmillan, 1883).

tioned reflexes,* the things that give the greatest pleasure will
become conditioned causes of acute fear and hatred if continually offered with a terrifying accompaniment. Both objective and subjective associations can condition stimuli that
provoke fear reactions to labor. I know single women who,
their natural longing for a child obliterated from their minds,
shudder when childbirth is mentioned. Associations of pain
and mental images of agony and death have become conditioned stimuli for such fear and abhorrence that these women
seek permanent refuge in virginity and spinsterhood. There
are some women who have had one baby who have been
known to refuse all marital relations forever after for fear they
should have to experience labor again. Even love for the child
cannot override the fear and pain that its arrival occasioned.
What devastation to homes, husbands, and children one ill-
conducted labor can bring!

Owing to the nature of Pavlov's experiments, the concept of
the conditioned reflex is often associated only with salivating
dogs, meat, and bells. But earlier writings, such as Galton's in
1883, made it apparent that the recurrent stimulus frequently
arises *within* the mind. The memory, or even the visualization,
of an incident may surround a natural and physiological
function with an aura of pain or pleasure so vivid that normal
reflexes are disturbed. Just as a colored light will produce
defense reactions of pain in a dog who was hurt when the light
appeared, so will the words "baby," "childbirth," "labor," or
even "motherhood" produce emotional states and their physical manifestations in women who suffered in parturition, and
every act that leads, in a normal sequence of events, to the
association of painful childbirth will give impetus to the primitive instinct to escape.

Fear of childbirth, then, becomes the great disturber of the
neuromuscular harmony of labor. I do not wish it to be in-

* Ivan Petrovich Pavlov, *Conditioned Reflexes; an Investigation of
the Physiological Activity of the Cerebral Cortex* (London: Oxford,
1928).

ferred that childbirth should be looked upon as a mental process. But obviously the mechanical efficiency of this function not only depends upon the structures and forces of the body but upon emotional stimuli, and upon the integrity of the influences to which the emotions are subjected.

SOURCES OF IMAGERY

Many young women from the age of puberty and even before have inquiring minds, particularly in relation to childbirth. Few hear much that is encouraging from girls of their own age, but, since the temptation to seek information is not curbed, again and again, drawn as if by sirens, they satiate their greed for knowledge by listening to voices that capture the imagination but utterly distort or destroy the truth. Too, the facts of childbirth may be withheld by the mother, the logical source, for the mother may have had such unpleasant experiences herself that she has no wish to communicate them to the child, who she believes will also suffer in childbirth. If, in a moment of confidence, she gives any information to her daughter, it is more likely to be fear producing than a stimulus to pleasant anticipation.

Thus the influence of too many mothers upon their daughters, either through the subtlety of their information or through the mystery of their silence, is a serious factor in producing a feeling of fear in regard to childbirth. Only too frequently, married women come into my consulting room entirely ignorant of the most elementary facts concerning childbirth. This series of events is frequently the origin, not only of an inherent fear of childbirth, but of physical manifestations of that fear.

We must remember, also, the influence of the friends of a woman about to have a baby. Wherever women are gathered together and the subject of childbirth arises, the general trend of the remarks is that childbirth is a kind of martyrdom, the suffering during which, though probably best forgotten, is satisfactorily recalled with obvious pride. Here it must not be overlooked that those who have suffered are justified in believing in suffering. There is no blame to be laid upon those who are honest in their opinions; neither was it their fault if they suffered. This does not, however, mitigate in any way the crime of their propaganda, for to produce alarm can never assist in the accomplishment of a task, however unimportant.

The influence of husbands is another potential source of anxiety concerning childbirth, if the husband has formed his opinions upon hearsay. His ignorance leads to an understandable anxiety over the welfare of his wife. Unfortunately, he communicates his anxiety to her, even though he is kept as far away as possible from the scene of her "ordeal" when labor is finally under way.

Apart from the more intimate sources of information about childbirth, women cannot escape the influence of the general trend of public and popular opinion. Constantly in contact with the modern foundations of both education and amusement, they read books, study papers, listen to radio and TV broadcasts, and see motion pictures. In far too many of these the same atmosphere is found: childbirth is an ordeal, essentially painful and dangerous to the life of the mother.

If the dramatist finds it necessary to increase the interest of the story by describing the events that occurred when one of the chief characters gave birth to a child, the incident is fraught with poignancy and tension, drama, suffering, and possibly death. As a student of human nature, the dramatist well knows that nothing is more likely to gain the attention of the reader. Do we often read of a normal character experiencing any happiness in childbirth, or see such a presentation on the screen? Similarly, the tense anxiety of the husband gives the author or producer a wonderful opportunity for drama—a young man may be seen walking up and down the room wringing his hands, perhaps drinking innumerable whiskies and sodas, looking imploringly toward a closed door or dashing hysterically at a bearded doctor. The company in waiting

registers a series of "expect-the-worst" expressions. Fortunately, this is sometimes so exaggerated as to become
laughable.

The daily papers are also printed in order to attract readers.
Unless it occurs in a taxicab or a telephone booth, the story of
a straightforward birth is not news, but the story of a mother's
death when a child is born is almost worthy of headlines.

HISTORICAL AND RELIGIOUS INFLUENCES

If we survey the history of childbirth in European civilization, we discover that suffering is often presumed, the minds
of both men and women being conditioned to the idea of
suffering as essential to childbirth. Since it is expected, it is
thus caused and aggravated. For generations the necessity of
pain has been accepted as a fact, even though the motivation
for earlier stories and dramas may have been to concentrate on
the negative in order to attract an audience, just as in our
day.

Ancient Practices and Pagan Religions

At the time of Hippocrates, four or five hundred years
before Christ, we read of a different outlook. Even prior to his
day, three thousand years before Christ, the priests among the
Egyptians were called to assist women in labor. In many societies witchcraft was resorted to, often very successfully, and
old writings suggest that herbs and potions were used to help a
woman give birth easily. In fact, it may be said with some
accuracy that among the most primitive people of whom any
record exists, help was given to women in labor according to
the customs of the time.

Hippocrates lived from 460 to 355 B.C. His aphorisms
should be read by every medical man. It was he who realized
that "our natures are the physicians of our diseases"; it was he
who recognized in the routine care of human ailments that

prevention was more important than cure. He emphasized that the daily discipline of a healthy person was to include diet, exercise, and fresh air. All the simple things of life to correct an illness were to be used before medicines, and last of all came surgery. It may seem strange to some of us that these things were written so long ago!

Today in the United States, England, and many other countries, everyone who qualifies to be a doctor has to take the Hippocratic Oath, an oath of allegiance to our science. This oath is a magnificent concept, to which one who is accorded the privilege of attending the sick should adhere, for it stands as fresh and noble as ever. Unfortunately, even today in my professional career, I have often seen only lip service paid to it and its tenets ignored. Yet it is upon the Hippocratic teaching that all modern medicine is based. If the principles of Hippocrates were reenacted today in all their simplicity and wisdom, they would undoubtedly alter the whole tone and tenor of our lives. Hippocrates made stern demands upon his pupils, but he always practiced what he preached.

There is no authority but *fact*, Hippocrates taught, and deductions are to be made only from facts. Since observation, common sense, and clear reasoning are not compatible with the speculative practice of medicine, a physician should be persuaded by no influence that cannot be justified by accurate observation. True science begets knowledge, but opinion, ignorance.

Hippocrates' teaching was largely based upon the laws of nature as they were understood in his time, that is, exploring the secrets of life, its origin, its maintenance, and its reproduction. He endeavored to organize and instruct midwives. He found no place for fear in childbirth except in the presence of abnormality, which may or may not have been caused by a faulty regimen in the life of the individual. Such confidence was placed in the ability of the natural law to carry out the work of reproduction that one statement was frequently impressed upon the students and doctors of that time: "We must refrain from meddlesome interference!" A statement particularly applicable to the care of women in childbirth. Indeed, it is important for us to realize that there is nothing *new* in the concept of natural childbirth. It is but a revitalizing and uncovering of that which conforms to the laws of nature.

Aristotle (384–322 B.C.) went further, and in some of his writings we find accurate and very desirable observations upon childbirth. He was probably the first man who ever urged *care of the mind* for a woman having a baby. A great naturalist, he was the first investigator of the development of the chick within the egg.

Followed by Aristotle and other great scientists, the Hippocratic and Grecian school of medicine held sway until after Soranus of Ephesus, who, living at the end of the first and the beginning of the second century after Christ, continued the emphasis upon the high level and humane principles of Grecian obstetrics. Writing a famous treatise on obstetrics in about A.D. 79, Soranus was quite possibly the greatest of all the ancient obstetric clinicians, and must be regarded as their leading authority upon childbirth and pediatrics. He denied the truth of certain superstitions about childbirth, and he stressed consideration of the *feelings of the woman* herself. He makes no mention of fear, and did not expect it to occur unless some abnormality disrupted the healthy function. His writings, as true today as nineteen hundred years ago, were collected by monks and, buried in the cellars of great monasteries, were soon forgotten, not to be rediscovered for many centuries.

Pain in childbirth has been recognized as far back as we can go in the history of man, but only in the presence of something contrary to the natural or physiological law, which then gives rise to fear. Fear is an emotion that, emerging from the primitive instinct of survival, is the natural protective agent prompting the individual to escape from danger.

There seems to be little doubt but that the unnatural, pathological, and destructive condition of fear in childbirth is found more intensely and frequently in the European civilization than in any other. Those of us who have traveled among groups who have not yet come into contact with European civilization have found that the presence of fear of childbirth affects only a small percentage of the population, confirming what we have read in the ancient writings, and those who do suffer from fear almost invariably have a reasonable cause.

The general tendency is to pass quickly from the discussion of fear to that of pain. But the origins of fear are important, because the association between fear and pain is very close. Thus it is necessary to draw attention to the influences of superstitions and religious customs, and all those things which pertain to ethical conduct and beliefs among various peoples. Fear produced by religious beliefs becomes an offense to the mental or physical integrity of childbirth. Unnecessary fear is a pathological condition.

Pagan religions demand an absolute belief in an outside controlling influence over the events of one's life. That control is exercised, directly or indirectly, by one's ancestors. All goes well with the individual, so long as he obeys the rules and does not offend his or her ancestors. It is the woman who carries, hidden in her mind, the knowledge of her disobedience of this law who becomes depressed and filled with fear during labor. She is anxious not only for her own life but also for the life and fitness of the child. Pain and suffering in childbirth then becomes the corollary to "the wages of sin is death," an idea common to all ethical teachings and religions. Thus if a dead or abnormal child is born, it is considered the reward of sin and disobedience of the law.

We found that some tribes in Africa go to extraordinary lengths to appease the wrath of their forefathers or their gods. When trouble arises in labor, as it surely does in the presence of this sin-born fear, free confession overcomes the trouble of a delayed or prolonged labor. This form of pain relief in difficult labor is well recognized among many tribes. When in the Congo we obtained first-hand evidence of the curative influence of confession as a means of palliating the angry ancestors or gods during labor. In the absence of abnormality, the baby was usually born soon after confession. Thus the ethical beliefs of an individual, and the consciousness of sin or disobedience in respect to these beliefs, do influence the course of labor, through the emotions.

The Middle Ages

It was about three hundred years after Christ that a big change in attitudes came about in Western civilization, due to a distortion of earlier Judeo-Christian teachings. It is generally accepted that the institutionalized Christian Church during this period, more than any other influence in the last two thousand years, retarded the progress of medicine and medical science. One of the principles of Christ's teachings is that we should visit the fatherless and the widows in their affliction, and heal the sick. But the priests of this early period—interpreting any efforts on the part of man to heal the sick as being presumptuous, placing oneself on an equal with, or even preeminent over, the God of Christians—went back to pagan practices, where prayer and fastings were the total remedies. If medicines or potions were used at all, they came from the monasteries through the Church, and it was the special prerogative of the priests to prescribe and distribute them. To study and believe in the laws of nature became an offense against the authority of the Church, and all books on medicine that had been written, including those of Soranus, were seized and buried beneath the monasteries. When the Roman Empire fell, all medicine reverted to the lore of superstitions, legends, salves, poultices, and talismen. The sick were no longer healed; they either lived or died.

With this as background, it is no wonder that the rites of paganism were relatively simple, pleasing, and acceptable when compared to some of the horrors to which women in medieval times were subjected, owing to the ignorance of those who were entitled to look after them in childbirth. During the thousand years up to 1520, the responsibility for childbirth was entirely usurped by the Church. No man was allowed to attend a woman in labor unless he was a shepherd or a man who looked after animals in sickness. Childbirth was considered the result of carnal sin, to be expiated by suffering in giving birth. Should the woman have trouble during labor, the Church, according to its ethics, demanded a live baby, whatever might happen to the woman in question. In fact, if a woman was dying it was not unusual for the baby to be taken from her through the wall of the abdomen, for which purpose men accustomed to castrating animals, usually hog-gelders, were employed.

The Sixteenth and Seventeenth Centuries

It was not until 1513 that a German, Eucharius Roesslin, discovered the hidden writings of Soranus and others. He wrote the first obstetric book in nearly fifteen hundred years, gleaning his manuscript from the works of those ancient, astute physicians, profound philosophers, and most accurate clinical observers the world has ever known.

The book of Eucharius Roesslin stood as a monument upon the high road of the development of care in childbirth. Nine years after its publication a doctor in Hamburg, thinking that too little was known about childbirth except through books, decided to observe the birth of a baby. Since no man was allowed to attend a woman in childbirth and the law was extremely rigid, he dressed as a midwife and joined the midwives at a birth. His observations were invaluable. Success in midwifery had begun to be established once more when he was deceived by a personal acquaintance and reported to the authorities. For that crime, that heresy, Dr. Weiss of Hamburg was burned at the stake. Only four hundred years ago!

It was not until 1580 that shepherds and herdsmen were prevented by law from attending women in labor, though physicians were still not permitted to assist midwives. Two hundred and fifty years ago physicians took over the work in certain cases, and later surgeons applied their skill, but even then little consideration was shown for the woman's feelings.

In the so-called ages of religious faith, the sixteenth and seventeenth centuries in England, if there was any difficulty in labor it was the custom, so that its soul might be saved, to baptize the child before it was born, the holy water being introduced onto the unborn child by use of a special instrument. The fact that the mother died still called for no remark.

I think we must all agree that there were reasonable causes for fear in relation to childbirth in those days. At the time of James I, when the Authorized Version of the Bible was translated into English, the first English book on midwifery had been published only fifty years before. Although several manuscripts on midwifery appeared, they were mainly for private circulation, and demonstrated little advance upon the works of Soranus of Ephesus. It was not until the nineteenth century that the foundations of our present knowledge were laid. We tend to overlook the fact that until 1847 no anesthetics or pain-relievers were used in childbirth, so that when a labor was abnormal the suffering was appalling.

The most important of all historical writings, and the most likely to be read, is the Bible. It is still the world's best-selling book. Many women read and study their Bibles—and many have been influenced to believe that childbirth is a grievous and painful experience because of passages in the King James Version like Genesis 3:16, which quotes the Lord as having said to Eve: "I will greatly multiply thy sorrow and thy conception; in sorrow thou shalt bring forth children." This passage has been known as the "curse of Eve," with its assumption that misery, pain, and sorrow automatically accompany every birth. Thus many still are of the opinion today that the teaching of natural childbirth is contrary to the Bible.

Nothing could be further from the truth! For those who believe the translators and others who compiled the various editions of the Bible were under divine guidance no argument will be of any avail, but if the Bible had divine inspiration, it is likely that the writers of the original manuscripts were inspired, and not the translators of the various editions in different languages.

If we put ourselves in the place of those brilliant classical scholars of the time of James I, from A.D. 1604 to 1611, the years occupied by them in completing this translation, we can see why their negative thoughts on childbirth were expressed in their translations. They used the word "pain" because they had no reason to believe any other term was applicable.

Recently biblical scholars have carefully reexamined the Hebrew and Greek manuscripts from which much of the Bible was translated, and have concluded that the words referring to childbirth do not signify pain, but refer to "labor," or to "a woman in childbirth."*

It is forgivable that the translators of three hundred years ago should interpret as they did, but I find it difficult to understand how these obviously controversial translations can continue to be accepted by many modern scholars of the classics, who copy and even intensify the mistakes, although they have many more manuscripts and advantages from which to deduce the significance of the words.

The Church must once again teach the beauty of childbirth and encourage confidence in normal, natural function, which is in harmony with the basic teachings of the Bible. We must not forget the significance of Christmas or the manger in the stable of a wayside inn. Five hundred million Catholics honor the Madonna and Child, and the millions of followers of the Protestant faith all turn to the spiritual associations of childbirth and motherhood.

In the meantime, let us assume as historical necessity the teachings of the past that emphasized the negative aspects of

* A more complete discussion of the Judeo-Christian concepts and biblical translations will be found in the forthcoming *Childbirth and the Family*, by Helen Wessel (New York: Harper & Row, 1973).

childbearing, keeping in mind that there can be no more horrible stigma upon civilization than the history of childbirth.

The Last Hundred Years

In 1847 a brighter picture began to emerge for women in childbirth, with James Young Simpson's discovery of chloroform, creating the beginning of the era of pain relief. Simpson was harshly criticized by the Church for giving women anesthesia in abnormal labor. A dignitary of the Church wrote in condemnation of his work: "Chloroform is the decoy of Satan, apparently offering itself to bless women but in the end it will harden society and rob God of the deep cries which arise in time of trouble."

That—in my father's time! But anesthesia had come to stay—and to such an extent that it was used in all labors, abnormal or not. Why *always* anesthesia, when in the natural state it is unnecessary? It has always been easier to utilize the pain-relieving discoveries of science than to investigate the complicated causes of pain. Since 1850 a hundred ways and means have been discovered to rid our women of the pain that has invariably attacked them, even when they most deserved the natural joy of their supreme accomplishment. Nevertheless, anesthesia, a gift from the gods, has been of the greatest service to women, and an important step forward in the development of humane care during childbirth.

In 1854 Florence Nightingale became the first person to make it widely known that cleanliness and fresh air were fundamental necessities of nursing. It was largely because of her work during the Crimean War that the standards of both the training and practice of nursing were raised. The gin-drinking, reprobate doctors who were found in great numbers at births both in hospitals and at home began to disappear. With their exodus, childbed fever occurred less frequently in maternity cases, but even so, women were still dying in hospitals at the rate of 12 to 15 percent of all normal labors. This means that one in every eight perfectly healthy women admitted died through childbed fever!

About this same time, Ignaz Philip Semmelweis, a nervous young man who was a physician at the Maternity Hospital in Vienna, came to the conclusion that the cause might be due to something arising within the hospital. He therefore made his students wash their hands in a solution of chloride of lime before attending women in childbirth. In one year, 1858, the death rate in his wards tumbled to 3 percent and soon afterward to 1 percent. This was the first great step toward preventing the attendant from taking death to the patient—but Semmelweis's only reward for his discovery was learning what the ancients had always preached, that to interfere with the law of nature was to invite the hand of death. For his success in saving lives Semmelweis was asked, for some made-up reason, to leave the staff of the hospital. He was told he had no right to require this washing, and was sent away. He returned to his home and died, a broken man.

Until 1866 there was no knowledge of asepsis. Hospitals were originally organized by priests whose humane intention was to move people from the hovels in which they lived to be cared for by doctors in hospital. In the homes a certain number died; those who went to the hospital for safety and good treatment died in much greater numbers. It is difficult to visualize the state of affairs that prevailed when limbs were amputated, abdomens opened, and Caesarean sections performed without any anesthesia and with an almost sure supervention of sepsis, giving rise to a high percentage of mortality in the simplest operations.

Probably all of us, if we are wise, pause to think sometimes how much harm we do in our efforts to do good, and how much trouble we cause when conscientiously endeavoring to prevent it!

In 1866, long after my parents were born, Joseph Lister first practiced aseptic surgery, and he continued to use antiseptics in spite of the opposition and ridicule of his colleagues.

Then Pasteur discovered fermentation and inoculation and Koch discovered bacteria, the two men becoming co-founders of the science of bacteriology. This is all recent change and innovation!

The care of women in childbirth benefited by the advance of these other branches of medical science, but in obstetrics itself little happened. At the beginning of the twentieth century the death rate from childbirth was lower, and severe pain was relieved, but still childbirth was an ordeal for a woman to face. Much pain still remained, pain that was unexplained and could only be obliterated by unconsciousness, which carried its own dangers. Was unconsciousness safe for mother and baby? It is incredible how pain was and still is accepted by many doctors and scholars, as an inevitable accompaniment of childbirth.

I cannot understand anyone who says women in childbirth should not be afraid, for who among us would not have some qualms about entering into an experience that we desired above all else, but that we believed must occasion severe pain, danger, possible mutilation, and even death to either ourself or our child? We know of only a few who have no fears: there are a number of women who faithfully believe in the rightness of their God and the sanctity of their bodies, and in my opinion there are also women who have an inborn belief in the laws of nature, not by formulating them to themselves, but because they are natural in their outlook and experience.

The extent and magnificence of the medical discoveries made during the last hundred years is beyond both praise and gratitude. Gradually truth has been discovered, and the safety of women in childbirth has been made an object of investigation, with results that would have been unbelievable when the mothers and grandmothers of many of us were born. But now that many of the troubles and dangers have been overcome, we must move on—not only to save more lives, but actually to bring happiness to replace the agony of fear. For although the consciousness of a woman's discomfort can now be dispelled, it is only at a price, for with it goes the awareness of birth and the joyful sensations and emotions that should accompany it. Now we must bring a fuller life, truer to natural law, to the women who are called upon to reproduce our species.

NATURAL LAW

I have chosen the term "primitive" in reference to woman in her original condition, as opposed to "cultured" or "civilized." It is obvious that such a term requires explanation.

"Primitive" is a word that is used very loosely, implying various meanings such as retrograde, relatively uneducated, and so on. But I am using the word to convey *primitivus,* which, like *primus,* means "first" or "original," for, in relation to *homo sapiens,* who is in a position to say what the original woman was like?

The use to which I have applied this word is not strictly accurate from the point of view of the anthropologist, but rather implies the relatively early stages of mankind in relation to mental development. That is not so much a matter of ages or years; we know nothing of the woman of the Glacial Age, and in fact have no records of the reproductive function of woman that go very far back beyond the age of civilization. Therefore I would like the term, for this particular purpose, to be accepted as indicating those women whose mental development has not attained a state of civilization. Women whose tribal lives and traditional limitations of experience have not allowed them freedom of thought or education of the imagination are, compared to the cultured women of today, primitive. The main difference is, in fact, in the development of the mental functions. There is very little evidence that modern woman is in any way less fitted to produce children painlessly than the woman without culture and without civilization. It may be that there are factors that tend to make the child relatively smaller among the primitive, but it is definitely open to argument whether or not the oversized child of the cultured woman is due to mismanagement of her pregnancy.

Woman, primitive or cultured, has before her no evidence suggesting that nature ever intended pregnancy to be an illness. The primitive woman continues her work—in the harvest field, on trek, in the rubber plantation, or wherever she may be employed. The child develops while she herself lives a full and natural existence. Muscularly strong, physiologically efficient, her mechanism carries out its normal functions without discomfort, difficulty, or shame. The child then is born easily, small and firm fleshed. Among cultured women we see this too—the athletic girl who continues her games, who hunts to the fifth month, who plays golf to the seventh month, who walks three or four miles a day to the full term of her pregnancy, who eats sensible food in a sensible way, who is not diverted from her normal routine by those who try to advertise special care, rest, diets, and enormous quantities of milk.

Such exaggerated concern is an offense against nature; it is a presumption that natural methods require unnatural fortification, and to those of us who believe in nature it is little short of inducing a pathological state into a very perfect physiological function.

Whichever of the many definitions of culture is adopted, one thing is certain, that culture is dependent primarily upon the activity of the mind. The more efficient the mental processes the more cultured the type. But, unquestionably, we have very largely lost many of the higher sensibilities that in the primitive state were essential to our personal survival. One has only to spend a few weeks with those who depend upon their wits for the supply of their food from natural surroundings to appreciate how soon we should die out if once again we were bereft of cultural attributes and were called upon to return to the primitive state!

From this the question naturally follows: to what extent can the culture of the mind have affected those functions which remain with us as primitive physical functions, childbirth in particular? The mind has developed, and the enormous fund of stimulus that passes from the consciousness to the autonomic nervous system has to meet new conditions. The lives of the cultured have gradually changed as civilization has developed. With repression, emotions of varying intensity have found new means of expression. The physician of today looks to the emotions and sentiments of his patients when endeavoring to find the original cause for many of their physical complaints, practicing "psychosomatic medicine."

Herein lies the fact of pain in childbirth. Modern woman is physically competent; modern childbirth is physically unaltered from primitive childbirth, but culture has brought to bear upon this function neuromuscular activities arising from the intensification of certain emotions that inhibit the progress of the birth and thus create pain.

But there is no reason why culture should be allowed to destroy all that is beautiful in the primitive! True culture should enhance original beauty and purify where contamination has crept in. If childbirth among the primitive races still persists today as a relatively painless procedure, it is indeed a slur upon our utilization of culture that the most dramatic, the most beautiful, and the most essential of natural functions should be made a terror, an agony, and a nightmare for so many.

A NEW LOOK

When we speak of normal, natural, or uncomplicated labor, we infer that the child is the right size and in the correct position to pass through the pelvic canal without undue strain or injury to the surrounding parts. In the majority of labors, everything appears to be perfect; the muscles contract well, the child is the correct size and in a good position, yet in spite of this there is pain. Why is this, when there is no other physiological function in the body that gives rise to pain in the normal course of health?

A close clinical study of natural childbirth has taught us much about the cause and origin of nervous impulses that are not physiological. *Fear* is a natural protective emotion without which few of us would survive. When through association or indoctrination there is fear of childbirth, resistant actions and reactions are brought to the mechanism of the organs of reproduction. This discord disturbs the harmony or polarity of muscle action, causing *tension,* which in turn gives rise to nervous impulses interpreted in the brain as *pain.* This is in keeping with the natural law of protection of the individual from abnormal or harmful activities in or about the body. Therefore, fear, tension, and pain are the three evils that are not normal to the natural design, but that have been introduced in the course of civilization by the ignorance of those who have been concerned with attendance at childbirth.

The fear of pain actually produces true pain through the medium of pathological tension. This is known as the "fear-tension-pain syndrome," and once it is established a vicious circle demonstrating a crescendo of events will be observed, for with true pain fear is justified, and with mounting fear resistance is strengthened. Thus the most important contributory cause of pain in otherwise normal labor is fear.

But fear also affects the circulation of the blood to and from the uterus, for persisting tension of the uterine musculature prevents complete relaxation between contractions. The great blood sinuses of the uterus are deprived of full expansion and the venous blood, replete with metabolites or waste products of muscular action, are unable to discard their contents as freely as they should. And further, stimulation of the sympathetic nervous system results in constriction of the arterial blood vessels bringing fresh fuel to the contracting muscles. As a medical student at Cambridge I watched Professors Langley and Anderson* stimulate the sympathetic nerves to the uterus. In a short time the organ became pallid, firm, and bloodless, but when the stimulation was removed it rapidly filled with blood and once again became an elastic, deep-pink organ. I have also seen, on more than one occasion, what is

* John Baxter Langley and Sir Thomas McCall Anderson, editors of *Journal of Physiology,* 1893–94.

known as a white, or *ischemic,* uterus. Because of urgent fetal distress, a Caesarian section has had to be performed, labor having been inhibited by strong but ineffective contractions. The women in these cases had no anatomical obstruction or *abruptio placenta* (premature separation of the placenta from the wall of the uterus), but uncontrollable fear had caused, through the resistance of the circular muscles, such tension within and ischemia of the uterine muscles that the baby, through excessive intrauterine pressure and restricted oxygen supply, was unable to survive a protracted labor and vaginal delivery. The white uterus persisted in spite of surgical anesthesia, which demonstrates the depth of fear that may remain within the psyche of the conditioned individual.

Sir Thomas Lewis* described the results of experiments dealing with the effect of partially restricted circulation upon muscle pain. He suggested that an impairment of circulation is a cause of pain because the blood flow is too slight to dispose of metabolites. These substances, which may be crystalline in form, when in high concentration irritate by laceration the inner walls of the blood sinuses and smaller vessels within the muscle fibers, so restricted circulation or relative ischemia could easily give rise to severe pain in muscle tissue. Not infrequently I have observed in the prolonged labor of frightened women a tenderness of the uterus; even gentle palpation of the womb through the abdominal wall gives rise to acute pain. A labor without disproportion or malpresentation of the baby is long because it is painful, not painful because it is long.

It is an indisputable statement that a very large majority of women today—however brave, however anxious to have a child, with whatever honesty they may say, "I am not worrying in the slightest"—have a background of fear in their minds that recoils from the ordeal they believe to be essential to childbirth.

* In *Archives of Internal Medicine* 49 (May 1932): 713.

A woman may be conscious of uterine contractions for hours, but have no discomfort until she is told she is in labor. This verbal stimulus to her mental imagery alerts her attention and anxiety. Although she may appear to be quite calm, a woman in labor has an inborn alertness to danger, and evidence of anxiety, however courageously suppressed, will forewarn her attendants of the special care she may need. In anxiety, the heart beats strongly and often rapidly, breathing is quicker and sometimes irregular, and is interspersed with a series of deep, sighing respirations. The nostrils may be widely dilated to facilitate the intake of air, and not infrequently the mouth is slightly open for the same reason.

Unless her anxiety is alleviated, the fear-tension-pain cycle is set in motion because of the stimulation of the sympathetic nervous system. The circular or inhibitory muscle fibers of the uterus are among those activated by this system, rendering the lower uterine segment and the outlet resistant to dilation. This rapidly produces tension greater than normal within the walls and cavity of the uterus. This excessive tension is recorded by the nerve endings specific for that form of stimulation and is correctly interpreted as pain.

One of my patients was a tall, athletic girl of twenty-two, being in every way what could reasonably be described as a fine type of British youth. But when her labor began I found a pale, anxious girl, whose natural sense of courage was being severely tested. Her mother resented what she described as my cheerful confidence—she took me aside and explained to me that she did not consider it a time for smiles. Since she refused to leave her daughter, I decided to go out of the house, instructing the nurse in charge to call me later. I heard nothing for five hours, so I telephoned and received word that progress seemed to be very slow. After nine hours, having heard nothing, I went back to the house.

There were no obvious signs of the end of the first stage, but the patient showed all the symptoms of fear. The distracted mother rushed out of the room with me—an opportunity for which I was grateful!—demanding to know how I could allow such agony. I pointed out to her that so long as she was in the room I could do nothing. Fortunately my advice prevailed, and she stayed away.

I made an examination, and found a loose, flaccid cervix, which I could dilate sufficiently with my fingers to feel the ears and nose of the on-coming head, indicating an *occipito-posterior* (face-up) presentation. As I examined—and it is not without interest that my examination occasioned no discomfort—a contraction occurred. The picture of agony was typical in all respects at the very earliest signs of a contraction. The nurse was clutched around the waist, the corner of the pillow seized in an agonized apprehension of pain. *The cervix tightened to a size no bigger than a quarter*. There was, of course, no advance.

I sent for an anesthetist. With the greatest of ease an *occipito-anterior* (face-down) presentation of the head within the pelvis was obtained. Under anesthetic the cervix admitted my whole hand with practically no tension. I did not apply forceps. The anesthetic was lifted, and within three-quarters of an hour a baby of seven pounds was born to a conscious and relatively calm mother.

I made full use of the third stage; the mother heard her child's first cry, and from that time all went well. Three years later I heard from abroad that her second baby had arrived. In three and a half hours she had produced a fine son weighing seven pounds three ounces. There had been no trouble. She had apparently suffered no pain, and no anesthetic had been given.

If women are to be taught to anticipate childbirth with relaxed confidence, it is necessary to eliminate the tension that gives rise to pain by removing the causes for fear. Those who seek to follow as closely as possible the natural law of childbirth should do everything possible to allay a young woman's anxieties and give her confidence by simple and truthful reiteration of the facts of natural childbirth.

Nothing can be of greater importance, both from the point of view of the mother, the infant, the family unit, and ultimately the social structure of the nation, than to persevere in the preparation of the woman's mind during the early weeks of pregnancy. By teaching the facts, thus implanting confidence, and by giving instruction in muscular relaxation, a state of anxiety may be replaced by a sense of well-being throughout the receptive months of pregnancy.

Prenatal preparation of the mind has been observed to have a close association with the pregnant woman's physical condition. A fear-conditioned mind often calls up physical complaints, backache or headache, dyspepsia or constipation, listlessness and muscular apathy, depression or weariness of mind and body. But many of these complaints, along with many persistent anxieties, will be removed by a psychological shift from the expectant mother's introvert self to her unborn child, particularly after she feels it moving within her. Her psychological constitution will become re-formed, and a more carefree state of mind will take the place of the anxiety tension to which she has been subjected for perhaps many years prior to childbirth. The imagery of childbirth will no longer be clouded by mystery and anguish for her, and she will be ready to have her baby in the happiest and most natural manner.

It is not only that we require, as obstetricians, to bring about an easy labor, without risk of injury to the mother or the child; we must go further. We must understand that childbirth is fundamentally a spiritual as well as a physical achievement and throughout this book it must be understood that the birth of a child is the ultimate perfection of human love, the culmination of the love between a man and a woman. In the Christian ethic we teach that God is love. The blessing of sexual necessity and pleasure is but an essential part of the love God has given to man and woman. It may be that in time scientists will be able to give such complete proof of the rightness of materialism that religion will become a weapon in the hands of the psychiatrists and the Church will be replaced by the clinic. But my close association with the birth of a child has led me to believe there is a limitation to science and that the extending boundaries of human knowledge have only reached the foothills of the towering mountains of Omniscience. This philosophy of childbirth is written, therefore, in terms of a belief in God.

For my own part, I stand in awe and utter humility before a woman with her newborn babe. There is so much to see and learn in their presence, so much that I am unable to understand or to explain, so much that makes me aware of the limitations of my own ability. It may be that among my colleagues there are those who feel the same. Obstetrics must be approached as a science demanding the most profound respect.

One woman who had feared, because of all the accepted causes, the arrival of her child, gained confidence and understanding before her baby was due; she had a natural and happy birth. Toward the end of the labor that produced her second, and much larger, child, she worked with tireless energy. "How many more?" she asked me excitedly, as she rested between the contractions.

"It will soon be here," I replied. "Why do you ask so anxiously? I hope you are not too weary."

"No, no, not that—but this brings back to me so clearly John's arrival. I can hear his cry and see his fat pink body in my hands. I'm longing for that heavenly feeling again—I simply can't describe it to you. It won't be long now, will it?"

Could we wish to blot out the mental imagery of her first experience? In the natural state the emotional experience of childbirth raises a woman to such delight and thankfulness that her mind turns to spiritual and metaphysical associations to express her gratitude and joy. Materialism and atheism are not included in the makeup of motherhood; neither can a robot lead a blind man across the road.

3

Education in Pregnancy

When a woman becomes pregnant, she should seek medical advice. When she does, she usually attends a prenatal clinic or visits a doctor. She wishes to know that all is well and to be in contact with some person from whom she can get advice upon matters relating to the birth of her child, and through whom she can arrange for a bed in the maternity ward of a hospital.

We overlook, perhaps, the excitement that attends these preliminary arrangements and the disappointment when preparations cannot be made according to plan. During the first pregnancy in particular, the average woman needs considerable support; she requires explanation of unfamiliar occurrences. The doctor, the nurse, and the prenatal clinic are responsible for her attitude toward childbirth, for these people are, in her eyes, experts on the subject.

To a young woman appearance, shape, and gracefulness are matters of serious importance. She is rightly proud of her figure; she demands to retain its beauty; she dislikes the ungainly spectacle of women whom she has seen in the later months of pregnancy; she fears swollen ankles, pigmented patches upon her face, white lines and stretch marks upon her abdomen, and development of the breasts. Attention needs to be given to these matters, along with explanation and care, by one who shows obvious interest in her well-being.

Of course she has her pelvis measured, her blood pressure taken, her abdomen listened to and prodded, the urine examined, blood taken for grouping, Rh factor, type, and complete blood count. But even if all is well, there is still need for a great deal more than just a few hints as to exercise and diet. However complete the prenatal care may be according to all accepted rules, it is lifeless if the mind is not cared for. And however carefully physical conditions are diagnosed and corrected, all these attentions may well be in vain if the emotional influences are abnormal. No woman should arrive at the hospital in labor without adequate preparation from qualified teachers.

Some women attend prenatal classes in hospitals or elsewhere, only to discover when labor begins that they have learned little that is of value to them *in labor*. There is nothing more disconcerting to a woman in labor than to find that she has been misinformed, or misled, concerning the part she must take in the process of childbirth. Untrue statements are worse than no teaching, for they add to the woman's disappointment a complete loss of confidence in her attendants.

We have to beware of those who aspire to teach never having learned! In such instances the approach to childbirth as a natural or physiological function will most likely be misrepresented, and a high percentage of failures earn a bad name for procedures that have been improperly employed. Intellectual information may be given concerning pregnancy and birth, but relaxation and correct breathing may be incompletely taught and their use as *essential* functions of normal labor not explained.

In other cases, a wonderful picture of positive painless achievement may be repeated at each meeting or class. But surely any teacher of experience knows that no one has the right to imply, without some qualifications, an invariable course of labor! A hundred possible variations of physical and emotional phenomena at the time of birth must be anticipated by the good clinician, and any that are harmful or threatening to the comfort or well-being of the mother or her child call for special attention and care.

Women inadequately trained for a natural birth have

suffered severe frustration and disappointment when deviation from the absolutely normal has to be corrected by assistance. Others who suffered more discomfort than they were led to understand might occur have hesitated to ask for, and even been unwilling to receive, pain relief, and by their refusal increased their babies' and their own troubles. Women improperly taught believe that pain relief by injections, drugs, or analgesics is evidence of failure and become morbidly depressed. I have too many reports from others who blame themselves because salutary scientific interference has been clinically indicated and skillfully employed. This is not the woman's fault; had she been properly and understandingly prepared she would have known the possibility that help might be advisable, and that birth can be made easier for both herself and her baby in these circumstances.

No woman unprepared for the possibility of rectifiable difficulty has been accurately taught the natural childbirth principles, for in these that possibility is strongly emphasized, in simple terms, enabling her to understand that modern science can help when trouble arises. Such knowledge gives courage and confidence, not fear.

Reproduction is a natural physiological function, not an illness. Our aim is to insure good health, both physical and mental, during pregnancy and so minimize the discomforts of labor and the necessity for interference, in order to assure the safe arrival of a healthy baby.

There are five specific objectives a conscientious physician may employ to help achieve these good results:

1. *To observe* the physical condition of pregnant women in order to prevent or diagnose as early as possible any abnormalities or irregularities that may disturb the health of either the mother or child during pregnancy, childbirth, or the postpartum period.

2. *To be forewarned* of physical or mechanical factors predisposing to a difficult labor, in order to avoid as far as possible emergent and unpremeditated interference.

3. *To educate* women concerning pregnancy and childbirth

so that the inhibiting influence of fear may be replaced by understanding and confidence.

4. *To instruct* women in each phenomenon of normal labor so that they may be prepared to interpret its varying sensations correctly, and meet its demands with discernment, patience, and self-control, assisting the natural forces rather than resisting them.

5. *To teach* women how to prepare themselves for the birth of the child in a manner that will enable them:

a. To have such *control of respiration* that they can breathe deeply, rapidly, or quietly when requested, or to hold the breath when called upon to do so by the attendant.

b. *To relax* when tension will cause resistance and pain, particularly during the inactivity of the first stage of labor.

c. To be *physically fit* in order to persist in the expulsive effort of the second stage of labor without undue exhaustion.

The first two objectives are in the province of purely medical attention rather than prenatal education. Therefore I shall not discuss them fully, because they are described in manuals and textbooks of obstetrics for the guidance of students, graduates, and postgraduates. It is numbers 3 through 5, and their application to the physically healthy woman who is well equipped to have her baby normally, that I propose to emphasize, with more details in later chapters.

When a young woman enters the consulting room believing, hoping, or fearing that she is going to have a baby, the physician's first investigations should be to confirm that she is pregnant. This may be ascertained by clinical signs, without an internal or vaginal examination at the first visit. Such an examination can be a severe shock to many young women and, apart from the discomfort it may cause, is an experience that frequently produces a lack of confidence in her attendants. If at thirteen weeks the uterus is not in the correct place and position, a vaginal investigation should be carefully performed for sound clinical reasons.

The doctor should then examine her attitude toward child-birth, both personally and generally. Close observation will unmask the true feelings of the prospective mother. We have all known the apparently indifferent woman, the enthusiastic, the alarmed, the radiantly happy, the angry, and the tearful. From such indications we may well mark out the psychological ground that has to be covered.

Many women consider that it is only right and proper that they should suffer certain discomforts in pregnancy. Pregnancy means morning sickness to some—indeed, morning sickness is one of the horrors of pregnancy to women of all classes of society, although when it occurs it frequently occurs in the afternoon! And the knowledge of that state acts as a conditioned reflex; having heard that it is one of the signs of pregnancy, they believe it to be a necessary accompaniment. They therefore start to have nausea and even vomiting as a subconscious justification of their state. It is Pavlov's story all over again—the association has become so definite from hearsay that the thought of pregnancy produces reflexes long conditioned in the mind. On two occasions women whose menstruation was overdue consulted me about their pregnancy because of morning sickness, nausea, and loss of appetite and weight. Neither was pregnant, and their symptoms cleared up as soon as they knew for certain that that was so! Conversely, it is frequently observed that the girl who does not know that she is going to have a baby does not have any of these symptoms.

Of course there is a percentage of women in whom nausea is actually caused by the chemical changes in the body that accompany pregnancy, but there are vast numbers of women who have felt neither sickness nor nausea during pregnancy. Women should be clearly told from the outset that nausea is not physiologically necessary, and that any tendency toward it can be controlled. It should be pointed out that the stomach should neither be empty too long nor overfilled; consequently, small, frequent meals are advisable until all tendency to nausea disappears. Very dry toast, or crackers, or small items for nibbling that can be carried in the purse, are all helpful, and fruit is best of all for some. If advice can be given to prevent or stop early sickness, a great step has been taken to gain the woman's confidence.

At the eleventh to thirteenth week, complaint is often made of frequency of urination. Perhaps the uterus is not quite clear of pressure at the brim of the pelvis; it may be slightly or completely retroverted. A vaginal examination at this time will afford an opportunity to lift a uterus that hesitates to rise above the brim. (Usually this condition corrects itself in a short time.)

The vicarious changes of taste and smell, and even sight and sound, are a cause of great concern to some. Those who have smoked may suddenly find themselves unable to feel comfortable in a room where others are smoking. Other women take a strong dislike to the smell of cooked meat. These changes—which are found in some cases to be due to a forgotten association—may be the cause of considerable anxiety if they are not discussed and their importance minimized.

Before the baby "quickens," the mother should be warned of it. She should understand that the first faint throbbings or regular tappings are movements of her child exercising its muscles and of its own initiative taking part in the perfection of its development. The child becomes a reality at this stage, and if the fetal heart can be heard clearly I give the mother a long stethoscope so that, if she wishes, she can hear the child's heartbeat. I explain that it is now about ten inches in length and weighs about one-half to three-quarters of a pound. Some women have complained of a disturbing regular throb in the uterus that goes on for half an hour or even longer; the possibility of the baby having an attack of hiccups interests the mother and gives her a sense of the reality of the child.

At some time during the first few months the question will probably arise as to the rights and wrongs of coitus during pregnancy. It is said that animals do not copulate when pregnant. I am not persuaded of the truth of that. In the later stages of pregnancy it may be true, but male rabbits, bulls, and rams do, and certainly the impregnation of hens does not deprive them of the attention of the cock.

Many women desire their husbands when pregnant, and in young people the bond of approaching parenthood often stimulates an irresistible affection that results in frequent and delectable copulation. During the early months a gentle performance of the act under the urge of affection is unlikely to be harmful. On occasion the wife may have no desire for it, just as when she is not pregnant. An understanding husband will respect her wishes, knowing that her mood will no doubt change within a few days.

A candid and sympathetic discussion of this subject is often a great relief to the young couple. The only medical contra-indication would be in instances where miscarriage is already threatening, and in the last weeks of pregnancy, shortly before birth.

If this intimate question or others arise early in pregnancy, it should not be difficult to discuss quite freely any doubts or anxieties arising in the mind of the expectant mother. The attitude of the obstetrician should be that of an impersonal but approachable counselor, and it is for this reason that it is best—in private practice—to arrange a fee inclusive of all visits during pregnancy as well as labor and the weeks following. This kind of arrangement leaves a woman free to see her doctor when and as often as she wishes, which is a great comfort to many. At a chosen moment, it is my practice to point out that I want my patient to know everything she wishes about childbirth, and that any questions in her mind should be put to me until the point is clearly understood: "I am far more concerned that you should have no doubts or fears in your mind than I am about your health. You are a perfectly healthy girl doing a perfectly natural thing. Your body is much less likely to mar your happiness just now than your mind is. If you cannot remember the various things you want to ask me, write them down as they come to your mind; we can probably settle them in a very few minutes. I am here to watch your physical development, to guard you against ignorance and misunderstanding and to be an adviser upon all subjects directly concerning your baby's arrival in a natural and healthy way."

Not infrequently, if the spirit of the occasion is suitable, I add some phrase to allay self-consciousness on the part of my patient lest I might think some of the questions foolish. Many women do not ask questions because they feel they ought to know the reply, and feel foolish mentioning a simple, but to them perplexing, subject. "Talk to me about it," I have frequently said. "We can say a lot in five minutes, and you are not wasting my time." And that is true. Blood pressure, measurements, hemoglobin, urinalysis, and abdominal examination can be conducted inside fifteen minutes if the consulting room is well organized. In a prenatal clinic, where the work is probably divided, five to ten minutes per patient is the maximum required for full routine examinations. It gives time for conversation, which, if it leads to important matters, can be prolonged.

But it is not the time that matters; it is the personal relationship, the friendliness of greeting, and the gentle care in examination that breaks down the barriers of shyness. Kindness can be dispensed as quickly as first aid, and a good deal more effectively, because its relief is permanent. Sympathetic understanding of troubles, both physical and mental, is an inexpensive remedy that often lifts a load of weariness and worry. Women are receptive at this time, and should be quietly guided to become interested in details.

But there is one physical condition for which the doctor must be especially alert, for it is not always given the attention its importance demands. What appears to be a poor attitude during pregnancy may be due to iron-deficiency anemia. I am not referring to the *physiological anemia* of pregnancy—that is, the plasma increasing in proportion to the number of red blood cells—which is compatible with good health. Nor do I refer to severe cases of *macrocytic* and *microcytic anemia*, or the "blood diseases," but to a shortness of iron apart from gross blood-cell changes. I have rarely seen a good example of natural labor in women whose hemoglobin has been allowed to remain below 70 percent from thirty-three to thirty-four weeks onward. I do not mean that their babies arrive with difficulty, but not infrequently labor is long, exhausting, and painful, with a slow recovery afterward.

The clinical aspect of anemia in relation to pain interpretation deserves some attention. In his article "Certain Aspects of Pain," Henry Head wrote: "Anemia is another cause of diminished general resistance to painful impressions."* Let us think for a moment of a woman who, tired in mind and body, short of hemoglobin, and forced to eat food she does not want, bravely faces what she believes she must endure. Labor begins—and soon she is in pain, a weary, weeping woman. Whether she was tired before she started labor or whether she is tired because of the expenditure of nervous and physical energy at the time is of no consequence. Tiredness of body intensifies pain. An ache becomes a severe pain; the mind is worn out and seeks only peace.

The percentage of hemoglobin should be estimated at prenatal visits as a routine; it is simple to do and takes very little time. If it is low, but follows during pregnancy the normal curve of variation—that is, falling slightly at about twenty-eight to thirty-two weeks and then picking up—it does not require special treatment. But if increasing tiredness, exhaustion after normal activities, breathlessness without reasonable cause, depression, and an absence of desire for meals is complained of, treatment is indicated. This is not to suggest that the woman feels ill, but she may say, as many do: "I'm feeling fairly well, but get so tired." The method of treatment will depend upon the diagnosis and judgment of the medical

* Sir Henry Head, "Certain Aspects of Pain," *British Medical Journal,* 1923 and also *Studies in Neurology* (London: Hodder & Stoughton, 1920).

attendant. One of the new preparations of iron often works like a charm, and with rising hemoglobin the patient will find new strength, spirits, and appetite, and will quite likely tell you she has never felt so well in her life.

As education in childbirth is largely concerned with protecting women against the evils of false suggestion, so helpful suggestion is used during the conducting of natural labor as a means of infiltrating the subconscious with truth. If those who attend women in labor view helpful suggestion with disfavor, must they continue to inflict strong and harmful suggestion upon women who would be willing to accept the truth?

For suggestion works either way, whether it is intended or not. The obstetrician who scorns the use of mental reinforcement has overlooked the fact that by his actions, thoughts, and sympathies he has unwittingly applied the most powerful negative suggestion. During pregnancy he has searched for abnormalities. He has suggested the possibility of illness and danger. By his promise of drugs and anesthetics he has introduced his own belief in their necessity, and therefore he has suggested that his patient will have pain to bear. By his manner he has conveyed the idea that he is her guardian against the assaults of mysterious and harmful eventualities. Further, the drama of labor is awe inspiring to the average woman who has not been educated in what her own experience in giving birth will be. When she enters the hospital, unprepared, the whole atmosphere may become a potent agent of harmful suggestion. The rubber gloves, expectant searchings down below, and quiet steps awaken in a woman's mind a host of fears and doubts. She may presume, and not unjustly, that the climax of all this must fulfill her worst and most vivid mental imageries. When she is taken into the delivery room, its polished furnishings, the instruments laid out in scintillating readiness before her eyes, the mask, the gown, all suggest that this is no simple affair. Her conscious mind remains alert, and her body misinterprets its sensations. Ultimately, these false suggestions are blotted out by anesthetics and drugs.

But if anesthetics are required to circumvent the prevalent

influences of false and harmful suggestion, why, in order to avoid anesthesia, is the use of true and helpful suggestion so often tabooed? The truth of natural labor is that there is no discomfort greater than healthy women are willing to bear. That is why women in labor are so susceptible to suggestion, if their prenatal education has prepared them for what to expect as a natural function.

We must also emphasize the *necessity for teamwork*. We cannot expect women who have been trained to carry out the procedures to be successful if, upon arrival at the hospital, a number is assigned to them and instead of a friendly greeting they are commanded to do as they are told in the "You-have-not-come-here-to-tell-*us*-what-to-do!" attitude. I do not wish to exaggerate this type of reception extended to both husbands and wives, but it does sometimes still happen.

As for the organization of trained teams, all those who educate or care for a pregnant woman should combine to follow the natural childbirth principles from early pregnancy through the weeks after the baby is born. The doctor, too, must carry through on this humane approach and should not be willing to interfere in a normal labor, or to do those things of which Aristotle so sternly warned us over two thousand years ago. If we interfere with nature there is a price to pay.

Of course, whether or not one is successful in protecting the woman from her fears or from other forms of pain, she must not be allowed to suffer. The scars of physical pain do more to ruin a woman's life, her marriage, and her motherhood than is generally recognized. It is necessary for a woman to have a scar from a Caesarean section, too often an emergency operation, but I would rather see the scar tissue of safe healing than the evidence of brain tissue incurably damaged by the shock of pain and terror.

Teamwork is essential, and there will be no good results without it. Today wives demand to be taught about childbirth and husbands are taking a great interest as well. All personnel involved in care of the pregnant woman also need to know what is to be expected of them. Today many hospital staffs are organizing classes for those whose children are to be born under their care; this serves not only to impart information, but to establish a rapport between the expectant couples and those who will be serving them later, when they return for the birth.

Education for childbirth should include the elementary facts concerning pregnancy, using diagrams, pictures, charts, and films as teaching aids. Basic instruction concerning clothing, diet, and hygiene should also be given. As the classes become more advanced, the phenomena of labor should take precedence in the discussion, and the women should be coached in learning correct breathing, relaxation, and the few simple exercises that will help them be in good physical condition for the birth.

It has become the custom in some childbirth classes to describe the various methods of inducing anesthesia or analgesia; different apparatuses are demonstrated and the women taught how they will be used. I have found that this introduces a serious fear that the rest of the instruction will be of no avail in labor. If the women are taught how these are to be utilized in labor and delivery, they expect that they *will* be required to relieve pain, and that the implication is that they will suffer.

But no difficulty arises if analgesia or anesthesia needs to be induced when a woman is in labor. A few words of advice and instruction at that time if she needs pain relief, and she quickly understands. Since over 95 percent of women who have been adequately prepared for a natural labor neither need nor desire such relief, there is no need to discuss the various means of pain relief. The risk of introducing fear during pregnancy to conflict with faith is unjustifiable.

I have never taught a woman during pregnancy how to use an inhaler for a whiff of anesthetic. I have never instructed a patient in the use of a hypodermic syringe and needle in case she requires an injection, *nor have I ever tied down a pair of hands and legs!*

These deflections from "orthodox" prenatal and obstetric procedures *have not prevented me, however, from eliminating all possible discomforts from normal labor.* Analgesia should always be available, for pain is the enemy of childbirth, *not* its natural accompaniment. It is, therefore, the first principle of an obstetrician to avoid or to overcome by the quickest and safest method any discomfort a woman in labor feels is more intense than she wishes to bear. The means of *preventing* pain from occurring in childbirth is the cornerstone of prenatal education; not teaching the necessity for pain and the methods by which it may be relieved. It is the quality of the instruction that makes these alarming demonstrations of pain-relieving apparatuses unnecessary.

Before we discuss briefly the teaching of relaxation during pregnancy, there are certain other considerations that demand attention. The attitude toward childbearing is variable; as obstetricians we must be conscious of what type or pigeonhole our individual patients fall into, and that is particularly important when we begin to teach them relaxation. Now, strangely enough, there are two types of women who are difficult or impossible to teach. Women who do not want their babies, who are bored by the whole procedure, and who feel they are merely doing a duty and are fed up at having to do it, very often avoid any practice of relaxation and become antagonistic to its teaching. Curiously, the other type is represented by the "plus" women, active, enthusiastic live wires to whom the application of modern science is all important. They are told the benefits of relaxation, but their reply is not infrequently that it would be quite unnecessary to apply it to them, as they will be able to control themselves when the time comes. They are sure that the whole thing should be conducted in a natural way and are preparing themselves along natural lines. Very often these women prefer the physical exercises, avoiding the careful practice of relaxation and assuming understanding, with no willingness to learn what they need to know.

But the majority of women are in the three types that are between the negative and positive extremes, all of whom willingly submit to being taught relaxation:

1. Those who are mildly negative, who are lazy and casual

in the conduct of pregnancy; they have to be kept up to the mark.

2. The real and natural mothers to whom all things to do with motherhood are inborn gifts and who are balanced in the exercise of their instinctive activities. They adjust themselves to the new rules of life without difficulty.

3. The slightly positive woman, who is so keen to do everything really well that she has to be gently restrained and very carefully educated.

Now, I am sure it will be readily appreciated by any experienced physician that a rule-of-thumb method of teaching relaxation is quite impossible under the circumstances. We have to use our discretion; it would be absurd to ask the negative woman to carry out, in exactly the same way, on the same principles, at the same times of day, those practices which we would invite the plus woman to carry out. If we are to get adequate results, we must balance our demands.

What, then, is relaxation in the sense in which we use the term? I suggest that for the purpose of its application in obstetrics, we consider relaxation to be *a condition in which the muscle tone throughout the body is reduced to a minimum*. We must remember that physiological reactions and reflexes vary, both in speed and intensity, with the fluctuations of neuromuscular tension. It is a quality that is susceptible to the moods and modulations of emotion in individuals, and there is *a direct relationship between the emotional state and muscular tone*. In fact, Jacobson goes so far as to say: "Present results indicate that an emotional state fails to exist in the presence of complete relaxation of the peripheral parts involved."*

In applying this to obstetrics, we can say that if the body is completely relaxed, it is impossible to entertain the emotion of fear. This is the important factor, for if fear is absent, then the overruling power of the sympathetic nervous system is absent

* Edmund Jacobson, *Progressive Relaxation* (New York: McGraw-Hill, 1929; rev. ed., 1938).

from the mechanism. I must remind you that this eliminates any excess of muscle tone in the circular fibers of the lower uterine segment, the cervix, and the outlet of the birth canal. Complete relaxation, therefore, offers the minimum of resistance to the muscles of expulsion in the birth canal.

I have found that complete general relaxation is the ideal to aspire to, but on the other hand it is astonishing how even imperfect relaxation may alter the whole course of labor. Possibly an expert like Jacobson might feel that some of our patients were not relaxing, according to what he believes to be complete relaxation. But if he saw a patient both before and after she had been asked to relax by her physician during labor, he would realize what a marked difference there is even if the performance leaves much to be desired. I have frequently been told how different labor becomes when the body is allowed to be "slack," and if women have tried to learn relaxation and are able to put it into effect, astonishingly gratifying results are obtained, for *the discomforts of labor vary inversely to the woman's ability to relax.*

I have been asked at what stage in pregnancy instruction in relaxation should be started. If there is the slightest tendency to nervous symptoms in the early months of pregnancy, such as morning sickness, salivation, or persistent frequency of urination, I embark on the early lessons of relaxation at once, providing there is no retroversion of the uterus or bladder irritation. The effect on nervous symptoms is very marked in some cases, and certainly worthwhile in all. If a woman is perfectly healthy and begins to feel, as she should, healthier and happier than ever before, I do not begin instruction in relaxation until the baby has quickened. There is a reality of pregnancy at that time that makes a woman anxious to do the things she is told will be of assistance to her and the child, and, if she is intelligent, can be taught enough in the remaining months of her pregnancy to enable her to get very good results from her efforts.

4

The Conduct of Labor

Many of my friends have asked me to give a detailed account
of the conduct of labor embodying the fundamental principles
of what has become known as "natural childbirth." It will be
necessary to begin by accepting the teaching of our great
masters of obstetrics so far as the ordinary routine of obstetrics is concerned. *The general principles of good obstetrics
must be recognized and practiced by all who undertake attendance upon women in labor.*

The obstetrician must be fully prepared to meet or provide
for all emergencies, and, since chapters on the conduct of
labor are usually concerned with the imminence of the unfore-
seen, it would be vain repetition to delve into the abnormal.
Let it be presumed, therefore, that all the sound general
principles are employed for the safety and care of women so
far as the purely physical process of childbirth is concerned.

Here we will examine the conduct of labor from the point
of view of the woman herself, her mental condition and
changing emotional state. This chapter is not intended as a
panacea for all the ills of labor, and will have but little influence in rectifying genuinely abnormal conditions or occurrences. But it does shed light on troubles that may appear to
be relatively unimportant but that in reality are the roots of
many serious evils.

Elation, relaxation, amnesia, and *exaltation* are the four
pillars of parturition upon which the conduct of labor de-

pends, each in its proper place maintaining, supporting, and controlling the impulses, both sensory and motor, upon which the neuromuscular harmony of the function relies.

Parturition is the great event in the reproductory cycle of woman. Although in recent years prenatal care has become increasingly important and its value fully recognized, labor is the real excitement for the patient and her attendants. But the nature of labor depends basically upon the efficacy of prenatal education, care, and, if need be, treatment, and the act of parturition should be complementary to the conduct of pregnancy.

ONSET OF LABOR (ELATION)

There is still some controversy on what indicates the establishment of true labor. The waters may leak for a number of days before labor starts—in fact, on several occasions I have observed that the water has stopped, the bag of membranes apparently closing. The "show" may appear some days before labor is established, but this sign is probably the most common of the three usual indicators of labor.

The recurrence of contractions or tightness of the uterus may be misleading, for some women who have not been prepared for labor and are still wrapped in anxiety may have contractions of the circular fibers in the lower part of the uterus for two weeks, three weeks, or even longer before the longitudinal fibers go into action and true labor starts. I have met women who believed in all seriousness that they were in labor from ten to fourteen days before the arrival of the child, but when the signs and symptoms that they had observed were discussed with them, it became clear that true labor had lasted for not more than twelve hours.

It is my opinion that the onset of parturition is best diagnosed by rhythmical contractions at shortening intervals, and a sense of generalized tightness of the abdomen without pain so long as the woman remains relaxed. The intervals will decrease from a quarter of an hour to five minutes or even less.

Women are all asked to go to the hospital as soon as it is established that labor is well under way. *Multipara* (women who have already had two or more children) recognize true labor contractions and waste no time, since they know how rapidly labor may develop under the influence of relaxation. *Primigravida* (women who are having their first child) have more time. My practice is to have them check with me on the telephone as to when to leave for the hospital.

To the Maternity Nurse

The arrival at the hospital should be a cheerful event, and it is essential that the nurses who greet patients know the value of maintaining an atmosphere of cordiality and confidence. After admittance procedures, the parturient woman is taken to a labor room and prepared for labor in accordance with instructions from her physician.*

Look upon fear as the great enemy of the patient; neither say, do, nor insinuate anything that will stimulate fear, or that may directly or indirectly mar the confidence which your patient has placed or desires to place in you and her doctor. Think, therefore, what does she fear? She fears pain and probably believes it to be essential. Her contractions are spoken of as "pains," and what are known as "pains" must be painful. *When will our nursing and medical professions cease to use this hideous term?* They are contractions, and if contractions, each becomes an effort to an end, each effort one more push that brings her baby nearer. Each contraction may be stronger than the last—therefore more effective, therefore more excellent—but if a "pain," the stronger it is the more intense the pain, and as the next one starts, the greater the expectation of agony.

* See *Standards for Obstetric-Gynecologic Hospital Services* (Chicago: The American College of Obstetricians and Gynecologists, 1969), pp. 28, 37 ff.

Stimulate courage in the patient by a quiet demeanor and your confidence in the fact that all is well; help her to relax from the beginning of labor; do not allow tension.

Not infrequently it has been noticed that an otherwise extremely skilled nurse has been unable to refrain from the temptation of advertising the relative superiority of her knowledge, and to call for full recognition of her professional efficiency. Small actions and large words have frequently destroyed the confidence of a patient that the nurse might justly have enjoyed. The maternity nurse may rest assured that until she has destroyed the confidence of her patient, she may enjoy it; that until she has advertised her efficiency, it is presumed; and that until she has called for consideration of herself, she has received it. Her attitude should be that of one who is present to support, not to interfere; of one who is there to advise, not to order.

Whatever you may think of the doctor in attendance, to your patient at least speak only in terms of greatest confidence and loyalty. It is not always easy to resist the temptation to insinuate mild disapproval of some action or word from the doctor, but remember it is the patient who matters. Not once but many times I have known a woman's confidence in her doctor to be severely shaken by a presumptuous attitude of disapproval she has discerned in the behavior of her nurse. Whether the nurse is right or wrong in her opinion of the word or deed of the physician in attendance, her duty to her patient is to place him on a pedestal that justifies complete faith in his conduct of the case.

FIRST STAGE OF LABOR (RELAXATION)

As early as possible after the patient's admittance to the hospital, my visit is made. This is not a hurried rush in and "Glad you've started! Get on with it—I'll be back in time" sort of visit, but a prolonged stay, possibly for an hour or more.

Elation, rejoicing, and a strong sense of contentment and

relief are the natural emotional reactions to the onset of labor, as was mentioned earlier. As her physician, be interested in her elation, encourage it, and mildly share it; she will feel that you are in harmony with her and will more readily accomplish relaxation of both mind and body as the contractions become firmer. Then as the spirit of jocularity wears off, as it will, the reality of her task will dawn upon her consciousness with a calm confidence.

It must not be overlooked that sometimes the most cheerful and apparently carefree woman may be very frightened. Beware of an excess of laughter between contractions; this is often a manifestation of tension of the mind and may well turn to tears when real effort and control become necessary in the later stages of labor. This anxiety or anticipation near the beginning of the final episode must be overcome by kindly but careful explanation of the sensations she is experiencing. During the visit a calm, reassuring, but firm kindliness is desirable.

If relaxation has been practiced and acquired as a habit, it will easily be accomplished during first-stage contractions. Complete relaxation of legs, arms, face, and therefore mind is the secret of a calm, quick labor. The points to remember are the few deep breaths as the uterus comes into action, and that the eyes should be open and the face relaxed—that is, no frown or puckered brow, no screwed-up eyes, no pursed lips or grinding teeth. There is no need for these exhibitions; they do no good. They are either demands for sympathy or manifestations of fear, and they increase neuromuscular tension.

How many doctors have been told, "Everything seemed much easier when you arrived"? The importance of the obstetrician's presence is not sufficiently realized, and one who fills this high office should be sure that he does not disappoint the woman who relies so implicitly upon his judgment, knowledge, and skill by appearing disinterested in her.

With the utmost patience, persevere until your patient is well relaxed during the contractions of early labor. Such patience will be amply rewarded. Speak quietly and with understanding; be honest in your advice and gentle in manner; point out once again the significance of these first-stage contractions. "They are pulling open the outlet of the womb. Step by step it expands and muscle is collected up and shortened, so that it cannot close again until the baby has passed through. The uterus must be left alone—it can do all this without any effort to help on your part. Consider it a machine apart from yourself, and in due course the dilatation of the outlet will be complete. There is no hurry—the door will open, but you must not make the work harder for the uterus by tightening the door. If you are rigid and squeeze up your face, then the muscles of the outlet will squeeze up, too. The uterus is astoundingly strong and persistent; the result of your resistance will be pain. But the more completely limp your muscles become, so much the more elastic will be the mouth of the womb, and so much less discomfort will you experience."

Women frequently comment on how different labor becomes once relaxation is obtained. They should be encouraged to maintain this state because it is common sense that an elastic opening is not only more easily but more quickly expanded. *Until a controlled relaxation is obtained by the patient the physician should not leave.*

A peaceful, confident atmosphere should be sustained and a close watch kept upon any untoward trend in conversation. The acute sensitiveness of women in labor must be constantly borne in mind. If you wish to try to deceive them you will fail. They miss nothing, and have a way of turning over in their minds the things they see and the words they hear. They are keen observers, not only of their own actions, but of the reactions of those about them to every fresh event or incident. This keenness of their perception must be appreciated; every expression, movement, and incident is observed, and no word or action passes unnoticed, for the occasion demands their fullest concentration. Any communication from those in attendance that can possibly be construed as disturbing their peace is harmful.

Nothing is more irritating than noise and restlessness when

relaxation is sought. Nothing is more exasperating than inconsequential chatter when the mind is occupied with an all-absorbing interest. Disturbing interludes of tune humming or muffled-up tap-dance rhythm on the bedside, frequent comings and goings, openings and closings, shufflings and solicitations, are thoughtless actions and indicate lack of human understanding. Women in labor also abhor loud voices, terse commands, and bright lights.

The patient's physical comfort should be attended to without ostentation. She should be reminded that the bag of waters in which the baby lies may break, and that this is perfectly normal. Many women have been terrified when, at the height of a strong contraction, the membranes have ruptured and they have felt a flood of warm liquid of which they had not been warned.

Care should be taken that adequate nourishment is given during the first stage of labor. It is a great mistake to leave a woman for ten or twelve hours without adequate nourishment. She is doing hard muscular work during this time and requires fortification, as we all do when we are occupied with physical exercise. Her hot or cold drink—whichever she prefers—may be given without demand for gratitude.

When the opening of the cervix is about two inches, or five centimeters, in diameter, a series of new sensations will be experienced, which will require explanation. It is not a question of physical pain that arises, but one of the emotional attack to which most women are subjected at this time. They wonder if they can possibly carry on; they feel the strain of labor, presenting an added impediment to complete relaxation.

This is *the first emotional menace of labor*. There are some women who, finding it very difficult to overcome this phase, become restless and, by their inability to relax, have a certain amount of real discomfort. A word of encouragement or explanation during this phase is of the greatest help, and should never be withheld. With the assistance of a nurse or medical attendant and husband who recognize the importance of this change, a calm and purposeful attitude toward labor can be reestablished. The contractions become stronger but the ability to relax improves. During and for an hour or two after this first emotional menace the woman should not be left.

Natural childbirth is not just sitting by and allowing what comes to take its course! The law of nature has a host of enemies not only in the mind and body of civilized woman but in the good intentions of those who are concerned with her well-being. An obstetrician should be a private detective who watches, guards, and unostentatiously accompanies a woman during her parturition. Should unpredictable emergency arise, he is able to meet it, fully equipped from the various departments of modern science with devices to overcome the misadventure, and safely deliver the woman of her baby.

At three in the morning we may be harassed by ruminations and imaginings that raise doubts in our minds and even warp our judgment. It takes a strong moral courage to be able to set out all the facts and review the situation with a calm, logical precision, particularly if the patient has detected a weakening in the support you have given her. During labor, a woman can spot a doubt in the doctor's mind as quickly as a falcon sees a rat in the stubble. However good an actor or however suave a humbug, confidence has no counterfeit. It is neither looks, words, nor works, but a special sense borne on the atmosphere of truth and inflexible honesty of purpose.

But always be on the watch. Concentrated observation need not be obtrusive, but it must be accurate and keen. You are more likely to find abnormalities by delineating the boundaries of good health than you are to find good health by concentrating upon real or phantom abnormalities. Your tranquility must be tempered with vigilance lest any harmful thing occur. It is astonishing how often patience will overcome difficulties and solve the host of mythical problems the long, quiet, waiting hours of night will create in fertile minds.

In general outline, I have drawn attention to some of the advantages of personal interest in a woman in labor, but the evils of its absence are not usually recognized. All sensitive women are hurt by friends who appear disinterested when friendship is most salutary. When, in times of anxiety, the support we expect of those in whom we have implicit faith is withdrawn, and when our self-confidence and fortitude are severely tested by the manifestations of a mysterious assailant, we long for the comforting voice of calm. However well-prepared and confident in her ability to achieve a satisfactory and natural birth a woman may be, *ultimately her success depends on each individual of the team of people* to whose influence she has been subjected during the changing phases of her reproductivity. She does not want to hear soft words and sob stuff, but explanation, instruction, and encouragement. She wants to hear that all is going well, that the baby is well and that she is conducting her job in an admirable manner. If she is left alone and not told these things, she may assume all is not going well and become alarmed with each new, though normal, phenomenon of labor.

Hospital organization, we know, makes constant attendance by medical personnel upon all women in labor extremely difficult, but *no patient should ever be left alone!** No greater curse can fall upon a young woman whose first labor has begun than the crime of enforced loneliness. Why cannot every obstetrician realize the enormity of this medieval torture?

Hear from women who have experienced this truly human attention what aid it gave to them; I suspect it will make you visualize their labors as something almost unbelievable. But observe as well whether your patient wants you there or not; some women dislike intensely the presence of anyone at all, and a good many do not want the doctor until they feel they must have him. Tactfully find out why, if you can. It may

* Ibid., pp. 40 ff.

teach you a lot about your patient that you had not previously suspected.

The Transition

During the latter part of the first stage it is of vital importance that nothing be said or done to allow tension. It is an interesting fact that neuromuscular tension is not relieved by analgesic drugs, for its influence emanates not only from the conscious but from the subconscious mind. Long after consciousness is lost the anesthetized patient will exhibit a picture of unrestrained anxiety; the reaction of muscular tension to a partially narcotized mind can be attested to by every medical student who has been called upon by the anesthetist to restrain the coal heaver, longshoreman, or powerful seaman during the early stages of anesthesia.

The final dilatation of the cervix is the phase that calls for the greatest control. At this time a woman demands that her courage be sustained, for real discomfort may be present in the most natural cases. Normally, a cervix is dilated much more rapidly from three inches to full than from half an inch to one and a half inches. The last few contractions increase the tension in the already well-stretched tissues of cervix and lower uterine segment, and the normal *nociceptors,* or pain sense organs, record pain stimuli as reactions to stretching and the small lacerations of tissue that may occur, for not infrequently such contractions are followed by a definite show of blood. Occurring in the area of the *sacrum,* or lower end of the spine, in about fifty percent of the cases, this tension is felt as an acute backache, and sometimes persists between contractions.

This discomfort is accompanied by a second change in the attitude of the woman toward her labor. Not infrequently it is the first time that she has been aware of any physical uneasiness, and it awakes in her mind many fears lest the backache resolve into a more severe pain. Fear definitely assaults the minds of many women just before full dilatation of the uterus, and is the *second emotional menace of labor*.

The backache, however, only persists for about nine to twelve contractions, a fact that a woman should be told, for a temporary discomfort is much more easily borne than one which is likely to persist. She should also be told to concentrate upon the depth and rapidity of her breathing. *It is possible to relax efficiently* in spite of the fact that respiration is quicker and deeper. The backache can be relieved by firm rubbing, or more often by really hard pressure on the sacrum.

If, at this stage of labor, there is pain anywhere else, it is probably due to some factor not usually present in normal labor. For instance, acute pain in the twelfth dorsal or upper lumbar region is not uterine in origin, but arises in the structures that take the strain of labor but that, if healthy, should do so without discomfort. Occasionally a woman will vomit during this latter part of the first stage of labor.

On one occasion I delivered a multipara, aged forty-two, of her second child, the first one having been born elsewhere some eight years before. She had accepted all the teaching she instinctively knew to be right, had practiced her relaxation to the best of her ability, and had taken a great interest in all the information I had given her upon the mechanism of labor. So little had appeared to be going on in her labor that I was not sent for for some time. When I arrived, I found her lying on her side, quiet and quite contented except, as she explained to me, for the considerable aching in her back. It was not a pain, she said, but a dull ache; it extended through to the front, and she felt it quite definitely along the lower backbone and above the bone in front.

When this occurs, I always do the same thing: I turn the patient over onto her back with pillows under her shoulders and the head well up, and during the next contraction I bring the knees upward and outward as far as possible; this almost invariably removes the pain in the front and relieves the discomfort in the back (fig. 1, p. 109). This is, of course, different from the sharp acute pain that the persistent occipito posterior will complain of just after full dilatation of the cervix. I explained to my patient the use of the gas apparatus, having placed it, as usual, in her hand so she could use it when necessary. She said there was no need for it, but it lay on the bed beside her so that she could use it if she wanted.

She told me that the pain in front disappeared after one or two contractions in that position, but that there was still a considerable ache in the back. She thought, possibly, that being forty-two her bones were a little stiffer than they should be; otherwise she felt quite convinced that there was no need even for the ache that she felt over the lower sacrum. She had not, up to that time, been using contractions very well, so I explained to her the best method of using them. "Wait," I told her, "until the contraction is at the top—you will understand what I mean—then draw a long breath and hold it. Do not push violently, but just lean on it." She did this and told me it was much more comfortable.

Her contractions came at about six-to-seven-minute intervals; in between them she slept. She was quite comfortable and controlled. When she awakened for a contraction, she said, "Now it is coming," and we lifted up her knees and let her push her feet against our hands. She hung onto her knees once or twice, but managed to do very well without exertion, and I told her not to press violently, as the baby would come easily. Her baby was born quite perfectly about an hour later.

On another occasion, on a Christmas morning a primipara was nearing second stage. She was getting good contractions; my opinion was that they were contractions that should have fitted in with the second stage, but she told me she had no inclination whatever to help them, and by relaxing in between times she was extremely comfortable, got on with her job in the most excellent way, and did everything she was told. She seemed very happy.

An hour later I was quite sure the contractions were second-stage ones, although she had no sort of urge to push down herself. So I told her to take a deep breath when the next one got to its height, and to "lean on it"; that is, to hold her breath and let herself contract in the upper abdomen so as to press down the lower. She understood that well, and told me it gave her a good deal of comfort; she liked the feeling, but her back was painful. Now, this pain in her back was not in the sacrum, the usual area, but was more in the region of the second and third lumbar vertebra. When I pressed on those, she said it relieved it a little but not altogether. She then turned over onto her back, drew up her knees and pushed against my hands— or, rather, my hands on one side and the nurse's on the other—held her knees and pulled on them, at the same time opening her legs as widely as she could. With the first contraction the baby's head appeared at the vulva, but after this progress became very slow. I watched several contractions carefully and could see no obvious reasons for the delay, but then I noted that she was arching her back when she pushed down. Since that is an unnatural position, I showed her how to round her back with her head forward. She said this was much more comfortable, and, indeed, seemed to work well. Suddenly, after three or four contractions in the rounded position, a loud, dull, crack sounded in her back. I asked her whether she had felt it and she said she had, and from that moment she had no further pain in her back at all. She herself said to me, "That seems to have cured the pain in my back." This was interesting, because I am persuaded that a good deal of the pain in the back during labor is owing to the posture in which the patient lies and the posture adopted during contractions. This particular patient had no pain whatever from that point on in any place at all.

Anesthetics and Analgesics

In childbirth there are two types of pain, each of which requires a different method of treatment. The first, which is unavoidable, accidental, and relatively rare, arises from abnormalities in the mechanism of birth, which require interference to rectify. This is true primary pain. The second, which is avoidable and relatively common, arises from the emotion of fear, which causes tension, which in turn causes pain—the fear-tension-pain syndrome we have already mentioned, which is responsible for nearly all the discomforts of normal labor. It is a vicious circle, for the increase of any one of them magnifies all three.

When a woman is in labor there should always be an anesthetic or analgesic apparatus at hand, and if necessary she should be instructed in its use. Throughout labor, if she appears to have any discomfort from which she desires to escape, her attention should be drawn to the available means of pain relief. It is interesting that women rarely desire analgesia under these circumstances; what discomfort there is does not justify its use.

When deep anesthesia is required a skilled and experienced anesthetist should be called in. The reagent to be used must be carefully selected after consultation between the obstetrician and the anesthetist. One method of pain relief is induced by deadening certain nerves in the pelvis with injections of anesthetic agents. When this method, in the hands of a highly skilled performer, is completely successful, it has certain physical advantages, but it has disadvantages that make unlikely its permanent or general place in normal obstetrics. It requires the constant attention of a specially trained and efficient staff, not only while it is being administered, but also after the baby is born. Apart from the possibility of physical injury there are serious risks to the mental processes of a woman who, although conscious, does not feel the sensations of childbirth. When she hears the first cry of her baby the normal flood of mother love is restricted by the absence of the pride of personal achievement. She may have a sense of failure and resent the fact that she did not take an active part in its birth.

Analgesia does not relieve severe physical pain. The milder

inhalants, such as Methoxyflurane (*Penthrane*—Abbot Laboratories), are used to relieve pain resulting from the influence of fear and tension in an otherwise normal labor. By their administration the senses are numbed and the pain-causing tension relieved. Such analgesia for short periods is the least harmful method of restoring confidence and releasing tension. If, however, too much is given or it is continued too long, risks are incurred both to the mother and the child.

One of my early colleagues stated that "the relief of pain by drugs is also a powerful means of conquering fear, and drugs are available which in my judgment provide a much simpler method. Incidentally, though the careful administration of drugs demands much sacrifice on the part of the doctor, it is probable that it is less exacting than the instruction in Read's technique, and that is a consideration to busy men and women."*

Does this really suggest that had I ever been unfortunate enough to be busy I would have learned that the easiest, safest, and simplest way to cure a poisoned mind is to poison the body as well? I have tried both methods, and find drugs more exacting, more uncertain, and less satisfactory. The women under my care have no doubt which they prefer. Let me summarize this matter:

1. For the perfect labor anesthesia is unnecessary because there is no pain.

2. The pain of labor should be *prevented* from occurring rather than obliterated.

3. Where the woman's ability to relax is absent and pain-producing emotions occur, analgesics should be used. Carefully administered pain relief during labor is one of the greatest gifts that our profession has made to civilization.

4. The misuse of drugs and anesthetics is the cause, directly or indirectly, of a large number of the complications of labor. It is the cause, not only of maternal and infantile mortality in

* Andrew Moynihan Claye, *The Evolution of Obstetric Analgesia* (London: Oxford University Press, 1939), p. 95.

many cases, but of ill health and domestic unhappiness in the lives of a great many women.

Anesthesia is only a veneer to cover up pain, trauma, and damage. It is sound and right in every way *if* used correctly in order to dispel pain. But if it is used in normal labor as a routine or to alter nature's intentions for either mother or baby, it is wrong—morally, ethically, and physically!

How much better it is for both mother and baby if the pain and damage can be kept from occurring in the first place. Professor Joseph De Lee, who taught at the University of Chicago Medical School during his lifetime, once wrote to me: "While I have not used pure hypnotism very often, I have used suggestion a great deal, indeed almost constantly, and I am irked when I see how my colleagues neglect to avail themselves of this harmless and potent remedy. It accounts for easily half of the success of local anesthesia."

The safest and most effective way to minimize the discomforts of childbirth is to enable woman, by preparation for, and understanding attention at, labor, to have her baby naturally.

SECOND STAGE OF LABOR (AMNESIA)

Sometimes a uterus calls for external help immediately after the cervix is fully dilated, but at other times the cervix may be fully dilated for some time without any reflex demand for assistance from the extrinsic muscles of expulsion, as in the cases mentioned earlier. Therefore it is advisable to introduce during the contraction a respiratory stimulus to this important reflex.

In the first stage, respiration is naturally free, increasing in rate and depth as dilatation progresses. From *twenty-four to twenty-eight full breaths* in a minute is normal at this time, *followed by one or two deep breaths* as the uterus relaxes, as occurs after the prolonged use or strain of any muscle in the body. But in the second stage, as a contraction develops to its greatest tension, a deep inspiration is made, and is held during the bearing-down effort. Now, if the cervix is dilated fully, the woman should be made to draw a deep breath and hold it at the height of the contraction. Not infrequently, after doing this once or twice she will begin to bear down, and will remark upon the satisfaction the effort affords her. Once the reflex is started in that way it continues, and the distinctive phenomena of the second stage become increasingly apparent. With the uterine contractions somatic relaxation is impossible, but between them it is easier than at any other time during labor; in fact, as the uterus works more violently in its effort to expel the baby, a relaxed sleep in the intervals between contractions is commonly observed.

If the woman's confidence has been maintained by a sympathetic comprehension of her reactions to psychical and physical stress, she will pass quietly into the second stage, with its lowered mental appreciation and its modified interpretation of sensory stimuli. As this *amnesia** occurs, she demonstrates the relative inactivity of her senses of discretion and discrimination; she becomes oblivious to her surroundings and careless of her appearance, expression, and speech. Normally—that is, in the absence of any dominating fear—she is devoid of any consciousness of herself and employs all her energies in the fulfillment of the immediate purpose.

Sit always at the *head* of your patient, for this is the center of activities. To sit, as is so frequently done, at the other end is wrong. Not only is your patient unable to see you, but she naturally concentrates her mind upon what is going on down below, feeling that you would not be there unless you expected something to happen. But in reality the doctor is frequently there long before he expects anything at all to happen at that end of the body that is worthy of his attention. Certain attentions may have to be made below from time to time, especially if preparation has not been efficient and complete, but surely a

* Dr. Dick-Read does not use this word in its usual sense of forgetfulness, but as descriptive of a relaxed inattentiveness.—Ed.

competent nurse in attendance can deal with this as satisfactorily as the doctor himself.

During the second-stage contractions, explain carefully to your patient how she can help her contracting uterus. This requires considerable experience. Do not allow her to be violent in the early part of the expulsive stage, because there is no need for such exertion. She must hold her breath in full inspiration and bear down when and as the uterus demands. With a first baby this is important, for unnecessary tiredness or fatigue, which should not occur, may create difficulty in the final dilatation of the outlet.

A patient of mine began labor with her third child. She had come to me rather late in pregnancy, telling me that she had had considerable trouble with her children before, and found it difficult to believe in the teaching of natural childbirth although, having heard of it, she wished to try. She practiced her relaxation assiduously, and did her exercises as well as she could, but she was stiff and rather tender in the back; she did not have what one would call a good obstetric back.

During her labor I asked her whether she would like me to sit in the room next to hers or whether I should be with her, and she was very emphatic about my not leaving her. She preferred absolute quiet and peace, and I must say that the nurse assisted me in that. There was not a sound of any sort—even walking was on tiptoe—and my patient relaxed beautifully during the contractions and slept in between them. Then I noticed suddenly that there was a drooping of the eyes and a slight listlessness. She was obviously passing into the second stage, but not before proclaiming that her back was extremely sore; there was an aching pain low down in the sacral region. This was relieved by pressure and rubbing, and we went quietly and patiently on. I told her that all that was required was patience and hard work, and that if she felt any pain I would certainly do something at once to relieve it.

And so, from the beginning of the second stage, she became

a typically amnesiac woman. She found it rather difficult to hold her breath and to—as I describe it—"lean on it," and also at first she quite definitely tensed her pelvic floor whenever a contraction started. The nurse, who was watching the contractions from below—as I naturally could not see—told me that there was definite contraction of the whole pelvic floor, the anus being quite drawn in when the uterine push was at its height. We overcame that with a little instruction, and got on well. The pain in the back became rather more acute. The patient could not get comfortable or get into a good position. As soon as she raised her knees she got a cramp, and so I decided that, since the head was obviously coming down well and there was slight distention of the anus already, she should turn onto her back and adopt the semisitting position I frequently ask patients to adopt at that time. As she did so, the very first contraction seemed to present a different picture: the head came down until it was visible, the pain in the back was much less acute, and after about four or five contractions at long intervals—ten minutes or so—the head was born perfectly.

I do not know the cause of that state in the second stage which dulls the conscious brain, but, from watching closely all the signs and symptoms, the first thing I should like to investigate would be the oxygen metabolism. The enormous muscular exertion must produce chemical changes altering carbon dioxide, oxygen, and lactic acid balance. On these lines the nature of the second stage of labor anesthesia can be explained. It is upon suboxidation that the conscious brain fades out and the instinctive reflex activities of the subconscious are made free to act. The ideal anesthetic state during labor is the subconscious, not the unconscious. This state is frequently present as a natural process in normal labor, and demands understanding, not narcosis.

For your patient's sake, be interested in her mental and physical well-being during labor; for your own sake observe closely her reactions to its demands. You are dealing with several different women during labor; she who is reacting to her social environment in the early first stage has little physical and mental resemblance to she who reacts to the uncontrollable neuromuscular energies of the late second stage. The old saying that women are always unpredictable is never more true than in labor.

The course and progress of labor must be watched and followed in all its stages, particularly at the end of the first stage, when the second emotional menace of labor makes its subtle attack upon a woman. And so it may be again in the latter half of the second stage of labor, especially if the woman, strong and healthy, is bearing her first baby. The thick perineum must gradually be thinned out by successive uterine contractions until it can allow the baby's head to pass. It is so slow—there seems to be no progress, no advance—the weary hours hang heavily upon the attendant's expectation. The woman, amnesiac and contented, is not aware of time.

When the head is in the midpelvic cavity—possibly the bag of waters or the baby's head is just showing—extra effort may be called for, providing that amnesiac rest and relaxation are obtained between the contractions. Waken the patient to the conscious reality of her surroundings and be alert to advise her on how to get a relaxed outlet and the best method of mechanical advantage for her efforts. But do not presume that she is unaware of what is going on. *She may appear to be asleep and behave in a dull and amnesiac state, but she is not asleep and will hear and understand everything as her contraction begins again.*

As the head advances through the birth canal and reaches the muscles that form the floor of the pelvis, a sensation of internal pressure is felt. Some women have described it as resistance, and it is the third occasion during labor when a large number of women feel a definite wave of fear and exasperation. It is at this time, when the baby's head may be only one inch from the outlet of the birth canal, that many women become frustrated and disappointed with efforts that they feel are of no avail. It is so marked that it has been termed the *third emotional menace of labor.*

The desire to escape, very largely exaggerated by the absence of discretion, may easily be misunderstood by those who have not examined this phenomenon closely. When a woman desires to escape from anything that she does not wish to experience, she may use all manner of wiles to obtain her object. Many will complain of agonizing pain while their pulse remains at seventy. Many will ask for anesthesia—not for pain, they will explain, but because they have "had enough." Some will say that they are completely exhausted and cannot possibly go on: "Will you please help me?" On occasions the attendant obstetrician will be told exactly what his patient thinks of him!

Great care is needed on the part of the attendant not to be misled by emotional exhibitions and not to mistake them for physical discomforts. Severe physical discomfort at this phase of the third stage of labor is extremely rare in a normal presentation of the child, a fact that has been told me after labor by a large number of women. Several women doctors, who have had their babies and observed the processes of physiological labor closely while they have been experiencing them and communicated their sensations to me, have explained afterward that in their opinion the most terrifying part of labor was the uncontrollable desire to *escape* at this third emotional menace. One went so far as to tell me that *I had not emphasized sufficiently the importance of this incident* and that, in spite of my reassurance, she had had considerable difficulty in accepting, at the time, the advice I gave her.

Now, this threat to a woman's self-control is in no way difficult to overcome. The method is that at the next contraction she should be told to *concentrate* and *push as firmly as she can*, for as soon as she exerts the maximum pressure all discomfort ceases and confidence is restored at once. The third menace of labor is negligible if it is met with a combative determined effort, for once the pelvic floor is adequately distended the head passes down the vagina rapidly and without discomfort.

Crowning

As the head comes down onto the vulva it becomes visible, and the patient should be told that the baby can be seen. This is a most encouraging moment, but she should *not* be told it will be there in five minutes. It may take half an hour for a baby to be born after the head is first seen at the outlet, particularly if it is a first baby.

The contractions now should be used fully. When the vulva is dilated to about one and a half to two inches in diameter the woman will feel the outlet stretching. This is natural, because the opening has to stretch. Since the sensation is one of burning, the woman must be forewarned, for it may be very frightening and may become acutely uncomfortable if not properly managed. *At this point all efforts to bear down should be stopped.* The burning varies in intensity but is rarely of such significance that the patient feels it desirable to resort to the analgesic inhaler. The sensation is intensified by an alarmed woman—she resists by squeezing up her pelvic muscles. An understanding attendant will overcome the slight and transient discomfort, as described below, and with full crowning of the head the sensation ceases.

This stretching of the vulva is rightly termed the *fourth emotional menace of labor.* Many feel that they must inevitably burst or tear and, in an effort to prevent this, will actually endeavor to contract the muscles of the pelvis in resistance to the oncoming head. Watch carefully the beginning signs of a contraction. If the patient automatically tenses up her pelvic muscles, if the anus is contracted and the muscles tense about the vulva, help her to relax. The woman must be reassured that she will not burst, but that she must relax and allow her baby to come in a quiet and controlled manner, without pushing, and that the sensation will disappear as the vulva is more fully dilated. I have wondered at times whether the dilatation of the vulva in some way or other does paralyze certain sensory nerves, for as soon as the vulva is nearly fully dilated it loses the sensation of burning and becomes quite anesthetic.

The absence of tension from the muscles comprising the floor of the pelvis, the relaxation of the vaginal sphincter, and, what is more difficult to explain, the apparent increased elasticity of the skin of the vulva, facilitates the passage of the infant through the birth canal. The uterus, of itself, will slowly urge the child forward. *During contractions the woman should be told to breathe in and out rapidly.* It is a comforting dispensation of nature that the pushing reflex can be overcome voluntarily at this stage of labor, and that a woman can breathe freely without giving way to the urge to bear down.

In this way the vulva is gradually distended—and it should be distended gradually without any violence, for tears of the skin and even of the muscles are frequently produced unnecessarily because a woman is encouraged to bear down violently.

Allow full crowning of the head and do not hurry by pressure from behind or efforts to stretch the vulva over the forehead; it will slide over quite easily without tear or injury if left to itself. Not infrequently a woman is unconscious of the birth of the baby's head. There is no doubt about the relative anesthesia of the perineum during the late second stage and for some minutes after the child has been born.

And again, when the head is born there is no immediate hurry if all has gone smoothly. It may cry before the shoulders arrive. Check the cord; a hand may be out of place; resist expulsion by violent contraction, or you may have a tear by shoulder or elbow. Support the head in the right hand and allow the child to awake its mother from her light amnesia. With the next contraction, the attendant may require gentle assistance from the woman and invite her to bear down. It is my custom to wait until pulsation has practically ceased before severing the cord, even if it is four or five minutes.

One of my patients provides a good example of several of these phenomena. Eight years previously, at eight months pregnancy, she had been delivered of twins by forceps. One had died, and the remaining twin was brain damaged. She had come under my care for this birth, and was very nervous and alarmed about it all. But her labor went well, and there was not much discomfort until near the end of the first stage. Then she began to feel a certain amount of discomfort low down in the back, which was different from any previous sensation. I pointed out to her that if she would put up with one or two of those twinges in the back—which, by the way, entirely disappeared when I pressed firmly over the sacral region—they would pass off quite quickly and that it was just a phase in the labor.

Then the really interesting part of her labor began. She had a prolonged and good contraction, lost her smile, and became a serious woman starting her second stage. She flung her head back, and when I looked to see whether there was any change at all down below, she said, "Oh, take off those clothes—it is quite impossible to be a lady now!" She lost all her natural reserve and shyness and the rather unusual refinement of speech that characterized her. She had one or two more similar contractions, and I said, "Now, I want you to draw a deep breath and find out whether you have any inclination to bear down." She tried this and found that it was not only pleasant, but that it was a distinct relief to her just to give a gentle push down when a contraction was at its height.

From that moment onward I saw one of the most perfect examples of what I have so frequently described as the amnesia of the second stage—the phenomenon I believe to be so important and to which so little attention is paid in modern obstetrics. She became an entirely different woman. Her natural, quiet voice and controlled self disappeared, and she seemed to alter in every way. She paid no attention whatever to the dishevelment of her hair, the position of her clothes, the position of herself. Her eyes were half closed; between the contractions she passed into a quiet sleepy condition, not answering when spoken to, and when a contraction started she suddenly brightened up and, saying, "Here's another one," grasped her knees, pulled her legs into the correct position, and helped for all she was worth. After a time she gave vent to an exaggerated groan, because it was nature's demand that she not relax the tension too quickly. I also pointed out that there was no need for her to suffer pain at all—I had already explained to her how to use the gas apparatus that was in her hand or on the pillow beside her—and she quite violently said, "It isn't a question of pain—it is this frightful bursting feeling. I feel I am going to burst down below." I assured her that she was not going to burst down below, and her reply was, "You don't know." She generally became an aggressive, different woman altogether, but still assured me that it was not a question of pain. As each contraction faded away she became listless, semiconscious, and sleepy.

The head came down nicely; the crown began to show; the membranes had ruptured previously. The second stage was only twenty-five minutes from beginning to end. When the head began to crown, I said, "Are you quite sure you are having no pain?"

She looked wildly at me again, grasped my arm, and said, "Pain? What do you call pain? The whole damn thing is painful—you ought to know it by now."

I said, "Why have you not taken your gas, then? It's there, and I asked you to let me know if you felt anything that hurt you, and you haven't taken it. Now, will you please take your gas, because it is not necessary for you to have pain. In fact, I object to your having pain."

And then, in quite a feckless way, she said, "Oh, it isn't really pain. Let's get the thing over—I'm sick of it. Can't you do something?"

I said, "No, certainly not—there is nothing to do. If you will do as you are asked now quietly, sensibly, and in a controlled manner we shall have this baby in a very few more contractions."

And she said, "All right, get on with it."

I said, "Won't you have some of that gas?"

"No, I don't want the gas."

The head came down and crowned, and there was a lot of scar tissue all around her vulva, and she said, "I think it is going to tear—it feels as if it is going to tear."

I said, "Does it hurt you?" and she replied, "No, it doesn't hurt me, but it feels awfully tight."

I said, "Very well—I think you had better have a few whiffs of gas."

So she put the mask over her face, and took a few whiffs of gas, and then said, "It doesn't hurt—what do I want that for?" And so on.

That was her sort of behavior the whole way through. She was certainly not a woman who was conscious of what she was doing entirely, and certainly not the Mrs. X I had known for five or six years as a rather mild, gentle, and refined woman in her manner. Here was the changed woman whose consciousness had been driven below the normal level, and whose powers of discretion and discrimination were dulled and whose sensory receptors were inhibited.

The baby was born naturally, and there was only a small tear—a little slit of less than half an inch long in the scar tissue that was kept together with one small stitch, the immediate insertion of which appeared to cause Mrs. X no discomfort.

When the baby arrived, it was quite an astonishing picture. Mrs. X came out of that amnesiac state, and I said, "Here is your little girl."

She looked at me. "That isn't true."

I said, "It's quite true."

Her eyes were half closed, and she continued to look at me in a suspicious way. The baby cried lustily, and I held it up.

She asked, "Are you sure it is normal?"

I told her, "There is nothing the matter with this baby."

But she said, sighing, "Ah, you don't know."

After possibly three or four very trying minutes, she took the child and held it in her hands. Then she seemed to cast her doubts and fears away; it was really a very dramatic picture as she suddenly cried, "Then I'll believe you!" In a flash her restraint disappeared and she was wreathed in the smile of incomprehensible happiness.

THIRD STAGE OF LABOR (EXALTATION)

Whether the first cry of a baby indicates its pleasure or displeasure upon arrival we are unable to say, but physiologically it is essential to the life of the child and extremely beneficial to the well-being of its mother. At the sight of her child the mother becomes an entirely different person. The amnesia has gone. Her happiness and the expression of delight are so dramatic that the birth of the child, which is the change from the second to the third stage of labor, has been called a state of exaltation.

There is a purpose in every natural phenomenon that occurs during labor. *This joy is not only the first flood of maternal love,* but, as has already been mentioned, in the more banal sense of physiological reaction it causes a violent contraction of the uterus, prevents any excessive loss of blood from the site of detachment of the placenta, and hastens the expulsion of the afterbirth. As a mother fondles and toys with the fingers of her child the great muscular organ is a hard solid ball of safety within her abdomen. I say "of safety," because from the obstetrician's point of view, should he have an anxious moment, it is when the uterus during the third stage of labor is flaccid and will not contract upon the afterbirth.

The child is placed in a warm crib beside the mother's bed, and the mother is given a hot or cold drink. After perhaps ten minutes, she will feel again gentle contractions of the uterus, or indeed the uterus may contract firmly without her being conscious of it. The attendant will know when the placenta has passed from the uterus into the vagina, and, about twenty minutes after the child is born, the woman may feel a definite desire to bear down and extrude the afterbirth. This is not done by the attendant, as it used to be years ago, for there is no necessity to help the uterus.

It should not be overlooked that many women believe the delivery of the afterbirth to be an event of considerable severity and discomfort. Therefore the care of a woman's mind during this twenty minutes or so is important. After a natural birth the attendant may be carried away by the atmosphere of happiness radiated by the mother, but the emotional changes of the third stage are quite definite, conforming to a miniature labor. The reaction to the first exhilaration may occur with the reestablishment of rhythmical uterine contractions. These are accompanied by slight drowsiness, which is disturbed by an irritated attitude toward the unexpected anticlimax of the recurrent uterine activity. The reestablishment of the expulsive reflex is received with satisfaction and success of the ultimate effort, a long persistent bearing down as the spongy mass is extruded. This is greeted with a sigh of relief and a feeling of final achievement. The delivery of the placenta is the end of labor.

If labor is conducted in this way you will be preventing many of those complications of labor which experience has led you most to fear: you will be surprised how seldom an occipito-posterior presentation delays labor; you will notice how rarely the placenta is slow to separate. A torn perineum will become to you a personal disgrace and not an unavoidable occurrence. And this kind of labor is more than parturition. Not only does the body of the mother suffer no damage, but her organs return to normal. Her muscles, uninjured, become reinstated; her nervous system suffers no trauma. We do not find the puerperal neurasthenia; we do not find the sleepless, wasting babies. The mother becomes again the wife, physically and mentally equipped to retain the affection and admiration of her husband. May the importance of this never be overlooked by the obstetrician who allows a torn perineum to go unmended, a pendulous abdomen to go untreated, and breasts to become straplike and unattractive. We are not so civilized that there is yet anything to take the place of sexual attraction in the maintenance of happiness in the homes of the people.

There is no more beautiful event in the life of a human being than the natural birth of a child. Subtract from modern childbirth the inflictions of ignorance, and it becomes a joy to the mother; protect a healthy woman from the influences of cultural contaminations, and parturition may be witnessed as a physiological masterpiece. Look with quiet, comprehending eyes at the miracle of nativity; each reflex is a reasoned part without which the intricate machinery would break down. No sound or movement of the newborn babe is without significance to its survival; already it is predisposed to a familiar pattern, but we see it suddenly possessed of individuality. It has not the ability to speak our tongue; its cries are not the tears of sadness but commands and demands for essential services. It looks at us and sucks its fingers; it sneezes and expands its lungs in physiological songs; it kicks and waves its arms; it urinates and grunts to expel meconium; within a few hours it learns the reward of importunity.

No science knows the origin or the nature of those forces which united in harmony to vitalize and perfect this new life, cast off from the uterus of a woman whose facultative genius has developed, nurtured, and ripened the physiological facsimile of herself. The cultural acquisitions of the human race are not yet comparable to the works of God.

5

Childbirth and the Family

Mutually well-selected pairs retain, or after marriage develop, a physical and emotional harmony known as love. This awakens in the man a desire for children by the woman he loves and in the woman the physiological preparedness for children and a possessive demand for the soul as well as the body of her man. These are healthy reactions to the natural and biological law, for they last longer and carry assets greater than sexual infatuation and physical satisfaction. Pregnancy sets the course of a woman for the fulfillment of herself. She expands her horizons and her ambitions, and if healthy in mind and body—the former is all important—she is no longer a woman in love only with a man, she is the mother of her man's child. She needs and expects him to join in her life for the sake of the baby that is their own.

THE HUSBAND

Not many years ago, in England and the United States, the idea of a husband being no more than proudly, but distantly, interested in the pregnancy of his wife was generally accepted, and in the mid-Victorian era women retired from public life as soon as they became "obviously with child." The relationship of the father to the family was less intimately companionable than it is today. But there is a change, and it is noticeable that during the last three decades husbands have demanded to know more about childbirth. In many other countries, however, the cooperation of the husband in pregnancy has long been recognized as one of the first essentials of family life.

During the 1920s I started a series of lectures for men's organizations because of requests I had received to instruct groups of young and expectant fathers in what I considered should be their attitude and behavior during the pregnancy of their wives. These talks were given almost entirely to the working classes of the suburbs around London, and one of the main features at such meetings was that, after I had spoken, an hour should be set aside for questions and discussions.

It soon became obvious that the ignorance of the average man in the street about childbirth was incredible. At that time I had the advantage of being the father of a growing family of young children and was closely interested in the question of the husband's role during both pregnancy and the early months of infancy of his offspring.

Some of the men whose wives had to work, whether they were pregnant or not, expressed very strongly the view that the local nursing associations should organize what they called "mother's helpers," who would be responsible for many of the domestic duties that normally fell upon the shoulders of their wives. They were concerned for the health of the prospective mother but at the same time expressed no desire to take upon themselves some of the extra duties that they considered were too much for a pregnant woman.

Others made it clear that the woman of the house was responsible for the provision of food and comfort that they enjoyed when they came home after a strenuous day's work, but many broke down the natural reticence of the Englishman and stated quite plainly what they thought, in some such terms as these: "I love my wife—she's got to have all the trouble and pain of giving me a child. My job is to go on earning a living to keep the home together while she is ill, but I want to do more than that and I don't know how to be of any help to her."

That attitude of the husband toward the wife was very prevalent, and I have no doubt that it was prompted by a deep affection and concern for her welfare. The general trend of my talks was to elaborate this aspect of the husband-wife relationship by giving the men a simple explanation of what went on during pregnancy, how the child develops, and the changes that occur during pregnancy in a woman's mind, particularly toward her husband.

During pregnancy a woman's activities, thoughts, and behavior need careful understanding and considerable tolerance and unselfishness on the part of the husband. There is, in return for this small burden that he must bear, a change in his own attitude, for pregnancy often intensifies his love for his wife. It creates in him an ardent desire to take care of her and attend to her needs and wishes with tenderness and consideration.

The importance of the husband's attitude toward, and understanding of, childbirth cannot be exaggerated. His words and actions, and even the atmosphere in the house that he may create in silence, have a profound effect upon his wife. Her health and happiness during pregnancy, and certainly her approach to labor, will be influenced for better or for worse by harmony or discord that she feels in her husband's mind.

The real joy of childbirth is most frequently experienced when husband and wife have mutual confidence, affection, and understanding, and have worked together in preparation for the arrival of their baby.

A man who knows nothing about these things will often sublimate his ignorance in irritability—preferring to succumb to the latter rather than disclose the former. He may even state dogmatically what is sense and what is nonsense. His urge to take care of his wife, whom he loves very dearly, easily develops into a rigid military-type discipline. Men often formulate domestic principles during their wife's pregnancy, and demand that they be meticulously carried out. Rest, diet, exercise, recreation, and even personal hygiene are matters in which they suddenly become expert without absorbing any authoritative teaching on the subject. If the doctor does not agree—the doctor is wrong.

This is, of course, a manifestation of conflict in a man's mind. Pride, anxiety, and tenderness get horribly mixed up, and that is one of the main reasons why some husbands suffer so much in childbirth. They need preparation and understanding just as do their wives. The surest way of being of assistance in the cause of peace and confidence, both in the home and elsewhere, is to urge, with quiet but kindly-stern authority, that the husband learn with his wife the phenomena and common sense of this natural human function.

During the last several years I have been gratified to find that the majority of husbands accept this advice—and what a difference it makes to obstetrics!

Let us, insofar as possible, give a few wide generalizations of the signs and symptoms of pregnancy, both physical and emotional, that will become apparent to an observant and attentive husband.

Conception is a supreme event in a woman's life—it is the beginning of that phase which represents the achievement of her physiological purpose. Conscious and unconscious experiences of her childhood and early maturity flood the vista of her future while being strongly influenced by the fantasies of the past. Every impression that she has received of childbirth shapes her acceptance of pregnancy. Each stress or strain that has caused her doubts or fears during those years when the small girl rehearses to her secret self what motherhood must be finds a place in her mind. As women vary in nature so do these psychological manifestations, but even more important are the different aspects of parenthood that arise from such considerations as: Is the baby wanted or unwanted? Was it planned or accidental? Is she longing for a child but her husband disappointed that she is pregnant?

Women develop, very early after conception, an acuteness of mind and thought that intensifies their appreciation of the words and feelings of their husbands. Although it is not necessary to explore more deeply the actual psychological basis for her reactions, it should be recognized that these are not just whims and moods but real mental states based upon sound psychological deductions.

Herein lies the responsibility of a husband to his unborn child. Happily, some men seem to have the inborn understanding of a woman's thoughts and needs at that time, and others wish to learn how they can be of service to the woman they love and admire. Husbands should take part in the intrauterine development of their children, learn and practice the important role of father. It is the most crucial phase in the life of a human being, for as the miracle of the child's construction progresses, the changing tissues, utilized in making the perfect form, may be deflected from the natural course. Therefore, the health of the mother is the responsibility of the father of the child and may thereby directly affect the quality of the baby.

There is so much more we need to learn of all these things. We know today that some of the things that happen during pregnancy may be attributed to superstitions that are not true (e.g., the child whose mother saw a horse stumble gets a wart on his neck!), but there may be something valid in some of the "old wives' tales." We are very unwise if we turn them down without a very discriminating investigation, especially those ideas which have stood the test of time.

I remember so well as a small child being told by my old nanny, "Don't you believe what the people say about the Master (my father) being able to cure warts." Of course he used to cure warts! He used to select the new moon and wave his hand over the lady and say, "Your wart will not be here when the next new moon comes." He did it "tongue in cheek," and he enjoyed doing it. But the warts disappeared. Today we know perfectly well that any minor hypnotist of strong persuasion can cure certain types of warts in the same way.* We are

* See *Time* Magazine, "Warts and All," January 4, 1971, p. 60.

beginning to learn that the fantasy of folklore is not so funny as we thought, particularly in relation to the unborn child.

We have come to realize that a child is nourished in the womb through its mother's blood, and that any emotional variations of the mother, in spite of constants, may in some way affect the nutrition and metabolism of the unborn child. I don't believe in biochemical constants; I don't believe even genes are constant. I believe there is something that flows in the mother's blood that varies according to her temperament. These substances, which come from the internal secreting glands and other structures that secrete or exude, vary as the physical and emotional state of the mother and are poured into the bloodstream that nourishes the baby. Thus the baby undoubtedly has its constitutional variants. We know today that by altering the emotional state of the mother we can record the concomitant changes in the pulse of the baby. We know that as the mother is, so at least is the baby directed in its development, particularly in its emotional development.

Let this postulate be examined in simple common sense. A pregnant woman's health has certain manifestations, but first and foremost she must be *happy*. This demands companionship and interest in her baby and all that concerns it. She can be happy only if her husband shares her hopes and anxieties, her laughter, and her waves of fear. He alone can be the safety valve of her unpredictable emotions and accept unmoved the explosions of her love, hate, fear, jealousy, and anger. The storms are usually followed by warm sunshine. But if she is alone and feels, justly or unjustly, that the baby she longs for has robbed her of her husband's love, serious temperamental and emotional states occur that set up local and sometimes general reactions within her body. A disturbed mind will upset the circulation of blood to certain organs of the body,* perhaps causing a serious deprivation of the oxygen supply within the body that is essential for the well-being of the small fetus in the womb.

* Walter B. Cannon, *Bodily Changes in Pain, Hunger, Fear and Rage*, 1929 (New York: Harper & Row, rev. ed., 1963), p. 93.

Therefore, throughout pregnancy the husband's part develops with the wife's. He reads and learns with her the dignity, the beauty, and the spiritual advantages of family union. To understand he must learn, and to be the pillar of strength his wife desires takes time, but nothing can be of greater or more lasting value to each member of the family unit.

But a woman does change when she becomes pregnant in some ways that are quite incomprehensible. She may discover that she has entirely new tastes, particularly for food, and she may eat things she has previously disliked or, more frequently, dislike intensely articles of food she had previously enjoyed. Some become pernickety, others voracious.

During the first trimester of pregnancy a woman who has usually been active, athletic, and untirable may be easily tired, complain bitterly of the weariness of the flesh, and have small urge either to be entertained or to entertain. This is not an unusual condition and does not indicate illness, for undoubtedly nature calls for a quieter life during the first three months of pregnancy. Twelve to fourteen hours of sleep is normal at this time, and should be encouraged. There are strange changes, too, in her attitude toward her husband, which are quite unpredictable. Some women cannot bear to have him out of their sight and overwhelm him with their affection and physical demands; others become cold and distant, quite unable to accept with any enthusiasm his wonted demonstrations of affection, and not infrequently the idea of any sexual life between them is temporarily repugnant. Such changes should be recognized and tolerated by the husband, who should exercise the art of kindliness and gentle persuasion to avoid any excess of either positive or negative emotionalism.

After three months, life becomes easier. Now the husband should learn with his wife what the succeeding phases of pregnancy will bring; he should be interested in her diet, her exercise, and her prenatal preparation for the arrival of the child.

Between eighteen and twenty weeks, when the wife has

become conscious that the small swelling in her pelvis is no longer an impersonal tumor, and the movement of the child is felt, she tends to become more interested in her baby as an individual. This is a time when the husband should tactfully intensify his interest in his wife, for there is a risk of her becoming too single-minded in her newfound possession to reciprocate his affection. By twenty-six weeks she will become noticeably pregnant, and should take particular care to maintain her appearance and her posture, and to dress in a becoming manner.

Happily, in these days of enlightenment women are proud of pregnancy and do not retire from the public gaze as many were wont to do in the past. The husband, too, very rarely shows embarrassment, which was not unknown in the time of our grandfathers; he tends to exhibit a laudable pride in her happiness and radiant good health.

Unfortunately, even today the misdirected prudery of authorities still exists in some places. A university with which I am well acquainted, where there are a large number of women students, many of whom marry before they have obtained their degrees, will not allow a woman who is known to be pregnant to continue her studies, as it is considered embarrassing for the young male students! In the same town, where a very high percentage of the women work in offices, those who become pregnant must immediately cease their employment. This gives rise to considerable agitation, and many of these women will suppress the fact of their pregnancy for as long as possible, since the money that they are earning is necessary in order to help the husband to obtain and furnish a home. Fortunately, this attitude toward motherhood is rapidly dying out, as indeed it must in a world in which it is necessary for women to work in order to supplement the earnings of their husbands.

During the last ten weeks of pregnancy the husband's lot is that of protector and guide for his wife. Her activities are limited, and, invariably, as the weeks creep on he will find it acceptable to his wife if he helps her in the domestic organization of the house, especially if there are already one or two small children in the family.

By this time he will have been wise if he has learned with her how the child arrives and the process of labor by which it comes into the world. He will also be familiar with the exercises she has performed to make herself physically fit, and he will assist her, and even practice with her, the arts of respiration and relaxation, and at the same time know clearly why they are so valuable a part of prenatal preparation.

A stockbroker, who did not come to see me until his wife was near term, and whose interest in her rose and fell with his stocks and shares, asked me resentfully: "Why should I know all about this—it's her business, not mine." I replied: "Oh, yes, she is excellent and with average luck should bear your baby with little or no discomfort, but I don't want you to have an unnecessarily distressing labor." This aspect of the situation appealed to him, and soon he was adequately informed. He was with his wife when their child was born, and it brought to them not only a son but something else they had never shared before.

Some years ago, a busy, erstwhile athletic attorney, who had become rather rotund because he had put in too much time at his work and not taken enough exercise, came in to see me with his wife, who was about thirty-eight weeks pregnant. She was extremely well and looking forward with absolute confidence to the arrival of their child. He remarked to me: "This prenatal preparation is wonderful—we do it together and I have not felt so fit in months!"

The signs and symptoms of the onset of labor were familiar to both of them, and the transport to the maternity hospital presented no difficulty, whatever the time of day or night it was required. They appeared to enjoy together a happy, confident anticipation of the arrival of their child and were both there to greet it when it came. I need hardly say that the arrival of their child was a pleasure both to them and to those of us who witnessed it. They organized things together for this event and the companionship of pregnancy was maintained.

When labor finally starts, the relationship during pregnancy of a husband and wife is made obvious by their behavior when they arrive at the hospital. It becomes almost possible to predict the nature and course of a woman's labor by the manner of their entrance to the labor ward.

Then the judgment has to be made by the obstetrician in charge: "Is this husband one who will be of help to his wife during labor, or will he not only be a nuisance to the attendants but also cause anxiety or even distress to his wife?" The totally unprepared man has no place at the birth of his child. The great question that has now occupied so much attention in so many hospitals, "Should the husband be present?" depends entirely upon the husband. If he has assured himself of adequate prenatal preparation and thereby obtained the confidence of his wife, and can be a support to her at that time, then, if she wishes him to be present, it is my opinion that he not only has the right but he *should* be with her. But if he has not occupied himself to become interested and have an understanding of childbirth at least equivalent to his wife's, he should remain absent until such time as the obstetrician requests him to greet his wife and their newborn child.

I have had many husbands present throughout the whole of the labor of their wives and the birth of their children. Each of these has stayed with his wife during the first stage, reminded her of the lessons they have learned together, and assisted her in breathing correctly during the succeeding phases of parturition and in relaxing when relaxation was indicated. He has remembered that uncontrolled fear in his wife can have a deleterious effect on her labor. I don't know of anything better than the good, honest, horny hand of a loving husband on the sacrum, to stop the backache most women have at the end of the first stage of labor. Many a woman has submissively loved her husband the most for the first time when those scratchy lumps of thumb and fingers have cured the threatening, aching fear by which she has been distressed. These men cannot be superseded in the value of their service by the most patient nurse or obstetrician.

As labor develops during the second stage, and the quiet, purposeful atmosphere of the room creates a calm and peaceful expectancy, the husband takes his place near his wife. If he shows signs of excitement, he is instructed to attend to his wife and to control his feelings, as the reality of birth is approaching. He understands the difference between physical effort and discomfort; he hears the explanation and admonition of the attendant obstetrician to his wife; he knows that she is being offered relief from any discomfort that she may consider to be more than she wishes to bear. He sees the analgesic apparatus ready for her use, but in such cases he almost invariably hears her retort that she would prefer not to be unconscious at this time. The directions of the obstetrician are intended not only for the wife but for the husband; the attending physician realizes that his concern is not only to see the child into the world but also to enable these two people to be united in the most wonderful, awe-inspiring experience that can possibly fall to the lot of wedded human beings. There is no drama or play-acting in the full recognition of the magnitude of this event to both of them. The first cry of the child is shared by both husband and wife in almost unbelievable ecstasy and relief from tension. The knowledge of its sex, the wrapping of the infant in towels, and the handing of it to a conscious, delighted woman present to the husband a picture of beauty that he describes in such words as "thrilling," "miraculous," "mysterious," and so on.

The full evaluation of this mutual experience is difficult to set down in a few words, but it is such that, when properly conducted, an association of marriage that is indestructible for all-time results.

I advocate strongly that all husbands should make the pregnancy of their wives a heaven-sent opportunity for an association in marriage of the highest level. Men who have been present at the birth of their children are unanimous in the sense of the "rightness" of their presence.

MOTHER—BABY

When a baby is born it should be put to the breast at the earliest possible opportunity—many of my mothers who watch their babies being born and take them in their arms wrapped in warm towels as soon as the umbilical cord is cut, notice the child is either sucking its fingers after it has quieted down from its first few lusty yells, or is mouthing when they stroke its cheek. A certain number of them have an immediate desire to put the child to the breast.

A newborn baby should remain with its mother, for she is its best nurse.* Even if she is one of those few who are not possessed of much intelligence she has the maternal instinct, which can often overcome many academic deficiencies. In the days following birth, after she is up from bed and moving about, she can look after the baby herself, learn its habits and its desires. This close association with the child will make her quick to appreciate when it is hungry or when it needs other attentions.

These "natural" children are different. They are not restless, they feed, they sleep, they do their duties according to the physiological demand. And what are the three things these children require and thrive on?

1. They are born to seek food at once from the mother's breast; they will not get it for the first two or three days, but they seek it at once and their importunity is rewarded.

2. They desire warmth from the mother's body.

And then, perhaps what is more important:

3. They need security in their mother's presence.

These three factors are the only provision that nature demands all children should have for their first weeks of neonatal life. Breastfeeding satisfies all three.

* See James Clark Moloney, *Child and Family*, April 1963.

A few women, for different reasons, cannot provide milk for their baby or, unhappily, have been given an injection to prevent lactation before they recovered the consciousness of which they had been deprived at birth.* We hear, too, that women are told it is "animal" to feed the baby from the breast, that what comes from the bottle is safer, it is better, it is prepared by science. This is happening today in thousands of homes of women who have a natural desire to nurse their baby and feel its warmth upon their breast, but someone whom they respect has told them it is better not to breastfeed.

No hot blanket, guardian nurse, or weaning bottle can replace the physiological character formation of the breastfed baby. There is no substitute for mother love. The relationship between those who love and those who are loved is not a sentimental association but a reality.

Man cannot feed the baby within the uterus. What justifies his presumption that he is able to improve upon the physiological provision because the child has recently left the uterus? We can fortify and reinforce with certain substances the adequacy of both the placental and the breast nutrition, but the basic natural nourishment supplies something no concoction can contain. And although skilled physicians can write prescriptions for mixtures upon which children may thrive, they cannot include the personality factor of successful mothering.

The child who develops on natural food becomes familiar with the comfort of being cuddled in soft warmth while it feeds, in the strong, possessive, and protective arms of its mother. In this way the earliest foundation of the mental stability of the child is laid, discernible in the ease with which it adapts itself to the new environment of extrauterine life. The absence both of frustration and of fear of insecurity can be seen in the placid, cooing child who lies awake in his crib

---

* Even if lactation has been suppressed in this way, the sucking of the baby can stimulate the milk supply. See *The Womanly Art of Breastfeeding* (Chicago: La Leche League, 1963).

and gurgles at the discovery that his fingers belong to him and he can make them do things.

Many psychiatrists have stated from time to time, not only that man relives the moment of his birth, but also that his mental development will arise upon his earliest associations with life. If this is true, the happiness radiated by the feeding mother to her child must envelop the infant in the aura of blissful associations with its earliest beginnings.*

The ability of a mother to feed her baby at the breast is commensurate with her ability to give birth to her child by natural childbirth. The mothers who witness the arrival of their babies and experience the sensations of relief, joy, achievement, and pride that are the natural accompaniment to the birth of a child invariably desire to feed their babies, and almost always are able to do so efficiently. We cannot disassociate breastfeeding from the manner of birth.

The profound importance to the baby of the first forty-eight hours of its neonatal life does not receive the emphasis many of us would wish it to have. For my own part I extend that thought to the development of the mother in the first forty-eight hours of motherhood.

In my own practice, where not more than 3 percent of the women who have normal labors accept the analgesia that is offered, 98 percent desire to be and become good breast-feeding mothers. We also find that, where women are subjected to interference either with regional or general anesthesia, the wish to feed their babies is less frequent. This could be put in another way: the nearer the birth of a child is to the normal physiological function, so much more likely is the continuity of the natural sequence of events of human reproduction maintained. When a mother takes her child to her breast immediately after she has witnessed its arrival, its contact stimulates, by direct reflex, strong contractions and retractions of her uterus. This activity hastens separation of

* Margaret A. Ribble, *The Rights of Infants*, rev. ed. (New York: Columbia University Press, 1965), pp. 131–145.

the placenta and the closing of the blood vessels in the part of the uterus to which it was attached.

The reflex action of the uterus and other structures within the pelvis continues after the placenta has been extruded, for each time the baby goes to the breast it stimulates retraction or shortening of the muscle fibers and diminution in size of the vast blood vessels that have been formed around and within the uterus during pregnancy. This process, known as *involution*, or restitution of the uterus to its nonpregnant state, is most satisfactorily completed under the urge of breastfeeding. In the first week or ten days after giving birth, the activity of the breastfeeding baby may establish within the maternal pelvis a healthy condition that will be a blessing to the mother for all time.

If, as we are led to believe, lactation and the flow of milk are associated with an outpouring of secretion from the pituitary gland, the stimulating influence of that secretion upon the pelvic organs is evident in a breastfeeding mother.

The feeding of the child induces certain conditions in the mind of the mother. There is a complacent, peaceful sense of achievement associated with the knowledge that she is giving herself to her beloved possession. Her pleasant physical sensations when the baby feeds not only give rise to uterine contractions, but to, a reaction closely akin to eroticism, which in many women stimulates contractions of the muscles of the pelvic floor and activates the glands of the vagina and vulva. I have heard it said that this intrusion of sexual feelings upon the purity of peaceful motherliness has so revolted some women that the conflict has inhibited the milk supply. In my considerable experience I have never met this psychopathic phenomenon. If a woman has accepted, for a variety of reasons, sexual gratification without love, I can understand the basis of conflict when, maybe at long last, she has learned the power of spiritual love for her baby. Love and sex can be two strongly opposing emotions.

It has been observed that a woman who has breastfed her

baby may require a smaller contraceptive diaphragm than was used eighteen months before pregnancy. I have no recorded case of this in a mother whose baby was weaned to the bottle from birth. The significance of this is clear to married people.

THE HOME

When successfully breastfeeding his child, a wife is supremely attractive to an affectionate husband. Sometimes when we are writing upon obstetric subjects we forget to call attention to the profound love for the baby that possesses many fathers. We do not remember how deeply they feel the emotional changes of their wives, nor the exaltation and personal satisfaction they enjoy when all goes well. The lack of a father relationship early in life can leave a painful gap in a child's feelings.* And husbands fail to realize what indignity their homes suffer from the alienation of mother and baby, if the infant is given at an early age to the care of a nursemaid, to be seen only for a few hurried moments in the evening before its parents change for dinner.

Of course there are those miserable creatures of society whose babies are due to arrive invariably at just the wrong time—who want a baby very much, but it *is* an awful trial and they are not at all sure what their husbands think about it. They would like to nurse the baby, but they have so many social engagements booked—things they do not want to do but must—that they are afraid they will not be able to . . . and so on, ad infinitum. Marriage itself, as it is understood in modern civilization, introduces complications into the mind of the young mother that never could have existed in the natural state of *genus homo,* when the instinctive desire of the male was reproduction, the reciprocal instinct of the female was parental, when the fullness of their mutual harmony was inspired by nature to the continuation of the species. Social

* Ibid., p. 101.

engagements, economic considerations, and procreation out of a sense of duty were limitations unthought of.

The care of the breasts is of far-reaching importance to a woman both as a mother and a wife. If she loses her figure and adopts an unbecoming posture it may affect her personality. Some women become self-conscious, develop a sense of inferiority among others, and an apologetic retiring manner, sometimes akin to shame, before their husbands. They blame lactation and even the infants whom they have breastfed, although these troubles arise after weaning to the bottle from birth more frequently than from breastfeeding. It is too frequently overlooked by those who attend child-bearing women that the breasts are reproductive organs. They have a sexual as well as a personality value, which subjects them to the buffetings of a variety of psychological assaults. For that matter, I know of no literature, except that which today is considered Victorian and grossly sentimental, that places childbirth itself in its true position and understands that labor is of love.

Perhaps it will be forgiven me if I issue a warning of the nature of things. Every act that leads, in a normal sequence of events, to the association of painful childbirth will become inhibited by the primitive instinct of escape. The chill of fear creeps into the warmth of love: the kiss becomes a mere peck and an established routine; the passion that was possessive and overpowering no longer binds life partners in the masonry of marriage. Coitus becomes an unjustifiable risk; its pleasures fade and disappear before the ever-present fear of impregnation. And so the seeds of domestic strain and misery are often sown by painful childbirth.

These feelings are often intensified during the first weeks a baby born so painfully spends at home, especially if the baby is not breastfed, for breastfeeding does not extend its benefits only to the mother and child. Many fathers are distraught with the troubles of their wives and cries of a restless baby who does not thrive. It is by no means infrequently the cause of one-child families, the father and mother agreeing that, quite apart from the trials that the labor brought to them both, they could never go through six or eight weeks of nerve-racking experience, physical weariness, and sleepless anguish that fell to their lot when the baby struggled to attain a standard of health and behavior in which the parents had lost all confidence.

Fortunately, the converse also applies. Some of those women who have experienced the happiness of their child's arrival say that they have never known the fullness of love until possessed by the irresistible desire to have more children. Again and again they recall and dream of that transcendental joy that shines like a persistent orb of light, illuminating the wonders of their new life of motherhood. Every act of love is enhanced; the physical and mental desire for the fullness of their husbands' affection perfects the mutual delight of their companionship. Restraint is flung to the four winds of heaven. As one they join together in the search for new and yet more delightful experience. Their coitus is a spiritual union blessed with profoundly pleasurable physical reaction.

The birth of a child is not a woman's monopoly. It is the major incident in the lives of three people—father, mother and child. Indeed, many husbands suffer more in childbirth than the women who bear their babies. To overlook or prevent the mutual companionship and assistance of husband and wife during pregnancy and labor is to show a grievous lack of human understanding.

The love of a woman for her child and the love of a woman for her husband have different foundations and manifestations. When a baby is born the first questions of a young mother concern the welfare of her baby. The first questions of a young father concern the welfare of his wife. This persists until the child is able to care and fend for itself. Experience has shown in the past, on many occasions, that in time of danger a woman will save her child before her husband, whereas a man similarly placed normally saves his wife first.

This does not mean that the wife has no love for the man, or that the man has less love for the child, but demonstrates the instinctive valuation of love between the three of them. This is well recognized in the traditions of the sea, where the shipwreck order is "Women and children first."

A woman should bear in mind that a little more tenderness to her husband after the child has arrived will strengthen the bond of affection between them. But this will not have the same effect if during the pregnancy the birth of their child has been the interest of only the mother and not of the father. Therefore the woman must interest her husband in pregnancy, must point out that it is his child as well as hers.

Most men want families and will love their babies in a man's way from the earliest age if they are encouraged or even allowed to learn. Paternal love is different from maternal love, but it is an equally deep emotion. Women must not pride themselves on being the only incomprehensible component of the human race; husbands are just as difficult to understand at times as wives. A man may consciously or unconsciously be confronted by dangerous reactions to his wife's pregnancy. He may fear for her safety or her health and beauty afterward. He may resent the child's arriving, being jealous of the love his wife will give it. He may desire her for himself alone and foresee a rift in the early companionship that they have enjoyed together. He may be disturbed by the immediate cost and future expense. It is thus we can say that the birth of a child may bind or break a marriage, and the possibility of these things happening therefore call for special attention on the part of the wife. She must take care of her husband, for above all things she desires to keep him for herself, and she knows that she and her child depend upon him.

Women, therefore, must share fully with their husbands the child that is born to them. The love of husband and wife, which gives them children, needs more care than the children that this love brings. It is a delicate and beautiful thing, fragile and sensitive. It must be nurtured, watched, protected, if it is to survive. It fades quickly if left without attention and must be looked after carefully as it strives to mature with the years. The husband must become interested in the affairs of the wife, which primarily concern the children and the care of the home. The wife must become interested, though not necessarily active, in the affairs that concern her husband, primarily the maintenance of the family and home.

From the foundation of a happy childbearing experience, shared by the mother and father, children can grow secure in the knowledge that they are loved and wanted. As boys and girls grow older, they will be prepared to learn and understand about parenthood. No prudery or lying pose of innocence will tarnish the personality of such educated, understanding young people. Thus it is that successful home and family life must become the ultimate objective of modern obstetric teaching.*

Let us suppose, therefore, that from infancy to puberty the sexual education of the child is carried out by the parents in the home. If parents wait longer than the immediate prepuberty years, or if the instruction is given over to others outside the family, then the child may be deprived of that security which is so essential to all the changing phases of development. In some ways this is comparable to the mother who is emotionally absent, and the father literally absent, from the birth of their child.

A similar series of events demands the closest maternal care and love during the premenstrual phase of a girl's life. I teach that mothers can make better mothers than those who are not mothers can ever make. I do not decry the work of those unselfish people who sublimate their own maternal love in an effort to fashion the lives of the young. But it is like breast milk as opposed to milk from a bottle—one is ever present, already prepared for immediate use when so desired, while the other is the acquisition of an unnatural regimen, satisfying the stomach

* See *Prelude to Action* (New York: Maternity Center Association, 1969), a report on the Maternity Center's fiftieth-anniversary seminar on childbearing and family life.

but never penetrating the deep and spiritual self within the consciousness of the child.

Human nature has not changed since the days of the Psalmist. The man who has a "full quiver" of children and an adequate income is the peace-loving worker whose presence in the community is an influence toward moderation and reason. But should his home be in jeopardy or his family in danger, he knows no fear, but flings himself into the fray with the violence of desperation. Is it for his own comfort or for his childless wife he fights to the death? Is it in the cause of justice among nations or is it for children who crowd his small home and climb upon his knee? From whence is the power in a man's arm? Let fathers of families answer, and husbands with good wives who mother their growing sons and daughters. The phylogenetic development of man has equipped him physiologically and mentally to fight for the protection of his children and their mother. Perhaps that is why peace-loving men who are forced into battle by an aggressive enemy fight with such fury that the professional soldier is amazed.

From my contact with men and women of all classes, I have been led to believe that it is for homes and families our people will cry out. The demand will be for parenthood, and for income from their work adequate to provide for children in health and happiness. Unfortunately, the prestige of a satellite in orbit around the earth is too often infinitely greater than the prestige of a revolutionary approach to the breeding of better human stock, or the founding of homes and family units of happy and contented people. The uninhibited development of a simple philosophy and sound physiques, which enable men and women to adjust themselves to an everchanging world, is allowed to occur where it may, if it will. Rockets and satellites, spaceships and hydrogen bombs, absorb thousands of millions of the wealth of nations, while the development of the human race to a higher standard of mental and physical efficiency is granted a disgraceful pittance. We do not demand greater numbers—the objective must be the *quality* of the child. As the quality of the mother, so the nature of the offspring will vary; the mother herself has been molded by the manner of her birth and the environment in which she was influenced by her parents as a small child. The bondage or the freedom of her puberty guides her to accept or to distrust the father of her own children, and so the cycle starts again in the birth of a baby.

6

Childbirth in Perspective
Harlan Ellis, M.D.

This chapter is written mainly for the medical student and/or the physician unfamiliar with the principles of natural childbirth. Having had the opportunity and good fortune to use the principles as outlined in the original 1933 text of Grantly Dick-Read for the past twelve years, I have been invited to present certain impressions and feelings about these principles as they apply today in the 1970s.

WHAT IS NATURAL CHILDBIRTH?

Natural childbirth is one part of a continuum of normal physiological events representing and illustrating the two basic laws of the continuance of a species, namely the law of reproduction and the law of maintenance of the species. Natural childbirth means normal physiological childbirth. When childbirth becomes associated with varying degrees of fear and therefore varying degrees of tension, it becomes in varying degrees unphysiological or pathological. Eastman and Hellman have stated in their textbook on obstetrics that to eliminate the harmful influence of fear in labor, a school of thought has developed emphasizing the advantages of "natural childbirth" or "physiological childbirth."[1]*

---

* References for Chapter 6 begin on page 142.

Natural childbirth as originally stated by Grantly Dick-Read has never meant that every woman will have a completely painless childbirth,[2] although it frequently produces no more discomfort than that which any woman herself wishes to experience, or is able to control by natural childbirth principles. Natural childbirth does not, nor did Grantly Dick-Read ever intend for it to, indicate that analgesics and/or anesthetics could not be used.[3] He specifically and continuously emphasized that anesthetics were always available if required, for he did not believe that any woman should be allowed to suffer pain.

The term "natural childbirth" has left a bad impression on many doctors because while in training at many teaching hospitals throughout our Western culture we frequently saw numerous examples of young women suffering through labor and birth with inadequate relief, which process was called, although incorrectly, "natural childbirth"; we seldom saw truly physiological childbirth during any of our medical training days, and, as a result, natural childbirth to us was synonymous with suffering and pain. Indeed, to many doctors, and to the general public as well, natural childbirth meant—and still means—simply childbirth without anesthetics or any kind of pain relief.

The suffering we continuously witnessed in childbirth so affected us that long before we completed our specialty training in medical school, internship, and three or four years of exposure in a residency, we became dedicated to the principle that when we had our own private patients we would never let them suffer in birth, believing as we did that without medication pain was inevitable. We determined that each and every one of our private patients would be entitled to some type of a regional block or general anesthetic. And so, after five, ten, or fifteen years of successfully using anesthetics for birth, it may still be that only a few of us had the opportunity of seeing a truly physiological or natural childbirth.

In this book I encourage each doctor to review the basic

principles of Grantly Dick-Read's original writing in 1933.[4] You and I may not accept every statement or criticism he has made of our specialty, but this must not allow us to be deterred from exploring this physiological and therefore most valuable way to handle the birth of a child.

If we believe that a physiological process, namely normal childbirth, must by its very nature represent suffering and severe pain, then we must review the following:

1. In no other animal species is the process of birth apparently associated with any suffering, pain, or agony except when pathology exists or in an unnatural state such as captivity.

2. There are certain "primitive cultures" where childbirth is looked forward to with joy and anticipation as something good. Here one finds little evidence of suffering, pain, or agony, again except when pathology is present.[5]

3. There is no other physiological process in our body that under normal conditions is painful except when complicated by fear or tension.

4. Experience shows that when a woman can be prepared so that fear and tension are prevented from occurring in labor, there is minimal or no suffering, pain, or agony.[6]

5. Childbirth education programs are starting up in almost every American city today, and thousands of women are learning the basic principles of natural childbirth.* Stories of good experiences are spreading by word of mouth, with the result that increasing numbers of women are discovering that natural childbirth is a more exciting and rewarding way to have a baby.

---

* Two significant organizations in the United States are aiding childbirth education groups at the local level. One is the American Society of Psychoprophylaxis in Obstetrics, which is devoted solely to the Lamaze-Pavlov method. The other is the International Childbirth Education Association, which encourages all groups devoted to childbirth education without regard to their specific methodology, and encourages the integration of childbirth and family-centered maternity-care concepts into programs of family and sex education. (See Sources of Information, page 401.)

The five points above indicate clearly that Grantly Dick-Read's original thesis was accurate in stating that when childbirth is normal, and therefore physiological, there is minimal suffering, pain, or agony.

Natural childbirth is, as we have said, a physiological birth, and when childbirth is not accompanied by fear and tension, there seldom will be more discomfort than any woman wishes to experience. *The problem is that it is not always a simple matter to have her enter the labor suite completely relaxed, calm, and competent.* Each woman is different, and each one may require varying amounts of preparation time and effort in order for her to arrive at this most advantageous condition. This book of Grantly Dick-Read's is aimed at that task. The rewards—for the patient, for the newborn, for the husband, and for the family as a unit—are great. The principles are correct, and today, in the 1970s, they do work clinically.

Each student, intern, and obstetrical resident should study in detail the principles of natural childbirth, noting especially the opportunities for preventive medical care. Throughout this book there are numerous instances where preventive medicine can be applied, not only in the interest of the baby, but in that of the mother, the father, and possibly even the environment into which the baby enters. There is a message here for those of us in obstetrics, that we can significantly contribute, not only another birth to our already overcrowded population, but a certain amount of quality in the birth process that may aid in some small way—or perhaps great way—our society in general. And we should always remember that childbirth to many couples is a very private event, and that to others it is also deeply spiritual.

NATURAL CHILDBIRTH AND PAIN

As stated above, natural childbirth does not necessarily mean painless childbirth. In the past, we and our textbooks in obstetrics have used the word "pain" to mean "normal uterine contractions" so often we ourselves began to believe that the pains of labor are the same as normal uterine contractions. Indeed, in the most current textbook on obstetrics, the word "pain" is used for contractions. Pain hurts, normal uterine contractions do not. In fact, uterine contractions will seldom give rise to any pain whatsoever if unassociated with fear and tension. Fear, of course, is followed by tension, and when cervical tension occurs in labor, the previously normal uterine contractions must overcome it. In their turn the uterine contractions get stronger, frequently to the point of producing varying amounts of pain, at which point they become pathological—that is, unphysiological—contractions.

As was said in 1920 by Rudyard Kipling, the *words* one uses are more powerful than any drug known to mankind. Thus it is important to realize the power of words upon the suggestibility of an obstetrical patient.

When we speak of fear or tension in connection with painful uterine contractions, we are talking about pathology. We are also talking about pathology when we speak of an *abruptio placenta* during a contraction; any degree of placental abruption, although minimal, causes pain. Another source of pathological pain during childbirth is contracting muscles fed by an inadequate supply of oxygen, as in angina pectoris. This condition can be caused by incorrect breathing. This demonstrates the importance of the natural childbirth principle of correct breathing during labor to prevent pain.

Still another area is involved in pain during labor, and that is the back. A back pain is most common with the first pregnancy, particularly toward the end of the first stage of labor. Note we are talking about pain *in the back*—the feeling a parturient patient has in the lower part of her back, usually over the sacral area—not about uterine contractions. In some this merely means a mild ache; in others it means more than mere discomfort; in still others it is severe pain. This discomfort can frequently be relieved adequately for many women by rubbing, for others by strong pressure from the heel of the hand or fingers of a prepared and trained husband (figs. 2, 3, 4, 5). Other patients may require a change in position to overcome the problem. Still others may even get in a "pelvic rocking" position (figs. 32, 33, p. 188) for a short period of time, possibly aiding in the spontaneous rotation of a *posterior occiput* position. Still others may require analgesics or anesthetics of varying amounts for relief.

Another source of pain is the pubic area, and, while such discomfort occurs near the end of the first stage of labor, as is also true of pain in the back, the pubic area usually does not produce as much discomfort as the back. Too, a patient does not usually experience both the back discomfort and the pubic discomfort at the same time. Gentle massaging of the area, changing to a semisitting position with her knees raised (fig. 1, below), and breathing techniques are all that a woman requires to control this type of temporary discomfort.

We, as physicians, have always used our anesthetics basically for pain at the actual birth because we have felt this must be the most severe pain of the entire event. Indeed, a woman unprepared for natural childbirth can have severe pain at this time—frequently, in this type of patient, hysterical in nature. She tightly contracts the pelvic floor in fear of the oncoming head, and this leads to severe pain as the baby emerges. With this type of unnatural birth, all of us would offer the appropriate amount of anesthetic. This, again, is not natural childbirth.

For the prepared patient, the birth itself usually means feelings of stretching, deep pressure, and, for some, discomfort—although seldom does a well-prepared patient feel any more discomfort at this time than she wishes to handle herself in order not to lose the more positive sensations of birth. But when the prepared woman who has just experienced natural childbirth is asked, "What is the most difficult part you experienced?" she doesn't mention the actual birth! She invariably replies, "The most difficult time came just before I was taken into the birth room," usually adding something like, "That back pain was really getting to me, but not the birth. The birth was exciting and I wouldn't have missed it for anything!" She felt the birth, yes, but, as an amazingly high number of women do, talks about it as a satisfying, exciting, good, thrilling experience. Even when asked in detail about the back pain, and why she would not accept anesthetics, she frequently replies, "Oh, it actually wasn't that bad," and adds, "Besides, I didn't want to take a chance on missing the experience of the birth."

As we know, there is a certain amount of risk involved with each anesthetic. Indeed, the fourth most common cause of maternal death in this country is related to the anesthetic administered.[7] Since we only use anesthetics for pain, a program designed to reduce the number of required anesthetics is a significant attempt to completely erase all avoidable maternal deaths.

In nothing he ever said or wrote did Grantly Dick-Read indicate that when a woman experienced pain it was simply

Fig. 1. Position for overcoming backache in late transition and early second stage.

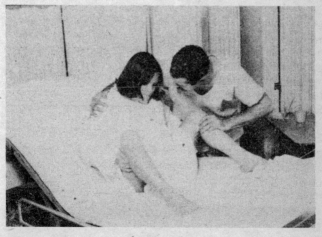

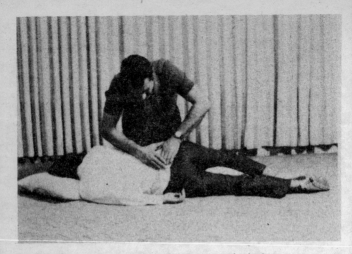

Fig. 2. Husband learning to use fingertips to overcome backache in labor.

Fig. 3. Husband using fingers to overcome backache in labor.

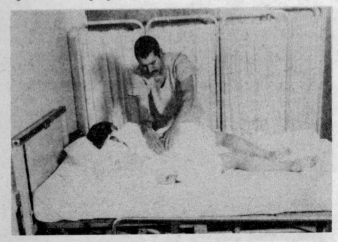

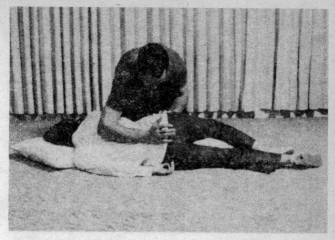

Fig. 4. Husband learning to use heel of hand for backache in labor.

Fig. 5. Husband massaging and applying pressure with heel of hand during labor.

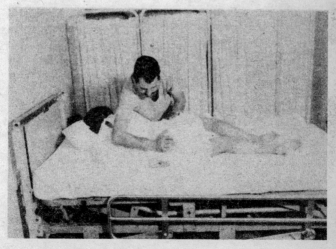

psychological or imaginary or "just in her head." He wrote and spoke only about prevention. He never implied that a woman could simply say to herself that she was not afraid and as a result was not going to have any pain. Unfortunately, it is not nearly that simple! But, fortunately, there is a proven way of pain prevention.

NATURAL CHILDBIRTH AND RELAXATION

The ability to relax during a normal uterine contraction is a basic principle in natural childbirth. For most women this must be learned, but for many the learning comes easily.

TO THE DOCTOR: Eastman and Hellman, after reviewing Grantly Dick-Read's work, admit that quite likely fear may exert a deleterious effect on uterine motility and cervical dilatation.[8] Thus you will discover that, if your patient knows and has the ability to relax at will, you can anticipate an easy labor and birth.

TO THE MEDICAL STUDENT: Be reminded that a tense doctor makes a tense patient and, in turn, a tense cervix. As we said earlier, tension of the cervix during an apparently normal uterine contraction produces an obstruction, which the uterine contraction must become stronger to overcome, producing discomfort. When the cervical tension is severe, the uterine contractions must become more powerful still—and certainly then they are painful.

TO THE WOMAN: Practice and learn complete muscular relaxation as if the ease of your childbirth experience depends on it, because it does!

Relaxation performs many benefits during pregnancy, labor, birth, and during the immediate newborn period, but its opposites, tension and anxiety, as Cannon[9] and others[10] have described in detail, produce many alterations of normal physiological processes throughout the body and work nothing but harm. If there is one characteristic that stands out above all others in an easy, nonmedicated spontaneous birth, it is the characteristic of muscular relaxation. But in most labor wards where the principles of natural childbirth are not practiced, exactly the opposite is obvious: patients hang on during a contraction, brace themselves, tense against each oncoming one. A patient preparing for a comfortable childbirth experience *must* learn relaxation. The avoidance of Grantly Dick-Read's fear-tension-pain cycle through relaxation is a basic principle of natural childbirth.

NATURAL CHILDBIRTH AND THE HUSBAND

In certain healthy Polynesian societies husbands play active roles in the care of their wives during labor (and here Margaret Mead[11] writes about women working, not screaming, during birth). In some cultures, the husband may actually assume direction and supervision at birth.[12] But in our society, when first discussing natural childbirth and the husband's participation during labor, and more specifically his presence during birth, the obstetrician should be prepared for the resistance of eight to nine out of every ten husbands to the idea of being in the birth room. It would seem that today most husbands expect the doctor and nurses to do all the work of helping their wives during labor and birth. Husbands report that they cannot stand the sight of blood or they cannot bear to see their wife in pain, which only further points out how uninformed the typical husband is about as basic a normal physiological process as childbirth. Those husbands who are invited to participate during labor and birth are taught that they are not to be there as an observer to see a birth. They can be shown a film for that! Nor are they there to assist the doctor or the nurse. Each is to be there for the sole purpose of assisting his wife and then sharing her joy in their child's arrival.

Husbands are taught in the preparation classes and in books such as this and others[13] that they have specific duties in the labor and birth room. They are taught, for example, to remain close by the side of their wives; to give her, repeatedly, instructions on relaxation, correct breathing, and proper position; to rub her back and apply pressure when she has back pain; and to give her continual emotional and physical support (figs. 6, 7). In the birth room it is the husband who takes instructions from the obstetrician, and it is the husband who then gives the instructions to his wife.

Following the birth, the husband has new responsibilities, not only in relation to his wife, but to his newborn. Husbands are taught that they must not wait until their child is five or six years of age to develop a relationship, but that they must do so from the moment of birth (fig. 8). An important part of the husband's new role is to encourage his wife's close relationship with the baby as well, including such things as skin-to-skin contact and breastfeeding, which are not minor matters but important aspects of the growth and development of the newborn. Indeed, much of the future of the newborn depends on the parents' attitude and relationship to him *starting at birth*.[14] A good experience for the husband at the birth of his child won't solve all future problems, of course, but it may provide the stimulus for a close relationship that will endure.

NATURAL CHILDBIRTH AND THE HOSPITAL

It is the opinion of obstetricians interested in the benefits of natural childbirth that hospitals are built in terms of the obstetrical patient as a sick person, thus providing separate care for mother and newborn. Work by such noted men in behavioral animal science as Konrad Lorenz[15] of Austria, or Harry Harlow[16] at the University of Wisconsin, as to the importance of the relationship between the newborn and its mother is too often ignored in hospital planning.

The administrator who is interested in the new and exciting methods of handling obstetrical patients would be wise to study more about what is meant by family-centered maternity care.[17] This is the trend of the future, and will make maternity suites built upon the older, conventional thinking obso-

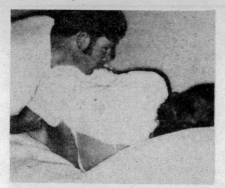

Fig. 6. Husband applying pressure with fist for backache.

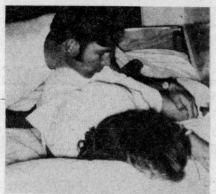

Fig. 7. Husband massaging back and giving emotional support.

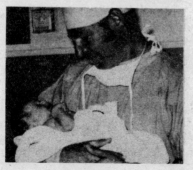

Fig. 8. Husband establishing his relationship with newborn.

lete. The new concept includes the principles of natural child-birth and rooming-in, as well as an interest in the family as a unit and not simply in the extraction of the baby from the mother.

As we look toward the future, here is a significant point. We do not want to discourage patients from hospital obstetrical care, and by so doing increase the desire for or the incidence of home births. This is already becoming popular among an important segment of the younger generation, in reaction to the inflexibility of much current obstetrical hospital routine. This trend toward home deliveries can perhaps be reversed if hospitals become more homelike and personal, while still maintaining high standards of hospital care.

Later in this chapter there is a discussion of an ideal family-centered maternity hospital, which could be constructed in the complete interest of the principles of natural childbirth.

NATURAL CHILDBIRTH: A TEAM EFFORT

It is the team effort that makes natural childbirth the success it is. This includes not only the patient and her husband, but the obstetrician and his prenatal nurses and childbirth training personnel. In the hospital it includes every individual that comes in contact with the prepared couple, from the admitting labor and delivery personnel to the postpartum nurses.

If your hospital is one of those that does permit husbands in the birth room as part of the obstetrical team during birth, then *permit only husbands who are prepared to give assistance.* It is the unprepared husband in the delivery area who leads to problems and brings unjustified discredit to this type of program.

The problems concerning husbands are few and infrequent. The often-heard comment that husbands tend to faint appears to be completely unjustified. The husband who is prepared and is active in taking care of his wife has little inclination to faint nor any opportunity to become "woozy." And to prevent him from becoming light headed from going long hours without food, at mealtimes trays should be ordered sent to him in his wife's labor room.

When the time comes to move into the birth room, the prepared husband can scrub and gown himself properly with cap, mask, and shoe coverings to keep from increasing the opportunity of infection. If he is not doing his job of assisting his wife, he should be asked to leave the delivery area.

It is my experience that husbands who are aware of the sincere interest of the hospital staff and obstetrician in observing all the safeguards for their wife and baby have little or no inclination to put blame on the hospital or doctor, even when the outcome is not a healthy, normal child.

When a prepared couple enter a hospital and the first question asked them is "How hard are your pains?" and this by a supposed hospital authority, they are certainly anything but encouraged! What a difference when one says, "How strong are your contractions?" Most sensitive husbands are very quick to pick up an atmosphere of negativity among labor and delivery room personnel, which may cause the experience to end up as a contest—hospital personnel versus husband. Because he is concerned for the welfare of his wife, he wants to protect her from negative influences and from interruptions that may disturb her relaxation and comfort.

It is important that medical students, interns, and obstetrical residents learn that they can tell *more* about the progress of the labor by a detailed observation of three or four uterine contractions than they can by three or four rectal or vaginal examinations. This does not mean that internal examinations are not important, for of course they are, and a certain number need to be done. One can frequently tell the sensitivity of an obstetrician, student, intern, or nurse by the care and expertise by which they do a proper painless vaginal examination.

Hospital personnel, as well as the doctor, must remember

that, since during a uterine contraction the husband may have his wife completely relaxed, this is not the time to interrupt in order to get a urine specimen or make some other routine examination. And it must also be remembered that there appears to be minimal value to perineal preps or routine enemas, which most women dislike intensely.

During the end of the first stage of labor, it is important to give continuous support to both husband and wife. The woman should not be transferred to the birth room during a uterine contraction. There is ample time between. As soon as the second stage of labor has begun and the bearing down starts, it is important that the patient be propped up adequately to get her in as much of a sitting position as possible. A primipara should remain in the labor room, propped up in the labor bed for pushing, until the birth is near. Sometimes contractions stop altogether for a time if she is rushed into the birth room too early in the second stage. A multipara should be taken as soon as the second stage begins, or even shortly before, in order to allow her ample time to get comfortably situated on the birth table, propped at the angle most suitable for her.

There are available natural childbirth backrests, which fit most birth room tables.* These can be elevated to almost any degree, and are indeed very helpful. With the patient prepared for natural childbirth, her husband at her side, the back of the table elevated, and the patient bearing down with each uterine contraction, there appears to be little question—and this is also the opinion of Atlee[18]—that the second stage of labor can be shortened. With such a wide-awake, cooperative patient, there is no need for such things as hands being strapped to the table (figs. 11, 12). While the patient is on the birth table the room must be kept absolutely quiet, so that she can remain deeply relaxed between uterine contractions.

The obstetrician's job at this time is to give further instruc-

* See *Sources of Supplies*, page 401. A little ingenuity can solve the problem temporarily if a backrest has not yet been ordered (figs. 9, 10).

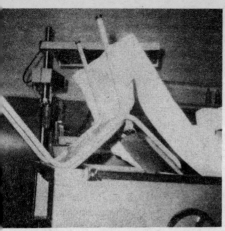

Fig. 9. Inverted chair used as backrest on birth table. Infant warmer in background.

Fig. 10. Inverted chair used as backrest for second-stage labor.

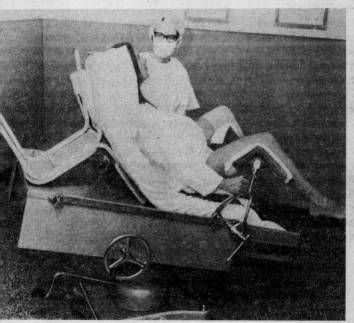

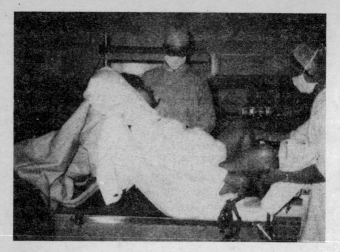

Fig. 11. Giving birth without stirrups, if desired, using them to lean legs against. Notice the draped, inverted chair used as backrest.

Fig. 12. Giving birth without stirrups, with husband and nurse supporting legs.

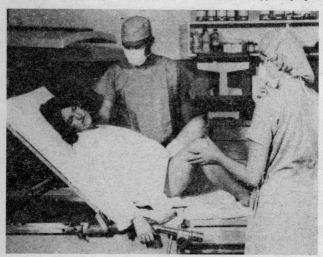

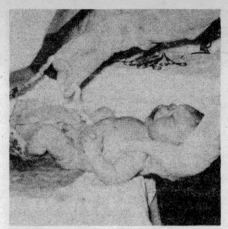

Fig. 13. Baby kept horizontal, cord not clamped until beating stops.

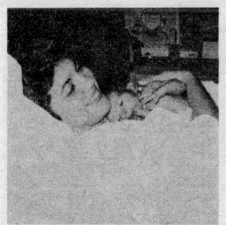

Fig. 14. Immediate newborn maternal closeness.

tions to the husband as the baby passes from the vaginal canal, telling him to encourage his wife to bear down during contractions, to breathe deeply once or twice, and then to relax between contractions. He tells the husband when to have his wife stop pushing and instead breathe rapidly through her mouth as crowning proceeds, so that pressure on the infant's head is slowly released as the head passes from the vaginal canal. Following the delivery of the head, the husband is now instructed to have his wife bear down in another effort, for the anterior shoulder need not be extracted by the obstetrician but can be delivered by the patient herself.

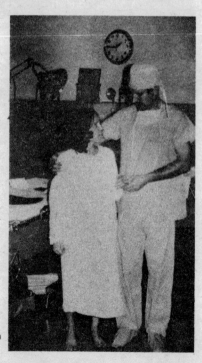

Fig. 15. Walking to room after giving birth.

Following birth the baby is not held up by the feet, for this increases the danger of intracranial pressure and may be harmful. He is laid at approximately the level of the undelivered placenta, in a horizontal position, not head down (fig. 13). If even minimal hemorrhages had occurred in the brain during birth, permitting the head to be lowered would have a tendency to increase bleeding that we might not be aware was taking place.

It is essential that the baby be kept *warm*, so during these first few minutes of life a warming hood* is immediately rotated over the newborn before the cord is cut. The cord is not clamped immediately, nor is it milked in an effort to force an unusual amount of blood into the baby. As soon as the cord has stopped beating, it is clamped.

The mother is shown the baby and allowed to discover the sex for herself. Since she is alert and observing this part of the procedure in the mirror, she sees her baby at once and hears his first cry. The baby is then given to the mother (fig. 14) for immediate newborn maternal closeness and frequently immediate newborn breastfeeding.[19]

During the next few minutes the eyes of the newborn are treated and he is tagged, weighed, etc., right in front of his parents. The only cleaning of the baby is the washing off of any blood or meconium. The normal *vernix caseosa*, the whitish, cheesy deposit covering the baby's skin at birth is not removed, nor is it to be removed later, since it may be of value in protecting him from skin infections. It is gradually absorbed into his skin like a vanishing cream.

The baby is kept in the birth room until the third stage of labor, the delivery of the placenta, has been completed. And before mother and baby leave the birth room, the father

---

* It is desirable for a hospital to be equipped with a type of newborn warmer (fig. 9) with a hood that can rotate over the mother and baby so as to keep the newborn warm. This type of warmer also makes it possible to keep the baby alongside the mother while the nurse tags the baby and cares for his eyes.

should have an opportunity to hold his newborn infant for a short period.

The mother is now returned to her room—or she returns herself, for in natural childbirth we find, surprisingly, that the vast majority of new mothers want to and can, with minimal assistance, get up from the delivery room table and walk back to bed (fig. 15). It may be debated whether this has any physiological advantage for the new mother, or for circulation in her lower extremities, but the psychological boost seems remarkable. In any case, upon her return the baby is brought to her for rooming-in. Postpartum education, concerning the newborn and the family, is continued until discharge.

From all this it is obvious that it takes a team effort. *If any portion of this team breaks down, it can be expected that the accomplishments will be proportionately less.*

NATURAL CHILDBIRTH: A CONTINUUM

Childbirth is considered one of the episodes that a conception goes through to become a child. There are many episodes from conception through pregnancy and on through the first year of life that are significant to the future growth and development of the child. What is wanted in childbirth is a spontaneous, unmedicated, easy, vaginal birth and, if possible, one that is thrilling and exciting—an emotional stimulus to both mother and father. With this as a beginning, we seldom hear from the mother following birth the statement, "Never again." A "never again" type birth quite possibly alters the environment that follows in an unfavorable way.

Natural childbirth is just one episode in a series of events that leads to the potential of any child. Education during pregnancy, an easy, spontaneous, nonmedicated childbirth, husband participation, immediate mother-infant relationship, rooming-in, breastfeeding, imprinting, and a close father-newborn relationship are the basis of what an educated modern childbirth can be expected to be, and are the principles of family-centered maternity care.

NATURAL CHILDBIRTH: THE PROBLEMS

At no time in the natural childbirth program are we interested in a patient simply being a "good patient" or a "quiet patient." She is not in any way to attempt something because someone else accomplished a certain feat. The success in natural childbirth is only a matter of degree, is only in relation to her own particular experience. There is no such thing as failure! When pathology is present, other methods of birth need to be considered, including anesthetic, instruments, and so forth. The principles of natural childbirth still aid in making whatever problem exists less significant. Having a patient relaxed, calm, and cooperative is a significant advantage in the case of an emergency Caesarean section or other form of emergency treatment. The essence of educated and prepared childbirth is for any mother to get the very best baby she can in the easiest way for herself.

When such conditions as transient hyperventilation are produced, one can only look to improper methods of preparation. Grantly Dick-Read emphasizes *never breathing any faster in labor than twenty-four to twenty-eight breaths a minute*. Deep, quiet breathing is to be maintained throughout the first stage. Pregnant women need to be taught to breathe slowly, avoiding high respiratory rates, for these may lead to hyperventilation. Persistent hyperventilation has been shown to increase fetal blood pH (acidosis).[20]

Other basic problems in natural childbirth are occasionally caused by the emotional instability of the mother and/or the father. When this is the case, making the birth pathological, it complicates natural childbirth just as physical pathology does. This type of neuropsychiatric pathology takes, if the patient is to have a fairly good natural birth experience, more patience and skill on the part of the physician and his assistants than would be required in other forms of childbirth using anesthetics. For in the latter case the husband can be removed and the woman sedated, although these procedures may compound their emotional problems afterward.

NATURAL CHILDBIRTH: SPECIAL BENEFITS

There are a number of contributions that natural childbirth can make in the area of preventive medical care today, one of which is in relation to premature labor. Premature labor today represents a forerunner of morbidity, such as respiratory distress of the newborn. In addition, immature development of the infant's neurological system is responsible for such pathology as mental retardation and cerebral palsy. In premature labor, how rewarding it is to have a well-prepared woman, calm, cooperative, understanding the process of labor, having an easy, nonmedicated birth. It is the pediatricians who stress the importance of a nonmedicated premature birth, for the potential of the child in question may be at stake relative to the outcome of premature labor. With 300,000 to 400,000 premature births in the United States yearly,[21] childbirth education and preparedness may be the most important aspect of prenatal care for any of these particular pregnancies.

The benefits of a childbirth education program for the unmarried pregnant girl or woman have been reported many times. Each year about 250,000 babies are born out of wedlock.[22] Childbirth education as part of a natural childbirth program offers a time of education and preparation for the unwed mother-to-be. It appears as well that with this type of program the incidence of repeat unwed pregnancies is decreased. Very valuable emotional and moral support, not given in the past in the usual prenatal care, is provided by natural childbirth instructors, who guide the young women to a new sense of self-worth. To consider the future of any particular conception, we must consider what the environment is going to be like into which that child will be placed. The unwed mother who is to keep her baby needs special preparation in how to raise a child without the influence of a husband. For the unwed mother who intends to give her child up for adoption, it is questionable whether the procedure of "completely" anesthetizing her with a general anesthetic in order to prevent her from ever seeing her child is in either the best interest of the unborn child or helpful to the mother as a person.

For patients who are classified as high-risk pregnancies, natural childbirth offers very special advantages. In a pregnancy complicated by pathology it is important to have a calm, cooperative, understanding patient who knows how to relax correctly and how to breathe to the most advantage for her labor. Because she has learned the value of lying on her left side, there is no problem in keeping her in the correct position during the different stages of labor. As a result, natural-childbirth-trained high-risk pregnancies require less analgesic and anesthetic, thus reducing some of the risk for the infant.

NATURAL CHILDBIRTH: A CHALLENGE

I would hope with these words to stimulate you again, as Grantly Dick-Read has in his original writing concerning "the emotional and physical potential of the pregnant woman and her husband," to study further the accomplishments a typical couple can achieve at childbirth when adequately prepared. I wish to challenge various disciplines of our society—not only obstetrics, not only pediatrics, not only psychiatry—but other disciplines of social behavior as to what pregnancy, childbirth, and the immediate newborn period means to any couple.

Psychiatrists, marriage counselors, pediatricians, nutritionists, even educators report on many things that happen prenatally, during, and immediately following birth that can affect the child all his life. With animal studies it has been learned that imprinting of the newborn may lead to lifelong abilities or disablties in the animal's ability to adapt to its social environment successfully.

The challenges represented by a natural childbirth program are as follows:

1. *To make childbirth an emotionally positive event.* Childbirth represents one of the most dramatic and emotional events of a woman's life. If this is so, and many think it is, then should we not spend more effort, time, and energy working toward making this an emotionally *good* event? A cross section of any group of women from almost any part of our society would indicate that a large majority associate childbirth with anything but an exciting and emotionally good experience.

I would hope that with these words one might get a response from psychiatrists as to what they think this type of experience might mean to any particular family. Are positive, emotionally thrilling experiences significant in relationships between husband and wife? Is it possible that many couples have too few emotionally good experiences in their married lives? I am in no way suggesting that this type of experience is going to mend previously torn or weakly held-together marriages, but I truly suspect it may add dimensions in an already successful marriage that are beneficial.

2. *To discourage separation of mother and newborn.* We need to learn how to apply many known and proven social behavioral animal attitudes to the newborn child. The behavioral scientists have written much, but it seems to me that because they are too timid to apply this data to humans, we therefore continue to ignore much of it. Does it not make any difference if we encourage the separation of the newborn baby from its mother? I am suggesting that we tend to do this even today, by the following methods:

   a. At birth, by quickly taking the newborn from the mother to a central nursery.

   b. By keeping it in a central nursery for twelve to fourteen hours after birth, permitting the mother and father only a few glances through a viewing window.

c. By implying to the mother in essence that it doesn't make any difference whether she breastfeed or formula-feed her newborn, thereby giving tacit approval to non-breastfeeding in a large percentage of women.

d. By not making rooming-in available to every mother, not only those with breastfed babies but with nonbreastfed babies as well.

e. By hospital nurses wrapping the baby tightly and snugly and keeping it that way when the mother holds her baby for the few minutes, every three or four hours, she is allowed to do so while she is in the hospital. This prevents the important stimulation of the infant in skin-to-skin contact with the mother.

f. By keeping mothers unnecessarily long in hospitals following delivery and thereby again increasing the time of separation between mother and child.

g. By implying that the newborn is very delicate and susceptible to disturbances, hence teaching that following hospital life it must still be kept sterile, quiet, and as untouched as possible at home.

h. By allowing no place for the husband to begin a relationship with his newborn for fear that he might drop or contaminate the new, delicate child, discouraging him from trying to start such a relationship until later in life.

It seems we have learned much about imprinting in monkeys, dogs, birds, and even fish, but what have we learned about the imprinting effect in the human newborn? What animal breeder would ever think of causing any type of separation of the newborn animal from the mother following birth? Only in humans do we teach them to do this. Is this, or could this be, the beginning of a nonimprinting environment in humans, which is believed to take place in the first four to six months of the newborn's life?[23] Could it be that some of our social ills actually take root at this time? In a society that seeks answers to many questions in our lives, particularly as to the causes of tension, anxiety, and depression, in addition to those related to the inability of parents and children to communicate with each other, it seems to me this period of time needs more attention. It may be that we should not ignore too quickly studies of so-called healthy primitive cultures that seem to be able to raise children with lower levels of aggression, anxiety, hate, and competitiveness;[24] that we should evaluate these to see whether there are not some principles of that particular type of care of the newborn that might apply, or could be applied to our culture. Certainly mother-child closeness is a constant finding in so-called healthy primitive cultures.[25] The absence of this closeness is more typical of the so-called unhealthy primitive cultures, and is also a frequent finding in retrograde studies by psychiatrists of deeply disturbed children.[26] The Rhesus monkeys separated from their mothers at birth show degrees of emotional disturbance later in life that are directly related to the degrees of early separation.[27]

3. *To update standard orthodox prenatal care.* Dare I suggest that we may some day find that the physical and emotional preparedness of childbirth may be as significant in maternal and newborn mortality and morbidity as routine blood pressure, weight, hemoglobin, and monthly prenatal checks are considered today?

Perhaps paramedical personnel can easily be trained to do much of the particular type of prenatal care that we as obstetricians do today, and that we accept as modern care of the obstetrical patient. If so, we would then be freed to spend more time with the high-risk obstetrical patient. It seems logical that these paramedical personnel could not only do much of our routine prenatal care, but in addition train and prepare patients for childbirth.

It is known that we have many problems in our urban cities that prevent or tend to discourage prenatal attendance, and it would seem that if we could make our prenatal care more meaningful to patients, perhaps by bringing in many of the considerations mentioned above, we would have a much higher percentage of attendance at prenatal clinics. The lack of prenatal care sought is related to location of the clinics, to the amount of prenatal personnel available, and to the attitude and quality of personnel who are available. Again, I am in no way trying to imply that we substitute our traditional prenatal care by something else. I am suggesting that we make our prenatal care more meaningful and more significant, with childbirth education and natural childbirth training an intimate part of it, and that much of it can be performed by personnel other than the obstetrician. In this way I believe we can make better use of the obstetrician's time.

THE NEWBORN POTENTIAL

Unfortunately, at the present time, evidence supplied by the world birthrate points to the population explosion warned of by Dr. Paul Erlich,[28] but hopefully it will, rather, fulfill the population theory of optimist Dr. Garrett Hardin[29] of the University of California at Santa Barbara. Then birthrates will come under control. Accepting Dr. Hardin's view, we should welcome the opportunity for a marked increase in reproductive quality. With increased reproductive quality all the way from genetics through the newborn period, we will be able to see an increase in potential in each newborn. What are we talking about when we speak of the potential of the newborn child? We are talking specifically about three things: physical potential, mental potential, and emotional potential.

Pregnancy is the best time to present this teaching because most couples are available to the obstetrician, receptive to his advice,[30] and most interested in this type of data, which they need to study and consider before birth if what they learn is going to be available for the newborn. It is obvious that the obstetrician is the best—and perhaps the only—person who can successfully initiate this type of program.

The task here is to stimulate couples during pregnancy by telling them about the great opportunities each has awaiting them with the newborn, rather than about the obligations facing them for the infant's care. If this is not done during pregnancy, few will find and study the appropriate material by themselves later.

Where do we find appropriate information on the subject? The book *Prenatal Influences* by Ashley Montagu[31] is one good source, since Dr. Montagu is aware of things that, if they are not prevented, can have significant effects during pregnancy. And if we review this same author's earlier book, *Human Heredity*,[32] we become aware of things that are already determined by the time pregnancy has occurred. Another significant book to review is *A Matter of Life,* by Dr. W. Coda Martin,[33] in which the author outlines a blueprint for a healthy family, including nutrition, prenatal care, and early relationships. Margaret Ribble writes on the early psychological needs and their satisfaction as the birthright of infants. She writes about the significance of oxygen, hunger, sucking, and breastfeeding, and what happens when these things are not present or do not occur.[34]

The following material is an example of the type of data that might be presented in childbirth education as part of a natural childbirth program:

1. *Physical potential.* A discussion can be held on the interesting values of early crawling and swimming in relation to future coordination and balance. The questionable practice of encouraging early sitting, early standing, and early walking should be discussed. It may be that these hinder rather than help future coordination.

2. *Mental potential.* Maria Montessori[35] writes that most of a child's ability to learn, and his pleasure in learning, is determined in the first three years of life. What ideas might be presented to couples along these lines? A newborn learns only through his five senses—seeing, hearing, smelling, touching, and of course tasting.

A discussion is needed of our usual practice of keeping the newborn quiet, separated, aseptic, and untouched. The reverse may be of more value for his future potential for learning. On this aspect, Joan Beck's book[36] should be reviewed.

3. *Emotional potential.* During pregnancy is the ideal time to present material that might help immunize their child against future emotional disability. There is much material available to tell prospective parents about a newborn's potential emotional growth and development. Newborn-maternal separation and its emotional effects should also be discussed, as outlined in the next few paragraphs.

In our hospitals, do we not tend to do just the opposite of what Margaret Ribble[37] advises, by separating the mother and the newborn child and thereby subtracting just a little bit of the potential of a child? We are not talking about extreme separation, in which children are separated from their mothers for months at a time. We are talking about what frequently goes on at the hospitals in our Western culture. The pattern continues afterward at home, where the infant lies isolated in crib or playpen while his mother works around the house. As Harlow at Wisconsin has pointed out in his studies with primates, it may not be the milk that is so important. But when he separates a newborn monkey from his mother for any significant period of time, he finds it does affect the ability of the baby monkey to develop in a normal psychological way.[38]

And what about the effects of imprinting that Hess[39] writes of in relation to human babies? Have we not learned much from Konrad Lorenz[40] about imprinting, the significance of early skin-to-skin contact and the importance of continued skin-to-skin contact? James Clark Maloney[41] writes about healthy primitive cultures in which the care of the newborn baby includes a continuous maternal newborn relationship. And it is a rare breeder of animals that would in any way encourage early separation of a newborn from the mother! Dog breeders who are interested in the temperament of the grown dog are emphatic about not separating the newborn from the mother until the seventh week. More information comes from studies by Pfaffenberger[42] and John Paul Scott and John I. Fuller in their book, *Genetics and Social Behavior of the Dog.*[43] Margaret Mead[44] also writes much about the so-called healthy primitive cultures versus unhealthy primitive cultures and the differences in their early child-rearing practices. This type of data should be presented, or at least discussed, when talking over the emotional potential of the newborn with prospective parents.

From what is said in the book *Childbearing, Its Social and Psychological Effects* edited by Stephen A. Richardson and Alan F. Guttmacher,[45] it is apparent that cultural, social, and psychological factors have significant influences on the course of the pregnancy, on the delivery, and on the outcome. The outcome, of course, represents the quality of the child. Dr. Norman Morris, professor of obstetrics from the University of London, stated at a New York Maternity Center Association symposium that if we could use pregnancy as a time for couples to learn what is known about the family and newborn growth, the repercussions on our society would be remarkable.[46]

Today we must be more concerned about the quality of the newborn potential, while at the same time controlling the quantity of newborns. It is far more significant that we have a quality explosion of a small quantity rather than a quantity explosion of decreasing quality! Pregnancy is a time not only for education and preparation for childbirth, it is also a crucial time for study and learning about the potential of the newborn.

NATURAL CHILDBIRTH: AN IDEAL PROGRAM

I wish to discuss briefly a type of overall program that would include the basic principles of natural childbirth and family-centered maternity care and have as its goal the improvement of the potential of the newborn child.

Personnel

Two groups of personnel would be involved in such a program: the obstetrician and his prenatal office staff, and the hospital and the staff of the maternity ward.

THE OBSTETRICIAN AND HIS PRENATAL OFFICE STAFF. The patient in her early stages of pregnancy would first be seen by the obstetrician, who then would outline his prenatal care as follows:

After a complete history, physical, and routine prenatal laboratory work, each obstetrical patient is assigned a pregnancy risk of low, moderate, or high. Risk, of course, means the probable outcome of the pregnancy of the mother or infant, which would then dictate the amount of effort, time, and laboratory studies that would be required for the particular patient. High-risk pregnancies would command a much greater amount of time, effort, and possibly consultation with other physicians relative to preventive obstetrics during the pregnancy. Low-risk patients would require a minimal amount of time spent by the attending obstetrician, possibly only two or three visits until the last month of pregnancy, other prenatal visits being carried out by well-trained paramedical personnel. Moderate-risk patients would then fit into an intermediate group, the amount and type of prenatal care for this group based on the judgment of the obstetrician in charge of each particular case. Nurse-midwives, registered nurses, and other paramedical personnel would carry out most of the routine prenatal care.

Risking a patient, of course, is well outlined in most general texts today and is a fairly standardized procedure. Not only would all patients get what we call routine obstetrical prenatal care in this ideal environment, but all patients would get childbirth education and a natural childbirth training program.

THE HOSPITAL AND THE STAFF OF THE MATERNITY WARD. The basic and most important point here is that the training program would occur in the hospital in which the patient plans to give birth, by the hospital personnel from whom she will receive care at that time, a concept designed to increase the confidence of the patient in the hospital and in the hospital personnel. What is required for training?

1. A room large enough to train at least fifteen couples at any one time.

2. A movie projector and such films as are available, to aid in childbirth education and training.

3. A blackboard.

4. A library adequately supplied with all types of childbirth education and training material.

5. Charts, such as the birth atlas.

6. Other available audiovisual educational materials.

7. Personnel who are actively working in the maternity ward areas of the hospital, including labor, delivery, and postpartum.

In addition, the hospital personnel would be assisted by the office personnel from the various doctors' offices. In this way all of the personnel who come in contact with the obstetrical patient would be intimately associated with the basic principles of natural childbirth and family-centered maternity care, producing a continuous line of care from the doctor's prenatal office through the labor, birth, and postpartum period.

The Natural Childbirth and Family-Centered Maternity Care Program

There are three distinct parts to this type of childbirth education: (1) *three two-hour sessions* that are given early in pregnancy, (2) *five two-hour sessions* that are given in late pregnancy, and (3) *two two-hour sessions* that are given during the hospital postpartum stay.*

CLASSES IN EARLY PREGNANCY. It is extremely important that childbirth preparation classes begin *early* in pregnancy, near the end of the first trimester, so the expectant mother can put into practice those things which will make for a healthier pregnancy as well as a happier labor and birth.

The first introductory session would include prenatal exercises, nutrition, and a discussion of breastfeeding. The exer-

*These are *minimum* requirements of time.

cises introduced at this time should include good posture, tailor sitting, the "pelvic rock" and the exercise for firming the muscles of the pelvic floor. (See Part II for a full description of each of these.)

At this session the importance of good nutrition during pregnancy should also be presented, along with what good nutrition means to the infant, not only during pregnancy, but also during the early period of its life. The discussion should include such subjects as the quality of the food we are eating today, particularly with regard to such things as refined foods and refined sugars, and the foods that lead to better health. Nutritionists write about the value of wheat germ, 100 percent whole wheat bread, and natural sugars, and if what they are writing is correct, there is no better time to educate young couples than when they are setting a nutritional pattern for their expected child *in utero*.

This first class session should also include an introductory discussion of breastfeeding. And there should always be reading material available to allow the prospective parents to study and investigate any of the subjects covered in more detail.

The second two-hour session would cover two vital subjects:

1. Teaching the patient relaxation. It takes considerable practice for some patients to learn how to control muscular relaxation. Others learn more readily. But for those who find it difficult, the additional weeks for practice can be of incalculable benefit during pregnancy as well as during birth. Once muscular relaxation has been adequately learned, it can be utilized for getting to sleep more quickly at night, and for gaining much more benefit from short times of rest through the day. Twenty minutes of complete muscular relaxation are much more refreshing than a two-hour nap.

2. Introducing the husband's role, not only for pregnancy and birth, but also for the first year of life. The husband can be awakened to the realization that he has a great opportunity to assist his wife during pregnancy, childbirth, and with their newborn child.

The third introductory session should present material designed to stimulate parents to consider factors relative to the emotional, mental, and physical potential of their newborn child. It is essential that this type of material be presented during pregnancy, early enough to give parents opportunity for further study on their own if they wish, in the quieter months before the child arrives.

With any of these classes there would be a movie and discussion, questions and answers. Young couples who are expecting for the first time are often excited about the prospect of parenthood, and are highly motivated at the outset of pregnancy to learn all they can. These sessions would therefore provide an ideal opportunity for pediatricians, psychiatrists, psychologists, sociologists, educators, and members of other disciplines in our society to be on hand for questions and answers.

CLASSES IN LATE PREGNANCY. This course would consist of five natural childbirth training classes, and would be the meat of the childbirth education program. The classes, which would train the couples to give birth as outlined in this text on natural childbirth, should start at approximately eight weeks before the expected date of birth, soon enough to prepare expectant mothers for a premature birth, if this should occur, yet late enough in pregnancy to keep the couples diligent in practicing the techniques that will be helpful in childbirth.

Prenatal education is incomplete unless it includes, during one of these late classes, a tour of the hospital labor-delivery area where the baby is to be born, so that when labor begins the mother will be returning to a familiar place. Each couple also should be told what to bring, where to park, where to enter the hospital, and how to enter in case of emergency so that there is no delay in attending the mother.

POSTPARTUM HOSPITAL CLASSES. The third set of classes include two two-hour sessions given to the couple in the hospital after the baby is born. The first class would include a discussion relevant to birth control in the future and family planning. The second class would be a discussion covering such subjects as postpartum care of the mother at home, care of the newborn at home, nutrition, and postpartum exercises.

In addition, during the day, under the supervision of a nurse, the mothers should be taught how to bathe, diaper, and otherwise care for their babies, and should have an opportunity in a group situation to discuss any problems concerning breastfeeding that may have arisen, encouraging each other under the guidance of one of the nursing staff.

NATURAL CHILDBIRTH: AN IDEAL EXAMPLE

A patient, having completed a natural childbirth training program, is now in labor. She is greeted as she enters the labor room by someone she knows, since one of the requirements for an attendant working on the maternity ward is that she take part in the childbirth education program. Because the patient and her husband have visited the hospital labor and delivery area enough times to feel comfortable with the surroundings, their entrance at this time does not produce the anxiety and apprehension that is so common when a patient enters strange surroundings and sees personnel she has never met before.

Ideally, a maternity ward should have a waiting room lounge equipped with television, stereo, magazines, and games. This waiting room would not be for husbands, but for couples in early labor. How often a patient is "not sure" if labor is under way, particularly if she has been so well trained in natural childbirth that she can feel the contractions, even though they are barely perceptible. She may arrive at the hospital in early labor, be admitted, put to bed in a labor room—only to be sent home several hours later when contractions cease, or prove to have been "false labor."

How much better it would be to have a comfortable waiting room lounge where those who think they "might be" in labor could come as guests, without being formally admitted. Husband and wife could then relax, watch television, play games, or read. If labor really proved to be under way this would be a tremendous advantage—no last-minute "rush" to the hospital would be needed. If not, the couple could return home later without having inconvenienced anyone, and without embarrassment. This lounge could perhaps also serve as the room where childbirth classes are held, and thus be a familiar, comfortable place.

If the patient is definitely in labor, she is placed in a bed in a private labor room, a room that has all the decor and atmosphere of home—which does not mean it has to lack aseptic conditions. The setting up of such a room may take a little planning and some imagination by interior decorators and architects, but basically it does not take elaborate or expensive equipment.

The room requires a bed that is firm, electrically operated, and that can also be used as a guerney to transport the patient if necessary. It must also have a comfortable chair for the husband to use before he becomes actively involved, as well as a straight chair for him to use beside his wife's bed later. The room should have lights that can be dimmed and a decor that is comfortable and relaxing. Harmonious colors and a few attractive pictures can make a world of difference.

The labor room bed should be one that has a triangular attachment, which, when added, will permit the patient to give birth on the same bed, turning the labor room into a birth room. With this type of attachment, the patient need only turn approximately thirty degrees to the bed to be in position for an easy spontaneous birth. A large number of women could give birth very simply by this method, without ever moving them into the birth room. The expense and cost of maternity care is diminished with this type of birth.

The labor room nurses who took part in the childbirth education program would, during this time, be readily available to help direct the husband in the proper labor coaching. The nurses' job is not to do the labor coaching, but to see that the husband does it.

When a natural birth takes place in the birth room, the patient's hands and legs should not be strapped (figs. 11, 12, page 120), and the stirrups should be of a type that allow her readily to adjust her legs as comfortably as possible. She is provided with a natural childbirth backrest, such as the Fitzhugh backrest, which fits on most birth tables and can easily be adjusted to any angle. The husband, who has previously scrubbed and changed into a gown, cap, mask, shoe coverings, and so on, stays continuously at the side of his wife, relaying directions to her from the physician.

During a labor in which fetal monitoring programs are carried out, there is no reason why the natural childbirth program cannot be used, an advantage being that the obstetrician attaching electrical scalp monitors to the baby would find his patient cooperative and understanding. At no time am I suggesting that we bypass any of the significant or important continuous monitoring of the patient during labor and birth.

After the natural labor is completed, the baby is cleansed and cared for and the mother returns to her room. In this family-centered maternity hospital care, the baby is carried to the mother's bedside in the rooming-in unit. Mother and baby stay in the hospital approximately forty-eight hours, and the father is welcome at any time to see his wife and hold his new baby.

It is during this postpartum stay that the two two-hour classes are presented by the postpartum maternity nurses. These nurses, having previously become acquainted with each patient, find their job more challenging and more rewarding as they conclude this final part of the childbirth education program.

CONCLUSION

Natural childbirth, of course, does not correct all obstetrical problems; we will still have many. Natural childbirth does, however, offer an opportunity for a high percentage of simple, easy, vaginal births. The essence of what has been written in this chapter was discussed and outlined by Grantly Dick-Read in his early writings of forty years ago. The only thing that time has done has been to prove his basic principles of natural childbirth, and what these principles mean to the patient, her baby, and her husband, and therefore to the family and society in general. For the magnanimous contributions that these natural childbirth programs have thereby made to happier childbirth, the art of obstetrics is truly indebted.[47]

BIBLIOGRAPHICAL REFERENCES FOR CHAPTER 6

1. Nicholson J. Eastman and Louis M. Hellman, eds., *Williams' Obstetrics,* 13th ed. (New York: Appleton-Century-Crofts, 1966).
2. Herbert Thoms, "The Preparation for Childbirth Program," *Obstetrics and Gynecological Survey* 10, no. 1 (1955).
3. Eastman and Hellman, *Williams' Obstetrics,* p. 411.
4. *Natural Childbirth* (London: William Heinemann Ltd., 1933).
5. Grantly Dick-Read, *No Time for Fear* (New York: Harper & Bros., 1955); Margaret Mead, *Male and Female* (New York: William Morrow, 1949), p. 238; *American Journal of Obstetrics and Gynecology* 84, no. 9: 1202.
6. H. B. Atlee, *Natural Childbirth* (Springfield, Ill.: Charles C Thomas, 1956); Helen Wessel, *Childbirth and the Family* (New York: Harper & Row, 1973); Thoms, "The Preparation for Childbirth Program"; Lester Hazell, *Commonsense Childbirth* (New York: G. P. Putnam's Sons, 1969).
7. Sol M. Shnider, "Obstetric Anesthesia Coverage: Problems and Solutions," *Obstetrics and Gynecology* (ACOG Journal) 34, no. 4 (October 1969): 615.
8. *Williams' Obstetrics,* p. 410.
9. Walter B. Cannon, *Bodily Changes in Pain, Hunger, Fear and Rage,* rev. ed. (New York: Harper & Row, 1963).
10. For example, Sprague Gardiner, quoted in Eastman and Hellman, *Williams' Obstetrics,* p. 336.
11. *Male and Female,* p. 238.

12. Helene Deutsch, *Psychology of Women* (New York: Grune & Stratton, 1945), p. 207.
13. For example, Robert Bradley, *Husband-Coached Childbirth* (New York: Harper & Row, 1965).
14. Victor G. Vaugham III, "Insight in Social Behavior," *Journal of the American Medical Association* 198, no. 1 (October 3, 1966).
15. In *King Solomon's Ring* (New York: Thomas Y. Crowell, 1952).
16. In "Love in Infant Monkeys," *Scientific American,* June 1959.
17. Niles Newton, *Family Book of Child Care* (New York: Harper & Bros., 1957); Ernestine Wiedenbach, *Family-Centered Maternity Nursing,* 2nd ed. (New York: G. P. Putnam's Sons, 1967).
18. *Natural Childbirth.*
19. Michael Newton and Niles Newton, "The Normal Course and Management of Lactation," *Clinical Obstetrics and Gynecology* S, no. 1 (March 1962): 61.
20. *Journal of Obstetrics and Gynecology* 76 (October 1969): 877–880.
21. Steer and Moore, "The Course of Perinatal Mortality: A Review of Etiologic Factors in the Sloane Hospital 1888–1967," *Obstetrics and Gynecology* (ACOG Journal) 34, no. 1 (July 1969): 116.
22. H. M. Wallace, "Teen-age Pregnancy," *American Journal of Obstetrics and Gynecology* 92, no. 8 (August 15, 1965): 1129.
23. Vaugham, "Insight in Social Behavior."
24. James Clark Maloney, *Fear, Contagion and Anxiety.*
25. Mead, *Male and Female.*
26. Margaret A. Ribble, *The Rights of Infants,* rev. ed. (New York: Columbia University Press, 1965), p. 4.
27. Niko Tinbergen, *Animal Behavior* (New York: Life Nature Library, 1968), p. 29.
28. In *The Population Bomb* (New York: Ballantine Books, 1969).
29. In *Population, Evolution and Birth Control,* 2nd ed. (San Francisco: H. W. Freeman & Co., 1969).
30. Thaddeus Montgomery, in *Controversy in Obstetrics and*

Gynecology, ed. Duncan Reid and T. C. Barton (Philadelphia: W. B. Saunders, 1969), p. 227.

31. Springfield, Ill.: Charles C Thomas, 1962.
32. Cleveland: The World Publishing Co., 1963.
33. New York: Devin-Adair Co., 1964.
34. Riddle, *The Rights of Infants.*
35. In Nancy Rambusch, *Learning How to Learn* (New York: Helicon Press, 1965), p. 18.
36. *How to Raise a Brighter Child* (New York: Trident Press, 1967).
37. Ribble, *The Rights of Infants.*
38. Harlow, "Love in Infant Monkeys."
39. Eckhard H. Hess, "Imprinting in Animals," *Scientific American,* March 1958.
40. *King Solomon's Ring.*
41. In "What Americans Can Learn from Healthy Primitives," *Unity* 149, no. 3 (September–October 1963).
42. Clarence Pfaffenberger, *Dog Behavior* (New York: Howell Book House, 1964), p. 125.
43. Chicago: University of Chicago Press, 1966.
44. In *Male and Female.*
45. Baltimore: The Williams & Wilkins Co., 1967, p. viii.
46. Norman Morris, *Meeting the Childbearing Needs of Families in a Changing World* (New York: Maternity Center Association, 1962), p. 14.
47. *American Journal of Obstetrics and Gynecology* 84, no. 9: 1202.

Part II

THE PRACTICE OF
NATURAL CHILDBIRTH

The following chapters spell out in more detail the specific instructions for the successful application of Grantly Dick-Read's natural childbirth principles.

The emphasis throughout his teaching is always upon naturalness, upon that which is most easily learned, practiced, and applied. The reader will discover that all the techniques he advocates one practice during pregnancy for comfortable childbearing are simple, everyday rules of good health. *Disciplined practice of these few basic techniques is essential for a happy outcome at birth,* but they are as applicable for healthful living at any time in our lives as they are for giving birth. There are no "tricks," no fancy ways of breathing, no difficult, unnatural, or complicated techniques to learn in his teaching.

Grantly Dick-Read's concern was with the whole of life, in which the birth of a child maintains a place as a positive and wholesome experience, contributing to the health and happiness of the mother and baby, and to the development of a happy family unit.

In our frantic, tense society, we would all enjoy life more and have better health if we would also faithfully practice and apply his simple but vital instructions for right eating, correct breathing, conscious control of muscular relaxation, and physical fitness through good posture and moderate exercise.

7

Prenatal Health

The general hygiene of pregnancy often brings to light much that surprises. Too many women of all income classes are ignorant of habits and customs they should have learned and practiced from early childhood. Women must associate the necessity for care of their own health with the health of their unborn babies.

DIET

There is little reason why a woman should alter the normal diet with which she has maintained good health. Her body is accustomed to it, and any sudden change may do more harm than good. It is well that she eat slightly less than usual, but skipping meals or going on crash diets to avoid weight gain is foolish, and detrimental to her basic health and vitality.

The Victorian idea that a pregnant woman eats for two people must also be dispelled. Excessive eating during pregnancy is even more harmful than at other times. If a woman is excessively fat, she should follow a carefully balanced diet prepared for her by her own physician, and under his constant supervision.

Vegetarians need not add to or change their food. They generally have less trouble with pregnancy and labor than those who are heavy meat-eaters, because the latter tend to skimp on fresh vegetables and fruits. If a woman is accustomed to eating meat, she would do well to choose liver, fish, and poultry more often than beef, pork, or lamb, and to balance it with salads rather than potatoes and gravy.

Fluids assist in the metabolism of other foods. An adequate amount of *protein* is essential, and is found in lean meat, eggs, milk, peas, beans, and nuts. Wheat germ is an excellent source of added protein and B vitamins. *Fats* are necessary as fuel for heat and energy in the body, and are obtained in cream, butter, cheese, and some of the fat meats. *Carbohydrates* are also energy making, and are supplied in sweets, flour, sugar, potatoes, milk, and rice. Unrefined natural sugars are probably the best source of carbohydrates.

Iron, calcium, phosphorus, iodine, and other *minerals* and *vitamins* are all necessary, and are supplied in a well-balanced diet containing fish and liver, milk, grains (100 percent whole wheat, barley, oats, etc.), vegetables, and fresh citrus fruits. Vitamin and mineral tablets as diet supplements are not necessary, unless the physician diagnoses some particular deficiency. Alcohol is best kept to a minimum, and smoking is not advisable.

CLOTHING

Psychologically, clothing has a much greater influence than is generally recognized. An expectant mother should look attractive, wearing suitable clothes, without trying to hide her shape or feel embarrassed by it. For her own composure she should realize that sensible people envy and admire a young pregnant woman.

After the first two or three months of pregnancy the center of gravity alters, so that it is safer to wear low heels. Many pregnant women fall downstairs or trip easily for no apparent reason, and although the majority of these accidents do no harm to either mother or baby, they are disconcerting and cause unnecessary anxiety.

After the fourth month there must be no undue pressure on the abdomen. Dresses and smocks should hang from the shoulders, and skirts and slacks should be adjustable to the changing shape of the body.

The breasts should be supported within well-fitting, rounded cups, with straps that lift them to the correct height upon the chest, but without any pressure whatever across the breasts or nipples.

Abdominal supporting belts are rarely required by a woman having her first baby, and those who have carried out their prenatal and postnatal exercises in order to maintain the tone of abdominal muscles do not require them for subsequent babies. But when a support is necessary, the general principle is that the uterus should be supported from below in a cup-shaped garment, with no pressure whatever on it above the level of the navel. Such a support helps keep the uterus from falling forward, and relieves backache by taking the weight of the developing uterus from the muscles in the small of the back.

PERSONAL HYGIENE

The Skin

It is not unusual, particularly for brunettes, to develop large areas of brown pigment on the forehead or cheekbones, or on other parts of the body. There is no way of preventing or curing this, but it does tend to disappear after pregnancy.

Sometimes itching is troublesome, probably due to stretching of the tissues. This can be relieved by keeping the skin clean and soft with a good alkaline soap or one of the many creams available for this purpose. Itching of the genitals arises from different causes, and should be reported to the doctor for his advice on treatment.

The Hair

During pregnancy there is sometimes a tendency for the hair to become rather lifeless, and to fall out. The hair should be given a good brushing, and a few drops of thin hair oil or lotion should be rubbed into the scalp. The chances are, if nutrition is adequate and the hair washed as often as is necessary, this bit of extra attention will help it keep its vitality and look better after pregnancy than before.

Fingernails

Fingernails can be kept from cracking by rubbing a little vaseline on and around them at night. To keep from harming the baby after its arrival, the nails should be kept short and clean.

The Teeth

As soon as a woman knows she is pregnant, she should have a thorough examination made of her mouth by a dentist, to see that no decay or sepsis is present. The teeth do tend to decay more while a baby is coming, due to the changes in a woman's own system, and not because of the baby's need for calcium. During pregnancy many women also tend to get red and puffy gums, which may bleed easily. A very soft tooth brush should be used and the gums massaged. This problem will disappear shortly after the baby is born.

The Breasts and Nipples

The nipples should be kept clean with warm water during the daily bath or shower, but no soap or other product whatever should be used on them. The softer and more elastic the nipples can be kept, the better for the woman who wishes to breastfeed her baby.

During the last ten or twelve weeks of pregnancy the breasts may exude a few drops of a very thick, yellow secretion called *colostrum*. If it cakes on the breasts, warm water will soften it, and, if it gets too thick, very gentle pressure at the base of the nipple with the thumb and forefinger will clear the little openings into the breast. This should be done extremely gently and without any force at all. Great care should be taken that the breasts are never handled roughly, or violently rubbed or massaged, as some erroneously advise.

If the nipple is slightly retracted and doesn't stand out as it should after warm bathing, this should be called to the attention of the doctor. He may advise wearing a breast shield during pregnancy to help the nipple come forward, so the baby will be able to nurse more easily later.

The Bowels

A glass of hot water, with or without a teaspoonful of honey stirred into it, helps maintain a daily bowel action when taken first thing in the morning. If constipation is a problem, stewed prunes, raw apples, figs, or raisins eaten with breakfast are helpful. No other tablets or preparations should be taken unless a doctor so advises.

8

Education

The human body is not a series of individual organs carrying out their allotted tasks unaffected by their neighbors. Our bodies are unified structures whose components exhibit the most perfect harmony that science has the privilege of investigating. Our organs and purposes are interdependent. No physical strain beyond our ability can be sustained without circulatory or skeletal injury, and no chronic fear or anxiety can be maintained in the human mind without the disruption of the normal physiological balance. The manifestations of such fear or anxiety may be either psychological or physical, for nature rebels against intruders upon its ordered processes.

It is important for women to understand the development of a baby within the uterus, for ignorance of these elementary facts may cause anxieties and doubts that are difficult to overcome, affecting her health adversely. Such complaints of pregnancy as persistent nausea, sickness, constipation, desire for unusual foods, excessive salivation, headaches, backaches, and a general feeling of weariness, may often be the physical manifestations of anxiety, which knowledge can help dispel.

FERTILIZATION

Nearly all animals, including human beings, have much the same principles of breeding. The female makes eggs and the male produces sperm. Eggs have to be fertilized by the sperm before they can grow into babies. Nature makes the process of fertilization pleasant to experience, because each race must go on reproducing itself or it will die out.

The female reproductive organs are located in the lower abdomen, below the level of the hip bones. In the center of these is the *uterus*, or womb, which in its nonpregnant state is about two and one-half inches by one and one-half inches by one-half inch. A small, muscular organ that weighs about one and one-half ounces, the uterus is shaped rather like a pear with the narrow end pointing downward, where it is attached to the upper end of the vagina. The lower, narrow end of the uterus is closed by circular muscular tissue called the *cervix*, through which a narrow passage opens into the uterus.

At the upper end of the uterus are two narrow tubes that extend out from each side, rather like arms extending out from the shoulders. Each tube is three or four inches long, and opens at the end furthest from the uterus into a shallow bell shape. Underneath each of these two bell-shaped structures is a small, oval organ called an *ovary*. Each of the two ovaries contain *ova*, or egg-forming tissue.

An egg (*ovum*) is developed and sent on its way by one of the ovaries each month, about ten days after menstruation. The ovum travels down the narrow tube from the ovary to the uterus, while the uterus prepares a lining of tissue to make a good "nest" to receive it. If the egg is not fertilized by a male sperm, it passes on through the uterus and is cast off. About two weeks later the lining of the uterus is also thrown off, and a new lining prepared for the next egg. The flow of cast-off, unused material is called *menstruation*.

A male child is born with testicles which, shortly before birth, have moved down from the abdomen into the scrotum, outside the body. In these organs *spermatozoa* are produced. It is estimated that each testicle contains over one mile of sperm-producing tubules, from the walls of which a healthy man may produce at each ejaculation over two hundred million spermatozoa.

The male sperm is ejaculated from the penis into the vagina of the female at the culmination of mating, or *coitus*. The mature sperm cell has a long, thin tail, which enables it to move toward the opening in the cervix of the uterus. It travels at the rate of about one inch in ten minutes. Considerable numbers find their way into the uterus and engage in what might be described as a race for the ovum. As soon as a sperm penetrates an ovum, making it fertile, the ovum undergoes an immediate change, which prevents any further penetration by another sperm.

The fertile egg moves on through the tube, becomes embedded in the wall of the uterus, and starts to grow. The lining of the uterus alters its character, developing the *placenta,* through which the mother nourishes her child. The placental site rapidly expands, its blood vessels and nerve fibrils bring vitality to the egg, and the growth of the *fetus,* the developing baby, begins.

DEVELOPMENT OF THE HUMAN BABY

Very shortly after the ovum is fertilized it starts to develop cells that are differentiated to form the various organs and structures of the body. Some of these become the mother cells of spermatozoa and ova, so that quite early in fetal life the sex of the child is determined.

During its growing life, the baby is protected by a "bag of waters," in which it lives. This protects the baby from injury if the mother is bumped or falls, keeps him or her at a constant temperature, and provides space for the baby to move about freely until the later months of growth.

The fetus grows very fast. At four weeks it is one sixth of an inch long, lying in a fluidlike sack about the size of a pigeon's egg. At the end of the second month it is about one and one-sixth inches long, and the arms, legs, and head are clearly distinguishable. By this time it has its own circulation of blood and its own nervous system.

It is now fed through its navel by a tube called the *umbilical cord,* which is attached to the placenta. This wonderful organ, the placenta, is attached to the inside wall of the uterus and filters from the mother's blood the substances necessary for the development of the child. Not only does it have the power of passing on to the child what it requires, but it also has the power of refusing to take from the mother's blood some of the substances that may not be advantageous to the child. By the time the baby is due to be born, the umbilical cord between the placenta and baby may be from one to three feet in length.

At the end of the third month the fetus is about three and one-half inches long, weighs approximately an ounce, and at the end of the fourth month it has grown rapidly to about seven inches and weighs about four ounces. Its heart can now be heard beating strongly, and it is possible to tell the sex of the child if it should be born at this stage. By this time the mother will have become conscious of the baby's movements. This is known as *quickening,* and it occurs at about eighteen or nineteen weeks after conception.

Out of all proportion to the skeletal growth of the baby is the development of its brain. From the earliest weeks, brain substance is present in the fetus. At three and a half weeks the brain can be differentiated into its three main divisions, and between three and five months it develops integrative cerebral function. One month before the baby is born its brain is perfected.

It is within the brain itself that the heritage of parental influence is most readily discovered. The baby's mental development is influenced, not only by heredity, but also by the nature of the mother's influence during pregnancy. The calmness or anxiety that affects her own nervous system may have an effect on the baby also.

At the fifth month of pregnancy the baby is almost ten inches long and weighs about one and one-half pounds. Occasionally one reads in medical literature of babies born at this age who survive. By the end of the seventh month, twenty-eight weeks old, the child is perfected. Although not fully grown or fully nourished, some twenty-eight-week-old children have survived well after birth.

At the eighth month the child is almost seventeen inches

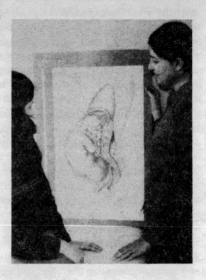

Fig. 16. Instructor showing patient diagram of baby at full term.

long, and has a very good chance of healthy survival. At the ninth month, or thirty-six weeks, the average weight is five to five and one-half pounds. The organs and functions are all well developed, and although children born now require more care than full-term children, they should survive perfectly well if born at this age.

At the tenth month, forty weeks—which is about the average time a child takes to develop—it should weigh about seven to seven and one-half pounds and be about nineteen inches in length (fig. 16), and it is in this condition that natural birth takes place.

THE UTERUS DURING PREGNANCY

The duration of pregnancy is counted from the first day of the last menstrual period. Most women suspect that they are

pregnant when the expected period does not arrive. They feel
perfectly well, unless for any reason they are anxious about
pregnancy. When about six or seven weeks pregnant, many
women will be conscious of sensitiveness and slight enlargement of the breasts. By this time the pregnant woman should
see a doctor, and keep in constant touch with him or a clinic
throughout the whole of pregnancy, and until at least six
weeks after the birth of the baby. These chapters are not
intended to instruct mothers in matters that are the special
province of medical advisers. There must be someone qualified to whom they can turn for advice upon any subject that
creates the slightest doubt in their minds.

With the growth of the fetus the uterus develops in size. The
muscle fibers become longer and more numerous. Fluid is
secreted into the cavity of the organ, which fills and expands.
After two months the pregnant uterus is about the size of a
large hen's egg. At the third month it can just be felt, in a thin
woman, above the pubic bone. At the fourth month it is halfway between the pubic bone and the navel. At five and a half
months it is up to the navel. At eight months it is about
halfway between the navel and the lower end of the breast-
bone.

Between the seventh and eighth month the baby's heart
beats loudly enough for the mother to hear it through the
doctor's stethoscope, although the doctor, with his practiced
ear, will have been able to detect it long before this time.

By thirty-five weeks the baby should have taken up its
correct position for birth, with its head downward and its back
slightly to the right or the left of center. At nine and a half
months, or thirty-eight weeks, the uterus reaches its highest
point in the abdomen.

At about the thirty-eighth week women who are having
their first baby will experience what is known as *lightening*.
This is the slipping down of the baby's head into the brim of
the pelvis. The baby's chin becomes flexed upon his breast-
bone, and the back of his head (called the *occiput*) slides

downward into the upper portion of the birth canal. The change is often felt in the abdomen. The uterus appears to have lowered, and this often gives the mother added freedom of movement and breathing. Thus at full term, or forty weeks, the uterus has dropped back one to two inches. The actual size of the uterus varies according to the amount of water in it and the size of the baby, but the levels in the abdomen at certain weeks of development do not vary much in different women.

The birth of the child may usually be expected within ten days or two weeks after this lightening occurs. With second and subsequent babies it may not occur, however. Not infrequently, in the easiest births of additional children, the head will remain quite high in the pelvis, or even above it, until well into the second stage of labor.

THE MUSCLE LAYERS OF THE UTERUS

When the baby is ready to be born, the uterus is a muscular bag about fourteen inches in length and not quite half an inch in thickness. It is well supplied with nerves that stimulate its muscles to contract, and it also has a plentiful supply of blood vessels, which are necessary to take fresh blood to the uterus and to carry away all the waste products of muscular activity. There are three muscle layers in the uterus (figs. 17–19):

1. The outer layer goes up the back, over the top, and down the front. These long muscle bands are found mainly in the middle and upper part of the uterus.

2. The middle muscle layer is a mass of interwoven muscles in which the big blood vessels lie.

3. The inner muscle layer goes around the uterus in a circular manner, and is found almost entirely in the area of the lower part of the uterus and cervix.

The outer muscles contract (shorten and tighten) to push the baby down, through, and ultimately out of the uterus. The middle muscles contract to squeeze the blood out of the walls of the uterus, and then relax to allow the blood vessels to fill up again with a fresh supply of blood.

But when the inner, circular muscles contract, they close the outlet, maintaining the uterus in its unemptied shape. Thus these inner, circular muscles *must be loose and relaxed* when

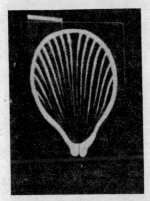

MUSCLES OF THE UTERUS

Fig. 17. Longitudinal muscle fibers.

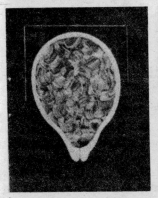

Fig. 18. Muscles interwoven with blood vessels.

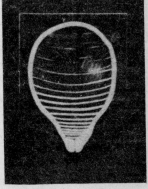

Fig. 19. Circular muscle fibers.

the long muscles contract to open the womb and push the baby out. If a woman is frightened during labor, this inner muscle layer contracts. Then the muscles that empty the uterus and the muscles that hold it closed are working against each other.

All through the body one finds examples of the harmony of muscles in polarity. For example, one's biceps relax when the triceps hold out the arm, but the triceps relax when the biceps pull the forearm up to the shoulder. If both sets of muscles are activated at the same time, pain soon results.

Whenever there are two big groups of muscles working against each other they soon begin to hurt, and in a short time the pain becomes very severe. We speak of this as the "fear-tension-pain syndrome" of childbirth, for a woman who is afraid is unconsciously resisting the birth of her baby by tightening the circular fibers, preventing the progress of the birth, and increasing the muscle tension within the walls of the uterus. This causes nearly all the pains and distresses in otherwise normal labor, which describes the labor of about ninety-five women out of a hundred.

FEAR-TENSION-PAIN

This fear-tension-pain series of events is experienced by everybody in circumstances very similar. The bowel is full, the desire to empty is acute, it pushes against our active restraint, but the time and place are not convenient. We are afraid to stop resisting even though it is uncomfortable and becoming painful, until there is the right opportunity to relax the outlet and let the contents be released. Again, we have a strong urge to urinate, but the right place is not available. We dare not relax the muscles that hold the bladder closed because of social and domestic repercussions, so we suffer increasing pain, sometimes agony, until the opportunity comes for the comfort of relaxing the outlet and emptying the distended, contracting organ.

This same principle is at work during the birth of a child. Fear of pain causes resistance to the working muscles of the uterus, increasing tension and causing pain. The muscles of the bowel and bladder are less powerful than those of the uterus, but even they become painful if their efforts to expel are resisted.

Fear is the natural protective emotion without which few of us would remain alive for many days. Its intensity varies from precaution and doubt to uncontrollable terror. Even mild anxiety can make a woman tense, thus causing the circular muscles to resist the expulsive muscles of the uterus. A tense woman has a tense outlet to the uterus, giving rise to the saying "Tense woman—tense cervix." A tense cervix means a long and painful labor in the majority of cases, for the mother is closing the door against the progress of her baby from the uterus.

By contrast, a relaxed woman allows the cervix, the "door" of the uterus, to open easily. If she understands what is taking place, is fully relaxed and confident, then the muscles that held the uterus closed during pregnancy will become loose and easily stretched open, when the long muscles begin their work of expelling the baby. The tension created by resistance to the birth will not be there to cause pain, and the baby will be born more easily and comfortably.

9

Breathing

The growth of the baby inside the uterus is maintained through the mother's blood. The wonderful organ known as the placenta, which develops along with the baby, is able to filter from the large blood vessels of the uterus the food required by the baby. This is passed to the baby through the umbilical cord to his navel. Through the cord the waste material of the baby is returned as well, to be disposed of by the mother. So it becomes clear that to have healthy babies it is necessary to eat and drink the right things.

One of the most important foods is oxygen. We cannot live without it, and whenever the supply of oxygen to the brain is insufficient for a short period of time, the brain becomes damaged to that degree. Adults breathe in oxygen through their lungs. The baby doesn't use its lungs for breathing, but takes its oxygen from the placenta straight into its bloodstream. Therefore, by breathing correctly, the mother can supply as much oxygen to her baby as it requires. During pregnancy it is of the utmost importance that as much fresh air as possible is taken into her lungs, and with the least effort.

Correct breathing is also essential during labor. The big muscles of the uterus are working to expel the baby, and when big muscles are used they require more fuel, just as a car uses more fuel to go faster or climb a hill. We don't feel our big muscles working if we are healthy, but we do breathe faster and deeper, and that is how they get extra fuel. During labor correct breathing is essential in supplying the necessary oxygen to the working muscles of the uterus. It also keeps the baby strong and in good condition while it is being born.

But in order for the breathing to help, the mother must also be *relaxed* enough during labor to allow the blood to circulate more freely through the middle layer of muscles in the uterus, thus replenishing its oxygen supply more quickly and plentifully.

No one can work to the best of her ability either physically ·or mentally if she does not breathe correctly; indeed, incorrect breathing is *the* bad habit that causes more illness than any other. It is surprising to learn that not one woman in fifty breathes properly.

The secret of correct breathing lies in the *control* of respiration—that is, control of breathing in and also of breathing out. Fresh air is taken into the lungs, which are like a very fine sponge made of minute air spaces and even smaller blood vessels. The walls are so thin that the oxygen from the air passes into the blood and the waste gas from the blood passes into the air spaces. By breathing we take in pure air and get rid of "waste" air.

Most people use less than four-fifths of their air space. To maintain a sufficient supply of oxygen, this means that they have to breathe five times for every four breaths taken by the person who breathes correctly. Breathing faster means more work for the muscles concerned with breathing, and more work for the heart to pump the blood around the body. In pregnancy this can become a strain and even a discomfort, the enlarging uterus causes discomfort to many women because they do not maintain good posture and breathe correctly. Therefore, during this time, when the oxygen intake is so dependent upon the correctness of breathing, these simple exercises should have priority over all other physical movements.

1. FULL DEEP BREATHING

Place your hands flat on your lower ribs, with your head up and shoulders back. Open your mouth and fill your chest slowly with air, filling in the upper part of the lungs as well as the lower, clear up under the collarbones. When you have breathed in as much air as possible, then let it out, slowly and completely. Lean slightly forward and force out the last possible breath. This will not cause any harm, so don't be afraid to take these slow, deep breaths.

Spend five or ten minutes each morning and evening breathing in and out, slowly and deeply, in this way. Many women are surprised at how much better they feel after only two weeks of practicing this simple breathing exercise each day. They quickly find themselves able to do more without becoming "out of breath." Rapid progress is made because there is usually so much room for improvement!

2. "WORK" BREATHING

When you have acquired the habit of freely breathing deeply, learn to breathe more quickly, but still keeping the breathing under control, while working around the house. Instead of seventeen or eighteen breaths a minute, gradually work up to *twenty-five or twenty-six times a minute*, but not faster. This "work" breathing supplies the extra oxygen needed for physical exertion, and is of great help in labor during the contractions near the end of the first stage. These in-and-out breaths, which are still to be taken deep into the diaphragm, should not be confused with shallow panting, which, since it tends to become too rapid, may lead to hyperventilation and may limit the oxygen supply to the uterus.

3. "SLEEP" BREATHING

Next, learn gentle diaphragmatic breathing, in a relaxed and comfortable position in a chair, or on the bed. This

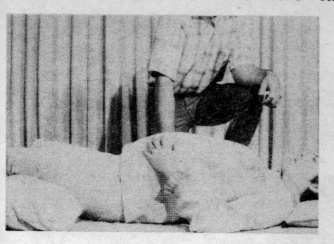

Fig. 20. Deep, quiet breathing—inhalation. Notice husband's watch is out of sight.

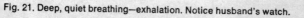

Fig. 21. Deep, quiet breathing—exhalation. Notice husband's watch.

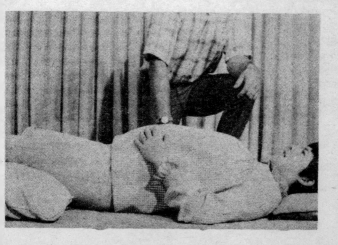

breathing is the normal breathing experienced in relaxed sleep, when an observer can see the lower diaphragm and the abdomen rising and falling gently.

Take a deep breath into the diaphragm, but not so deep that it also fills the upper chest. As the diaphragm gently expands, the abdomen can be seen rising (fig. 20). Slowly let the breath out again, letting the abdomen fall gently (fig. 21). After a few such slow, deep breaths, a person often yawns, showing that this breathing is a real aid to relaxation. As this quiet, slower breathing deep in the diaphragm is continued and the person becomes more relaxed, the breathing itself becomes automatic and no longer requires attention to continue.

This relaxed, natural "sleep" breathing is invaluable during pregnancy for falling asleep at night, and is most helpful in providing comfort during the first stage of labor by making relaxation more effective.

Some women push up the abdomen with its muscles while breathing in, but this is a mistake.* The abdominal muscles must stay completely slack, the abdominal wall rising and falling of its own accord as the air is taken deep into the diaphragm and released.

4. BREATH-HOLDING

Take one deep breath, let it all the way out; take another, let it all the way out. Then take a full breath and *hold it*. In your mind count up to ten, then let the air out through your mouth, not in a rush, but with control. After holding your breath, again take one or two deep in-and-out breaths to clear the lungs of stale air and replenish the oxygen supply. Practice

* Grantly Dick-Read's breathing technique is often confused with that of Helen Heardman, as outlined in her *Physiotherapy in Obstetrics-Gynecology* (Edinburgh: Livingstone, 1951). She taught a form of abdominal breathing in which the breath was held for long periods —one or two breaths a minute. This method is foreign to Dick-Read's approach! —Ed.

the breath-holding as the weeks go by until you experience no difficulty in holding a full breath for half a minute. (Remember, always take one or two deep in-and-out breaths both before and after holding the breath.)

Learning to hold the breath makes the work easier in the second stage of labor, when each contraction of the uterus needs you to hold your breath and push down to help the baby through the birth canal.

5. RAPID BREATHING

Learn to breathe short in-and-out breaths with the mouth open, but *not more than thirty-five to forty a minute*. This is necessary just as the baby is being born, since it keeps the mother from pushing down as the baby's head emerges slowly. It helps prevent any sudden and excessive pressure on the outlet, and thus helps avoid tearing its edges.

This more rapid breathing should be practiced just enough to learn how to do it. It is to be used in labor *only* to keep from bearing down, and under a doctor's continual supervision.

10

Relaxation

It is necessary for a woman carrying a baby to have a certain amount of rest, even if it is only for half an hour a day. Physical tiredness may become embarrassing in the later stages of pregnancy if the habit of rest is not acquired in the earlier months. Learning to relax properly makes this rest more effective.

Thus relaxation is of great benefit during pregnancy. Half an hour's relaxation is worth more than twice that time in sleep. It releases states of tension that a woman might unconsciously develop, and so helps avoid all manner of aches and pains. It introduces a calmness and helps establish confidence, which, in a state of tension, is practically impossible to do. Tension is caused by anxiety, and relaxation helps overcome anxiety by relieving tension of the mind as well as of the body.

Relaxation is also of the greatest possible assistance to a woman during labor. If she is able to become completely relaxed *during* the contractions of the first stage and *between* the contractions of the second stage, she will find that normal labor has no unbearable discomfort from beginning to end.

But relaxation is not only of value for pregnancy and labor. If it is continued, it lays a foundation for good health afterward also. We all live under considerable stress, and there is more emotional as well as physical weariness than is usually recognized. Such tension undermines both health and happiness in the rush of modern living. A woman who practices relaxation enhances her natural beauty, is more poised both with friends and with strangers, and is more at ease with her newborn and her husband.

The teaching of relaxation should be begun about the time that the mother is conscious of the quickening of her child. Most intelligent women can learn enough in the remaining months to enable them to get very good results in labor.

Muscular relaxation is a condition in which *the muscle tone throughout the body is reduced to a minimum*. When muscular tension is absent, emotional reactions and even thought patterns fade. Thus a completely slack body during labor eliminates any excess of muscle tone in the circular fibers of the lower uterine segment, the cervix, and the outlet of the birth canal. And this is not all. In a state of complete relaxation and mental calm, the sensations of uterine muscle activity during labor are interpreted in their true sense, just as the contraction of the biceps in the arm might be interpreted.

PREPARATION FOR RELAXATION

Draw the curtains and darken the room slightly—bright sunshine makes relaxation more difficult than shade or soft light. Before starting to relax, eyeglasses and dentures, if any, should be removed. The bladder must be completely empty so that the pelvic muscles can safely be relaxed.

It is important that the person relaxing be in such a comfortable position that she feels no need of support to remain in that position without moving. She should be on a very firm bed or couch or on the floor, with a folded blanket under her on the floor if it seems too hard. Two pillows are needed, one under her head and one under her knees. Her head should fall slightly to one side on the pillow and her arms should lie a few inches from her side, with the elbows half bent outward and the hands half closed. Her knees, supported by a pillow, should be slightly separated, her feet falling outward. It is important to have *all joints in a semiflexed (i.e., slightly bent) position,* for joints as well as muscles must be completely relaxed.

RECOGNIZING TENSION

When we speak of muscle tension, we are referring to tension in the muscles attached to the bones—the skeletal muscles. These are all under the control of the will. With practice they can be tensed or relaxed when so ordered by the mind. While the involuntary muscles of the intestines, blood vessels, heart, lungs, stomach, uterus, etc., cannot be directly relaxed by the will, they are all profoundly influenced by the complete relaxation of the skeletal muscles, which enables them to carry out their respective functions more efficiently.

One cannot be conscious of muscular relaxation unless he is able to recognize muscle tension. This is usually quickly done. I tell my patient to let her arms and legs lie as loosely as she is able to: "Try and avoid moving your toes, and do not wiggle your fingers. Just lie absolutely still and loose on the couch. Now let me have your right arm and let me have it *entirely.* Do not try to help me raise it, because any effort you make to help me is going to do more harm than good."

I then take hold of her elbow and wrist and raise her arm just off the couch. I explain that I want her hand to drop so that there is no "life" in it at all. It is astonishing how many people cannot drop their hand! Because of unnecessary muscle tension they slowly lower their hand, and then wiggle a finger or a thumb.

I continue testing her elbow and wrist until complete relaxation of the hand is obtained. I say again, "Now I am going to lift your hand, and I want you to let it drop absolutely as if it had no life in it at all." This sometimes takes quite a long time to do. Then I put my finger across the back of her hand and say, "Raise your hand very slowly, and at the same time you will feel my finger pressing it down. When you do that, realize what muscles are trying to raise your hand."

At the first movement of the muscles of the forearm in the effort to raise her hand I usually say, "Let it go," or "Relax." We do this several times, and I point out that it is the muscle of the forearm that is trying to raise the hand. Not infrequently my patient observes that as soon as the effort to lift the hand is made, she can feel the muscles tightening.

This instruction is then extended to groups of muscles, allowing them to become slightly tense and then definitely relaxed. It is amazing how quickly the average woman is able to relax her arm, once she understands the muscle tension and the "pull" of the muscle in action, but it takes considerable practice before she becomes expert at releasing this tension. I then ask her to do the same thing with her left arm, and on to other parts of her body.

Instruction is given in a quiet voice, slowly and clearly. "Take a deep breath through an open mouth; curl up your toes and tense the muscles of one leg." Pause. "Release your breath slowly and relax the whole limb. Compare in your own mind the feelings of tension and relaxation." This exercise is repeated, followed by the same procedure with the other leg.

The instruction is then extended to other groups of muscles throughout the body, allowing them to become alternately tense and relaxed, thus discovering what tension of each muscle feels like, and then how it feels to release that tension and relax the muscle. This applies to the chest, back and abdominal muscles as well as the arms and legs. When learning to relax the abdominal muscles, particular attention should also be called to tensing and relaxing the muscles of the pelvic openings, the vaginal and anal passages.

Relaxation of the face is extremely important. A woman who screws up her face in labor is not sufficiently relaxed in other parts of her body. There are about sixty facial muscles that can be tensed, and a woman must be trained to "let go" this tension. It must be remembered that a woman does not look her best when her face is relaxed. I always point this out and tell her that I have no desire for her to look her best, but I want her to *be* her best. I find that the face is probably the most difficult part of the body for a woman to relax.

But women must be taught to release the tension in muscles around their eyes, cheeks, mouth, and especially the eyelids. After a time she who acquires good relaxation of the face finds it very much easier to eliminate tension from her whole body. Any woman who is capable of relaxing her facial muscles at will can go through labor with the maximum ease that the absence of tension makes possible.

As time passes during a period of relaxing, the weight and heaviness of the limbs will be realized. Only with considerable difficulty can one leg be raised slowly from the bed. Recognition of tension versus relaxation will be assisted if the contraction of muscles in the leg is noticed before the heel is raised from the bed. The thigh muscles and those down the front of the leg will produce a distinct sensation of tension if the movements are made sufficiently slowly. The same may be tried with the arm. From the shoulder start to lift the arm—not the hand, but the whole arm—from the bed. The strain upon the muscles will be felt long before there is sufficient force to raise the limb. These tests must be carried out thoughtfully and *very slowly*. Violent and sudden flinging of the arm or the leg into the air will undoubtedly be easy, but it will teach nothing of the sensations of relaxation and early tension. Having raised the limb one or two inches from the bed, let it fall. In this way a consciousness of muscle tension will be developed, which makes the practice of deep relaxation much easier to recognize and practice.

When a person becomes physically relaxed, the mind takes care of itself. Several patients have told me that it is very difficult for their imaginations to become quiet. All the events of the day are vividly recalled as soon as they try to relax. This is, of course, an indication that their relaxation is incomplete. But they should not be urged to avoid thought in any way, because the attempt to stop thought is one of the most *active* mental exercises! Instead, it must be remembered that no emotional state can be present if there is real relaxation of the muscles of the body. Thought is to be concentrated on relaxing these muscles. As the muscles relax, the mind itself will automatically become quieter, until thoughts fade.

PRACTICING RELAXATION

It is not necessary to tense the muscles of the body each time in order to relax, once one has learned to recognize the *difference* between tension and relaxation in any part of the body. For each practice session, the following procedure may be carried out:

1. The bladder should first be emptied, so that the pelvic muscles can be relaxed with safety. Then stand and stretch the whole body, breathing in deeply through the nose to full lung capacity. Then exhale, allowing the shoulders to drop and the head to fall forward as the lungs become empty.

2. Lie down on a wide couch, the floor, or a hard bed, with a pillow under your head *and the upper part of your shoulders* (fig. 22). Another pillow should be made into a roll and placed under your knees for support, so that both knee and hip joints are slightly bent.

3. The feet should be about six or eight inches apart. Arms should be eight inches to a foot away from the body, with the elbows flexed outward, the hands with palms down and fingers curled slightly inward. The head should be allowed to fall gently to one side on the pillow, with the chin slightly raised as the head falls back.

4. Take three or four slow deep breaths and, on breathing out each time, let every muscle in the body become limp and still. Think of the shoulders as "opening outward." Feel the arms hanging from the shoulders and the hands lying heavily on the bed. Fingers and thumbs must not move. There will be a sensation of sinking into, or even through, the bed. The feet fall outward upon the heels, and the knees are carried outward by the weight of the feet (fig. 23). There must be no movement of the toes.

5. The head and shoulders are to be so completely sup-

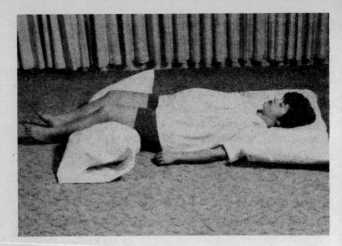

Fig. 22. Relaxation on back in earlier pregnancy. Pillow under head should be down under neck and shoulders, as shown here.

Fig. 23. Note the excellent relaxation of legs and feet, knees falling outward, feet inward. Head is incorrectly supported, neck bent forward because the pillow does not come down under neck and shoulders as in Fig. 22.

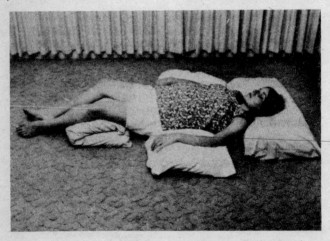

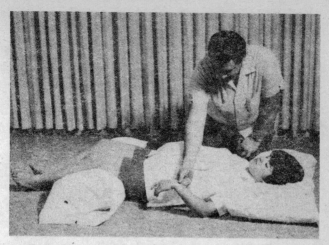

Fig. 24. Husband checking limpness of arm muscles, flexibility of elbow, wrist, and finger joints.

Fig. 25. Husband checking limpness of thigh and leg, flexibility of hip, knee, and ankle joints.

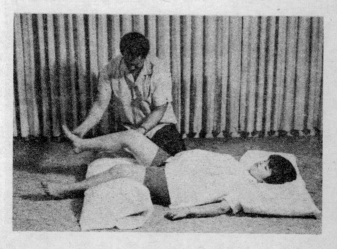

ported upon the pillow that the muscles of the neck are absolutely loose. Let the eyelids half close of their own weight.

6. Concentrate briefly on each arm without moving or tensing it, to be sure it is not being held stiffly in any part, that the muscles are not twitching or the fingers fidgeting (fig. 24). Do the same with the legs, buttocks, and back. Note carefully the muscles of the back. If they are relaxed, there will be a sensation of pressure upon the bed or floor from the weight of your body.

7. Relax the muscles of the face, the brow, eyelids, cheeks, and the muscles around the mouth. Think of your head as making a dent in the pillow. Particular care must be taken not to blink the eyes or move the eyeballs within their sockets. The muscles of the face will be felt hanging loosely from the cheekbones, which causes the jaw to drop slightly and hang loose.

8. Release any remaining tension in the abdominal muscles and pelvic floor muscles. Take two or three breaths deeply into the diaphragm, letting the chest and abdominal wall collapse with its own weight slowly as each breath is exhaled. Allow the breath to leave the lungs through the mouth without controlling or impeding it. Do not force it out. After each expiration, pause for two seconds (or until you want a new breath) before inhaling into the diaphragm again, deeply and gently. With each outgoing breath, relax the abdominal wall more fully, and "let go" tension in the pelvic muscles, as if opening up down below. Remember to keep your lips parted and your cheeks and jaw "hanging loose," to help relax the pelvic area. If your mouth is tense, you will be tensing the pelvic area, too. As relaxation deepens, the "sleep" breathing will become very gentle and quiet, as if you were really asleep. It is not necessary to remain conscious of the breathing pattern once full relaxation is achieved.

9. Let all the joints of the body relax a little more with each outgoing breath until they seem to be detached altogether (fig.

25). Note the train of sensations in the limbs—usually heaviness followed by lightness or "floating"; faint, transient pins and needles in the hands; feelings of warmth passing up from the extremities.

10. A pleasant, daydreaming state generally ensues (as in sunbathing) and any tendency to directed thinking should be deliberately diverted into a daydream. Remain in this relaxed state for about half an hour. (The sense of the passage of time is often lost or blunted.) Sleep is not the aim, and for most patients muscular relaxation without falling asleep seems to be more refreshing. But relaxing again in this way at night will help many insomniacs put themselves to sleep.

11. *Get up slowly.* Jumping up suddenly may cause faintness or dizziness. Take two or three deep breaths, bend the knees and arms once or twice, and then slowly sit up. Take two or three more breaths before standing up. Stretch the body once more, and then normal movement may again be safely resumed.

BREATHING

Breathing can be demonstrated to be either tense or relaxed. If too deep a breath is forced, or breathing is too rapid, certain tensions become apparent in the diaphragm, the ribs, and elsewhere. In relaxed breathing, both breathing in and breathing out should be without tension. "Sleep" breathing—that is, drawing the air into the lower diaphragm rather than the upper chest—aids in achieving relaxation more quickly and deeply. As the person relaxes, the abdominal wall will gently rise and fall. But as relaxation becomes deeper, breathing becomes perfectly smooth and in many cases almost inaudible, for less oxygen is needed during relaxation than when in a state of tension or movement. This quiet breathing is quite adequate to carry on all respiratory functions in labor during the first stage, without any necessity for shortness of breath, panting, or occasional deep breaths or sighs. All these breathing variations are signs of tension and incomplete relaxation, which will cause the contractions to become uncomfortable.

POSITIONS FOR RELAXATION

1. *On the back*. This position has been described above. However, after eighteen to twenty weeks of pregnancy many women have difficulty being comfortable in this position.

2. *Reclining chair position*. The body rests at an angle of 45 to 50 degrees, the forearms relaxing on the arms of the chair and the knees relaxing on the lower portion of the chair, tilted slightly higher than the hips. The head should be supported and fall slightly to one side, so that the neck muscles are slack and no part of the body requires any muscular effort to remain in its position.

In the hospital, this same position can be attained by raising the head of the bed to the proper angle, and either placing pillows under the knees to elevate them, or raising the bed under the knees, if it has that kind of mechanical flexibility (fig. 26). Pillows should be placed under the elbows to simulate the arms of a chair, and the head and shoulders should be so well supported that the neck muscles are fully relaxed, with the head falling slightly to the side and backward.

3. *Lateral position*. This is a most important position, and should be learned as an alternative to the other positions in early pregnancy, even though it may not be necessary at that time. In the later months, when the uterus is large, it is usually uncomfortable to lie flat on the back, for this interferes with good circulation and, because of the pressure of the uterus within the abdomen, makes breathing difficult. The lateral position is most helpful during labor.

Lie on the bed or floor on the left side, with the left arm behind the back and lying relaxed alongside the body. The right shoulder should be dropped, or supported by a corner of the pillow, and the right arm flexed slightly at the elbow and resting loosely on the bed alongside the pillow (fig. 27). It is important to either support the right shoulder or make sure it drops forward, as there is a tendency for muscle tension to hold it up. The head should be resting on a pillow, face turned toward the right shoulder, the chin slightly raised to make breathing easier, lips parted, and jaw slack.

The left leg should be stretched out on the bed, but bent slightly at the knee to relax the knee and hip joints, and the right leg should be drawn up until the knee is on a level with the upper abdomen. A large, firm pillow should be placed under the right knee and thigh to give it support, so that the knee and hip joints are fully relaxed and loose, and the muscles of the upper thigh, abdomen, lower back, and pelvic area can hang completely slack (fig. 28).

Two or three deep breaths into the lower diaphragm should be taken, and the whole body made to "let go" more fully with each exhalation. A sense of comfort and support will be felt immediately, if the position is right (fig. 29). The uterus will be supported upon the bed without pressure, taking the strain off the back muscles. Free movement of the diaphragm and abdomen is obtained during breathing.

During early pregnancy this position may also be used while lying on the right side. Relaxation is equally effective while lying on either side, but in later pregnancy, and when in early labor, the *left* lateral position is the best position (figs. 30, 31).

RESIDUAL TENSION

The difference between simply lying still and true neuro-muscular relaxation can be recognized, by a competent observer, in indications of residual tension. A rapid pulse rate and certain nervous reactions and reflexes are the result of tension. But the physician can also diagnose tension by listening to the breathing of a woman, for any irregularity in her breathing is evidence of imperfect relaxation. The flicker of an

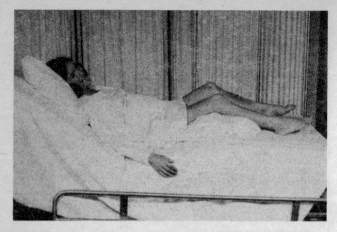

Fig. 26. "Reclining chair" position for relaxation in labor. Pillows under the forearms (not shown) may be helpful in keeping arms limp.

Fig. 27. Left lateral relaxation. Lie on left side, left arm and shoulder resting on floor, arm bent at the elbow. The corner of the pillow on which the head rests is to be brought down under the right shoulder and forearm also, so that they are fully supported by the pillow, and completely relaxed. The right forearm rests on the floor, not on the pillow.

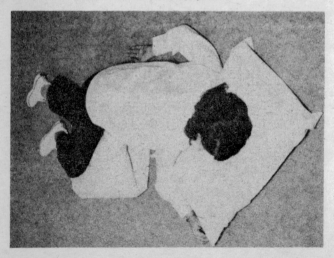

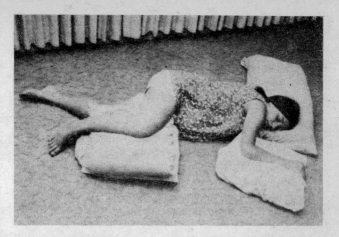

Fig. 28. Left lateral relaxation. Lie on left side, left leg bent at the knee and resting on the floor. Bend the right knee and draw it up toward the body, placing a pillow under it. The right upper thigh and knee must be *fully supported* by an ample pillow, so that all the leg and back muscles are completely relaxed (slack).

Fig. 29. Husband learning to check relaxation during a contraction.

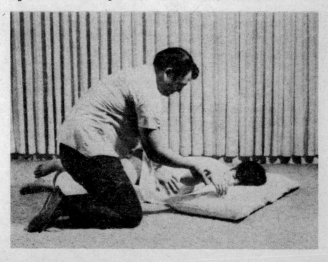

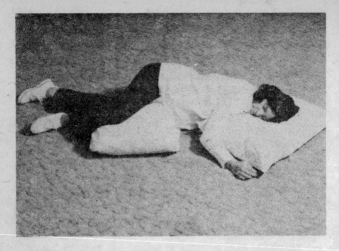

Fig. 30. Practicing relaxation in left lateral position during pregnancy.

Fig. 31. Relaxing in left lateral position during first-stage labor.

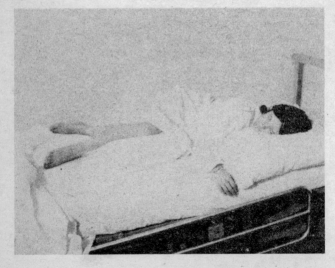

eyelid, moving of her eyeballs in their sockets behind closed lids, shifting of a finger or toe, or swallowing, all demonstrate the presence of residual tension of which the woman herself is not aware. If, in the silence of a relaxing class the instructress makes a sudden slight noise, she will notice those who react immediately to this disturbance.

The aim should be to train women to relax until all residual tension is eliminated, but at the same time realize that the instruction received at prenatal classes alone is not enough to achieve this desirable state in every woman. Those who do overcome residual tension are usually the perfect obstetric patients, providing they have no disproportion and the baby is lying in the normal position. But every woman benefits by the measure of relaxation she learns, for any lessening of tension in labor lessens discomfort by just that much. The experienced obstetrician will realize that no one can prophesy with certainty the conduct of any woman in labor, although it is possible to detect those who appear likely to do well, and to predict those who are more likely to find relaxing difficult.

Perhaps I may add that the obstetrician himself would be very well advised to become adept at relaxation. Not only would he be more competent to teach his patients or train instructresses, but he would find himself retaining his energy during those long hours of waiting. His mental acuity and manual dexterity would be more efficient also, than if he had remained tense with anticipation during his attendance at the labor.

11

Physical Fitness

There is no reason why a woman has to become fat and ungainly in order to become a mother; indeed, there is no reason why she should not have an even better figure after she has borne a child than before, for the benefits derived from exercises are the same whether a woman is pregnant or not. When exercises are undertaken seriously, the physical condition rapidly improves and a sense of well-being takes the place of the lethargy so frequently found among people whose lives do not include enough physical activity.

Certain movements associated with the mobility and flexibility of the muscles and joints of the pelvis are valuable during labor and delivery. Others assist in the depth and control of breathing. When we visualize the course of normal labor, we realize that the first stage must be without muscular effort on the part of the woman, while the second stage may require an hour or two of physical effort, in the case of first labors, to help the uterus expel the infant.

But we must not exaggerate the importance of exercises for childbirth. They make the mother feel fit and help correct breathing and relaxation, but a woman with a well-trained mind who knows how to breathe and relax correctly, but is unable for some health reason to do any exercises, can still have a good birth experience. She will have her baby much more easily than will a woman who has a highly trained athletic body but who knows little or nothing of how to cooperate with nature in giving birth. Indeed, some of the most perfect labors I have witnessed have been of women with groups of muscles partially paralyzed below the waist. They had suffered from accidents or polio, and their crippled bodies, which they swung from the hips on crutches or walking sticks, could not be physically trained.

I am anxious that this be understood, for the exercises described in this chapter are not to prepare mothers for an athletic event, but for a natural, common-sense experience in which a certain degree of physical fitness has advantages. These exercises represent the most elementary practice of physical training, but they are enough. Anything more than sufficient has been shown by experience to make *no difference* to the course or comfort of labor. Anything less deprives a woman of advantages she might more easily have enjoyed by being in better health.

POSTURE

Correct posture enables a woman to move gracefully and to breathe freely. A straight line from the ear to a point just in front of the heel on the sole of the foot should pass through the center of the shoulder and the hip joint, enabling the muscles of the limbs to work to the best advantage in all directions and retaining the abdominal organs in good position within the pelvic cavity. Holding the head at such an angle avoids round shoulders and the poking forward of the chin, and holding the body in this position makes breathing free, deep, and effortless and gives one a feeling of well-being and cheerfulness, which is important.

A woman can adopt the correct position by standing near a mirror and picturing the imaginary line just described. Her head should be carried as though slightly above her height. She should check her posture in this way periodically through pregnancy, for the alteration in the shape and weight of the body during pregnancy will unconsciously lead to stooping unless attention is paid to it. There is nothing more attractive than a young pregnant woman moving freely and maintaining her personal appearance in good posture.

EXERCISES

The following exercises are to be done slowly, remaining deliberately aware of each movement. Breathing and muscular action are to be coordinated in an easy rhythm without holding the breath, except in one exercise. All the exercises are simple, and no strain is required to do them satisfactorily. No exercises are done with the arms above the head. Shoulder height is the maximum to which the arms should be raised in any prenatal exercises.

Exercise 1: Pelvic Rock

This loosens and mobilizes the lower spine and pelvic joints. It prevents and sometimes relieves backache.

On hands and knees, place the hands about twelve inches apart and the knees about nine inches apart, keeping the knees directly in line with the hips. Let the back sag, at the same time raising the buttocks as high as possible (fig. 32). Take a deep breath in this position.

Slowly raise the back, allowing the breath to be expelled as the back arches (fig. 33). At the same time, squeeze together the muscles of the buttocks and pelvic area and tighten the muscles of the upper legs.

Return to the original position and *repeat ten times,* slowly and firmly.

Exercise 2: Squatting (with Variations)

These exercises loosen the knees and the hip joints, tone up the muscles of the legs, and stretch the muscles on the inside of the thighs. This exercise parallels the best position for delivery of the child, for in the squatting position the pelvic diameter is enlarged to its maximum size.

Stand on the toes, and then sink down to a position of squatting or sitting on the heels, still balancing on the toes. Place the palms of the hands on the knees and stretch the legs wide open, keeping the back straight (fig. 34). Rise to a standing position and then lower the heels to the floor. If the balance cannot be maintained, hold on to a support with one hand. *Repeat five times.*

VARIATION (a). For those who find the squatting too difficult or too strenuous, the same exercise can be simulated while lying on the back, with the knees drawn up toward the chest and pressed together (fig. 35). Allow the knees to fall outward, pressing them widely apart with the palms of the hands, the soles of the feet pointing inward (fig. 36). *Repeat five times.*

VARIATION (b). Sit on the floor Indian style, with knees outward, the soles of the feet placed together. Grasp the ankles with each hand, lean forward and place the forearms on the lower legs, then gently press the knees apart with the elbows (fig. 37). *Repeat five times.*

VARIATION (c). Sitting Indian style as in variation b, grasp the ankles but keep the arms straight. Let your husband or an attendant push down against the knees while you try to *push* up against the pressure of his hands (fig. 38). (Important note to husbands: Do not force too hard! Crunching her knees to the floor may cause damage.) *Repeat five times.*

VARIATION (d). Sit Indian style (fig. 39), crossing ankles, often during the day for quiet work, reading, sewing, or watching TV. Try relaxing occasionally in this position, letting the elbows rest on the knees, the back sag, and the head drop gently forward, eyes closed.

Exercise 3: Firming the Breasts

This exercise increases the circulation to the tissues under the breasts, strengthens the muscles supporting the breasts,

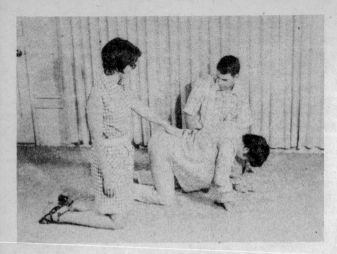

Fig. 32. Pelvic rocking. Let back sag, keeping elbows straight, knees directly under hips.

Fig. 33. Slowly raise small of back as far as possible, keeping legs from knees up at right angles to the floor.

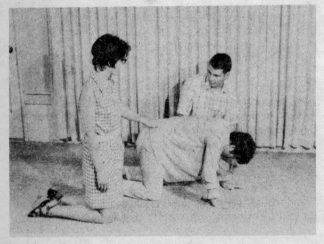

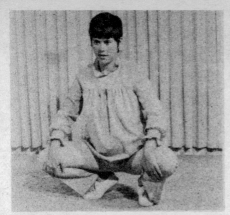

Fig. 34. Squat, balancing on toes. Press knees open with hands.

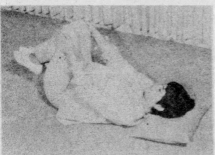

Fig. 35. Draw knees up toward chest, press together with hands.

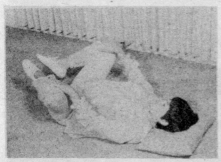

Fig. 36. Press knees as far apart as possible with palms of hands.

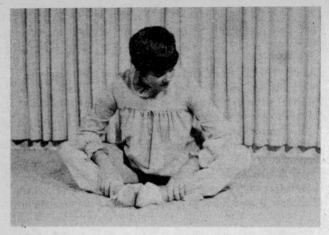

Fig. 37. Soles of feet together, press knees apart with elbows, grasping ankles.

Fig. 38. Soles of feet together, push knees up against husband's hands.

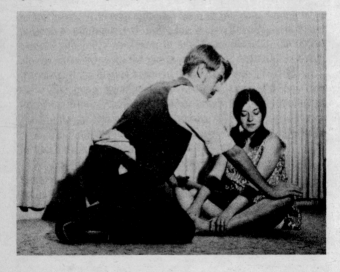

and also seems to help in establishing an adequate milk flow for breastfeeding. This is the only exercise that also gives practice in holding the breath.

Grip each arm firmly behind the wrist and raise the arms to the level of the shoulders. Push the skin of the forearm up, tightening the arm muscles and the muscles of the chest (fig. 40). When done correctly, one can feel the breasts lift. Relax and repeat.

Now take a deep breath, and hold it while doing this exercise *ten times,* taking about ten seconds. Relax. This time is to be gradually increased until the breath can be held comfortably for twenty seconds, which is a considerable help in the expulsive stage of labor, while the mother pushes, before she can exhale.

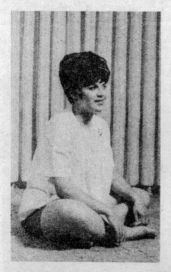

Fig. 39. Sitting Indian style.

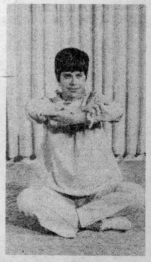

Fig. 40. Exercise for lifting and firming the breasts.

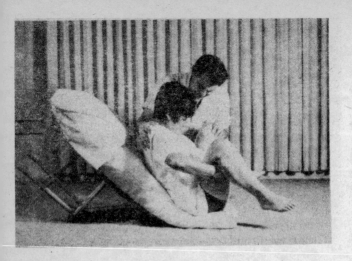

Fig. 41. Practice position for bearing down.

Fig. 42. Bearing down with contractions in second-stage labor.

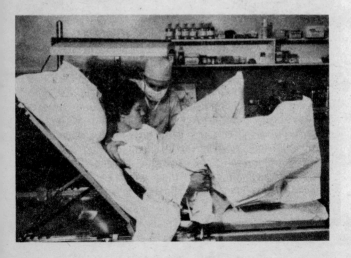

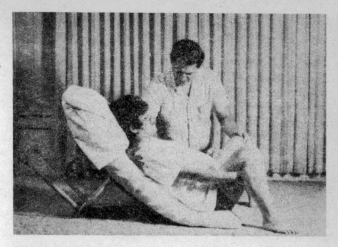

Fig. 43. Practice rest position in second-stage labor.

Fig. 44. Relaxed and happy between pushing with second-stage contractions.

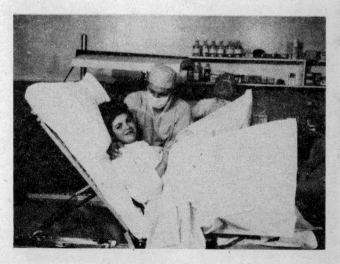

Exercise 4: Labor ("Work") Position

During the last two months of pregnancy this position should be practiced, as it is the most comfortable and advantageous while giving birth.

Rest with the back on an inverted chair padded with pillows at an angle of 40 to 45 degrees to the bed or floor. Draw the knees up to the sides of the abdomen toward the shoulders, grasp under each knee with the hands, bend the head forward and pull the knees up and *as widely apart as possible* (figs. 41, 42, 43, 44). When the knees are at their widest, the soles of the feet will be turned partially inward toward each other.

Exercise 5: Firming the Pelvic Floor Muscles*

This is the most important of all prenatal and postnatal exercises, and requires some explanation in detail.

The anus, vagina, and urethra are the three openings in the female pelvis. The anus is the end of the bowel; the vagina, the end of the birth canal; and the urethra, the end of the urinary bladder. When standing, the force of gravity places an immense strain upon the muscles that support the floor of the pelvis and close the openings.

Contract the anal and vaginal passages firmly and at the same time tighten the buttocks. Close the anus until the sensation of drawing it up into the rectum is felt. There is no need to move the legs or buttocks, as this distracts attention from the important area. When the anal sphincter is completely closed and retracted, the vaginal sphincter, the *levator ani*—a large internal muscle—and the sphincter of the urine outlet are also tensed. Each of these openings is surrounded by fibers of muscle arranged as a double figure eight; therefore all three

---

* Arnold Kegel, M.D., gynecologist at the University of Southern California, has perfected and promoted pubococcygeal exercises in the United States so extensively that they are often simply called "the Kegel."

outlets are closed by what is virtually one muscle. Squeeze these muscles as tightly as possible, hold for a definite pause, and relax *slowly*. By relaxing slowly, one learns how to "let go" tension in these muscles. Do this exercise at least *twelve times, twice a day*. It can be done any time, anywhere. As the uterus grows, the blood vessels multiply in number and increase in size. If the tone of the outlet muscles is below normal standard, control over them is lessened. Urine may leak, particularly during laughing or coughing. Similar defects may arise in the anus, as well as the development of *hemorrhoids*, or *piles*—varicose veins of the anus. If the muscles of the pelvic floor and outlets are exercised and kept in tone, these troubles will occur less frequently.

This exercise also facilitates the restoring of the stretched and dilated openings to normal size and tone after labor, and prevents some of the minor discomforts of aging. The feeling of firmness underneath has a marked influence on a woman; she will move or stand in a more confident posture.

Controlled activity of the vaginal sphincter and the static tension of the pelvic floor are also assets of considerable domestic value. Coitus can be performed satisfactorily for both husband and wife when the wife has learned conscious control of the vaginal sphincter. Rather than the too-frequent complaint that intercourse is uninteresting after a woman has had a baby, I am told from time to time that this natural marital function is performed more satisfactorily than before.

This simple exercise is a panacea for many ills and should be taught to and performed habitually by all women—whether pregnant, postparturient, or just woman!

12

Labor: First-Stage Labor

Two hundred and eighty days is an arbitrary figure for the length of pregnancy, calculated from the first day of the last menstrual period. (The average actual length from conception to birth is estimated as 267 days.) But a baby may be full term and quite normal if it arrives at any time between 265 and 290 days. It must not be thought, therefore, that a baby born ten days before the expected date is necessarily premature, or ten days after is postmature. A woman under my care had all three of her children on the three-hundredth day from the first day of her last menstrual period. She had very easy labors, and there was no evidence that any of the children were overdue. When a baby is "ripe" and ready, labor will begin.

ONSET OF LABOR

There are three signs that labor is beginning:

1. *Rhythmical contractions of the uterus.* These are felt as sensations of tightness without discomfort in the abdomen. The uterus becomes hard and tightness can be felt all over the organ. The importance of the sign is in the *rhythm* and not the contractions. A pregnant woman may have definite contractions for some weeks before her baby is due, but, if a regular and continuous rhythm is not established, they do not usually indicate the onset of labor. True labor contractions may start once every ten or fifteen minutes, or even at longer intervals, but gradually the interval decreases until they come every

three or four minutes. There is no pain as long as the abdomen is relaxed.

2. *Leaking of the waters.* The bag of waters may leak slowly, or it may suddenly burst and the waters flow out in a gush. This occasionally occurs before the uterus starts its rhythmical contractions, but this is true more frequently with subsequent babies than with the first. There is no pain when the bag of waters bursts, though it may be startling. It is wise to notify a doctor immediately. Rhythmical contractions may begin in an hour or two if they have not begun previously, or they may not begin for two or three days. But it is an indication that labor will soon be under way, so the woman should be under her doctor's advisement.

3. *The show.* A slight discharge of blood and mucus, known as "the show," may appear. It usually occurs after uterine contractions have begun to dilate the cervix slightly, thus dislodging the plug of mucus that kept the cervix sealed during pregnancy. This is positive evidence of the onset of labor.

Any one of these three major signs usually makes it easy for a woman to realize that her baby is on the way. She should get in touch with her doctor, even if there is some doubt in her mind, and follow his advice on when to leave for the hospital.

EARLY FIRST-STAGE LABOR

Once labor has begun and the doctor been notified, "plenty of time" should be the motto, with no hurry or anxiety unless the hospital is a long distance away. Small chores can be attended to around the house in preparation for leaving. Often there is excitement and relief that the day has come, which gives rise to a flurry of last-minute activity. This distraction helps the uterus settle down to its work without too much attention until labor is steadily under way. The doctor will advise when to go to the hospital, probably not, for a first baby, before contractions are five to ten minutes apart.

Upon arrival at the hospital (figs. 45, 46) the mother is

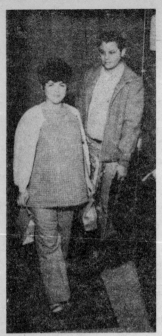

Fig. 45. Arrival at hospital in labor.

Fig. 46. Being greeted by receptionist.

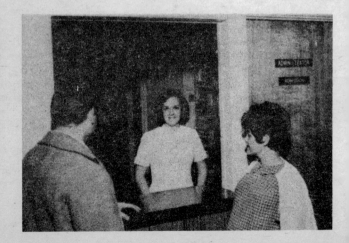

greeted by a receptionist and taken immediately to a labor room if labor is progressing rapidly. If not, she is identified by her prenatal records and admitted according to the usual obstetric routine. She is weighed, her blood pressure taken, and a specimen of urine examined.

Once in the labor room she is prepared for an examination by her doctor or a medical attendant. This preparation must be in keeping with the written instructions of her own physician. No enema, perineal shaving, analgesics, amnesics, sedatives, fluids or oxytocics are to be given except on his written orders specifically for her.* During the medical examination the physician will determine how far along she is in labor, listen to the baby's heart, and determine its position by examination of the abdomen.

I do not advise that during the first stage of the average labor a woman should be asked to relax the whole time unless she wishes it, unless she has overcome all the difficulties of progressive relaxation and is adept at the art. In the ordinary labor I prefer the woman to be awake to her general condition, able to listen to instruction and learn what is going on, and able to recognize the encouragement given her by those in attendance. But as soon as there is a sign of a uterine contraction, she must at once apply herself and relax to the very best of her ability.

A quiet restfulness between contractions is sufficient. Many women read or sew duing the earlier part of the first stage (fig. 47). Some prefer to walk about, if the waters have not yet broken. Undisturbed peace should characterize the first stage of labor—without mental or physical tension, with every happiness that a woman can be given, and with every encouragement to be confident in the right outcome of her labor.

Sometimes, when labor is slow in making progress, a mild sedative may be beneficial to help her rest peacefully or sleep.

* See *Standards for Obstetric-Gynecologic Hospital Services* (Chicago: The American College of Obstetricians and Gynecologists, 1969).

A few hours' sleep, particularly at night, during the early dilatation of the cervix evades the weariness of mind and body that causes a woman to begin to interpret any sensation as painful. This therapeutic common sense should not be confused with the use of drugs to relieve pain. No woman should have to go without sleep for fifteen or twenty hours of a slow first stage.

Adequate nourishment through liquids is also important during the first stage of labor, to sustain her energy and avoid fatigue. Milk, orange juice, tea, and other liquids should be given in ample amounts. During this same period of waiting, the husband should be given full meals at every mealtime, without his leaving her bedside (fig. 48).

When the first stage of labor is well established, a woman should be in a room with a nurse or physician in constant attendance. The companionship of her husband is also invaluable at this time, particularly if he has been trained in helping her remain relaxed and comfortable (fig. 49).

As rhythmical contractions of the uterus increase in intensity, gradually dilating the cervix, there is a demand for patience. If the training that has been given in deep, quiet breathing and complete relaxation is well and truly carried out during contractions, this period of waiting is much less taxing on a woman's patience. The routine of becoming *completely flaccid*, especially in the abdominal and pelvic area during a contraction, will help her improve her skill as time goes on.

When the opening of the cervix is about two inches, or five centimeters, in diameter, most women will begin to feel the strain of waiting, becoming impatient with contractions that seem to be doing no good. They may become restless, not relax as well during contractions as before, and thus begin to have some discomfort. A nurse or medical assistant should recognize that this is a typical emotional reaction, and make every effort to reassure the patient by explaining what is happening, and coach her carefully in reestablishing adequate relaxation and controlled deep breathing with each contraction, until she is comfortable once more.

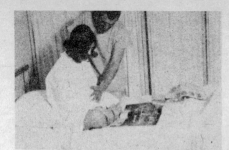

Fig. 47. Quiet activity during early first-stage labor.

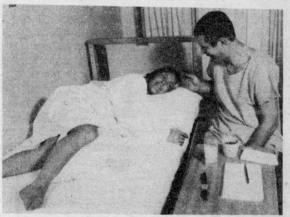

Fig. 48. Husband in constant attendance. Notice his watch, pen, and paper for timing contractions; his coffee (or meals); liquid for the wife.

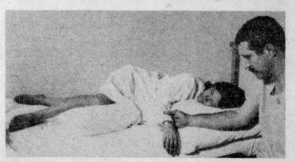

Fig. 49. Complete muscular relaxation during contractions of first stage.

At this time the woman should lay aside any other work such as reading or sewing and assume the labor position most comfortable for her (either the "reclining chair" or the left lateral* position). She should remain fairly relaxed between contractions in order to deepen the level of relaxation *during* each one. Her husband will be a most beneficial influence in helping her become comfortable, as they begin to practice together in earnest what they have learned she is to do during labor (figs. 50, 51, 52, 53). Thus as the contractions become stronger and closer together her ability to relax improves and discomfort fades. But even though she has overcome this first period of anxiety and is relaxing well, she still *must not be left alone.*

LATE FIRST-STAGE LABOR

Position

As labor progresses and the contractions come more quickly and become stronger, the woman should assume the left lateral position for relaxation, as described earlier. It is important that the patient lie in the *left* lateral position, and that she never lie flat on her back during labor, or during late pregnancy. The supine position interferes with adequate circulation.† Before assuming this position, she should make certain that her bladder is empty. All her joints must be loose and bent slightly, her knee and upper thigh firmly supported by a large, firm pillow. She must consciously "let go" all muscular tension in the upper thigh, lower abdomen, and

* "Angiographic studies have visualized occlusion of the vena cava, as well as displacement and partial obstruction of the aorta, almost consistently in the supine position during late pregnancy." From J. Bieniarz, *et al.,* "Aortocaval Compression by the Uterus in Late Human Pregnancy. IV. Circulatory Homeostasis by Preferential Perfusion of the Placenta," *American Journal of Obstetrics and Gynecology* 103 (1969): 19–31. Reprinted by permission.

† See *American Journal of Obstetrics and Gynecology* 103: 19–31; *op. cit.*

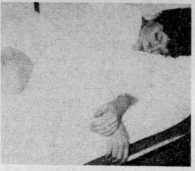

Fig. 50. Relaxing on left side rather than left lateral. Pillow between knees.

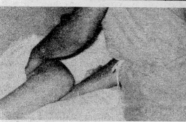

Fig. 51. Husband checking relaxation of right leg.

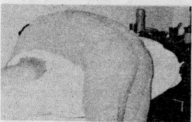

Fig. 52. A long reach for a massage of backache!

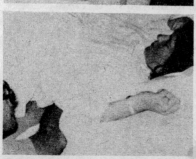

Fig. 53. "Reclining chair" position, husband still massaging backache.

lower back, and relax the pelvic area so completely that the outlet seems to be falling open of its own accord. Her husband, and an attendant as well, should test her right knee and hip joint for looseness and flexibility throughout this area.

Breathing

During labor the control of breathing plays a large part in avoiding discomfort and assisting the uterus to carry out its work. As the contractions of the first stage increase in intensity, breath is taken *more deeply* into the diaphragm but still quietly and smoothly, lips parted. *Twenty-four to twenty-eight deep breaths* may be taken in a minute (one in-and-out breath every two or three seconds, *but not more*).* The reason for this is that the uterus, which is a large, muscular organ, not only uses a great deal of oxygen to maintain its activity, but has to get rid of the carbon dioxide, the waste product of energy. Since we take in oxygen and throw off carbon dioxide through our lungs, an increased intake and output of air is an obvious corollary to uterine action.

A husband can give valuable assistance in coaching the breathing, reminding his wife to breathe deeply enough to expand the lower diaphragm and abdomen during a contraction, letting it rise and fall gently with each breath until the contraction ceases. This can be as effectively done in the lateral position as in any other. He must make sure that her breathing does not become irregular, rapid, or shallow. Such unnatural breathing patterns are signs of tension and anxiety that deprive the uterus of needed oxygen and cause discomfort. A watch with a second hand will help him keep her breathing under control. After each contraction, he should remind her to take one or two full, deep breaths, to cleanse the lungs of "used" air.

The points to remember for comfortable contractions are to

* Faster breathing techniques may lead to hyperventilation.

keep the abdomen, pelvic area, hip and thigh muscles and joints completely slack, while lying in the left lateral position. As the uterus comes into action, deep in-and-out breaths are to be taken, causing the abdomen to rise and fall gently. And while the woman should keep her eyes open so she can follow instructions, her face must remain relaxed, her lips parted, her jaw slack. There must be no frown or puckered brow, no screwed-up eyes, no pursed lips. There is no need for these exhibitions, for they do more harm than good and cause tension elsewhere, with consequent discomfort.

Relaxation

Relaxation during the first-stage contractions has the most astonishing effect. If the patient has been sympathetically treated and well instructed, she should have no difficulty whatever in avoiding all pain during the first stage of normal labor. It may be that it will not be easy for her, during the last part of the first stage, to avoid discomfort, but the calmer she is the more relaxed she will become. It is difficult to relax when under the influence of strong emotional disturbance.

When a physician has acquired for his patient some degree of relaxation, he should remember not to be too ambitious and expect too much of her. But occasionally he will have the absolute delight of finding a woman who becomes adept at relaxing. When he does, if everything else is normal, he should call in his medical friends, gather the students around, collect the nurses, and let them come and see a real natural labor. I have had many such cases. Some of them have appeared to be lying as if in a daydream from the beginning of their labor until the end. Their relaxation was so complete that they became almost oblivious to the fact of parturition, and, at the end of the first stage, relaxation during the contractions of the so-called pain period of labor enabled them to pass through it without discomfort. They then automatically brought into play the muscles of expulsion as the second stage began, but continued to lie in a completely relaxed state when not pushing.

The idea of pain-relievers and pain to such completely relaxed women is quite absurd. It does not enter their minds. They have no desire for it, for they do not have pain. But they understand what is said to them, listen, and carry out instructions in full cooperation.

Discomfort

No woman should be allowed to suffer greater discomfort in labor than she is willing to endure for her child's sake. In my experience the use of anesthesia presents no difficulty. If there are clinical indications, the signs and symptoms determine the most suitable method of pain relief. But even with the array of simple and effective methods of pain relief available, considerable experience is required in order to obtain the desired results. It should not be overlooked that if any re-agents are used contrary to clinical indication, or at the wrong time in labor, serious trouble may ensue. The most important factor, therefore, in the use of analgesia and anesthesia in childbirth is the skill, experience, and judgment of the attending physician. Without these nothing is either safe *or effective*.* No reagent of any kind, of course, should be given without the doctor's written order, specific for that particular patient.

TRANSITION

Just before the cervix is fully dilated, that is to say, stretched wide enough to allow the baby to pass through into the vaginal portion of the birth canal, certain changes occur. In about 50 percent of women the ultimate stretching of this

* Bowes, *et al., The Effects of Obstetrical Medication on Fetus and Infant.* Monograph of the Society for Research in Child Development (Chicago: University of Chicago Press, 35, no. 4, 1970).

rim of muscle tissue at the outlet of the uterus gives rise to a backache over the sacrum or bottom end of the spine. The pain is caused by the stretching of the tissues but is referred to the lower back and felt as backache. This ache can be relieved by firm pressure of the hand of husband or attendant, or by slow, heavy rubbing over the lower back and sacrum.

The contractions are strong at this point, for it takes powerful contractions on the part of the uterus to pull the circular muscles completely back over the baby's head. Yet this is a most important time for the mother to be able to relax with each contraction and not oppose it.

The temporary discomfort of the backache often is accompanied by a second change in the attitude of the woman toward her labor. Not infrequently it is the first time she has been aware of any physical uneasiness, and it awakens in her mind many fears lest this backache resolve into a more severe pain. Fear definitely assaults the minds of many women just before full dilatation of the cervix.

This backache, however, only persists for about nine to twelve contractions. A woman should be informed of that, for a temporary discomfort is much more easily borne than one which is likely to persist. She should also be told to concentrate upon the depth and rapidity of her breathing, breathing through her mouth, her face relaxed. It is possible to relax efficiently in spite of the fact that breathing is quicker and drawn deeper into the diaphragm.

Now for the first time vague signs of pressure, those early symptoms of the second stage, appear. Even a well-prepared woman can be confused. She needs guidance, coaching, encouragement. She needs the skill of her helpers in controlling her deep, even, breathing as she relaxes with each contraction. At this point, it is more comfortable for the patient to turn onto her back and be propped up in the reclining chair position, her back raised, and knees raised and resting on supports. Her head and shoulders should rest on a pillow, her neck relaxed and head turned slightly to the side and tilted back a bit, her arms and legs remaining completely limp during contractions.

As this transition from the first to the second stage of labor develops, there may come an irresistible desire to bear down and push the baby from the uterus. If the desire to push comes during a contraction, the patient should remain relaxed and pant softly or blow out through her mouth to keep from pushing, until the desire passes. *She should never bear down until she is unable to avoid it.*

Summary of First-Stage Labor*

I. Onset of Labor
1. Rhythmic contractions. Leaking of waters. The "show."
2. Expectancy, exhilaration, and animation.
3. Doctor is called. Any normal, desired activity is continued, relaxing just during contractions. Go to hospital when doctor directs.

II. Early First-Stage Labor
1. Cervix dilates to 3/5ths.
2. Cheerfulness, followed by temporary anxiety. Desire for companionship. Labor taken more seriously.
3. Relaxation in any comfortable position during contractions, "sleep" breathing, ample liquid intake, rest or sleep as desired.

III. Late First-Stage Labor
1. Cervix dilates to 4/5ths, contractions stronger, more frequent.
2. Temporary anxiety again, caused by strengthening contractions. Can be overcome by reassurance and careful coaching.
3. Complete relaxation in left lateral position during contractions, allowing "sleep" breathing to change to slightly deeper "work" breathing, evenly and quietly, not more than 24 to 28 breaths a minute. Complete relaxation between contractions.

IV. Transition
1. Cervix dilates to completion.
2. Acute sensitiveness to words and noises, bright lights, or other disturbances. Backache in over half the women, causing some anxiety. Relaxation gradually becoming difficult, with the change in breathing required for expulsive contractions causing some confusion.
3. Some relief of backache, achieved by firm rubbing of the sacrum. "Work" breathing kept at an even, moderate pace.

* Key: (1) Physical symptoms; (2) emotional symptoms; (3) position and aids to comfort

Change made from the left lateral to "reclining chair" position, sitting with the back at a 45° angle, knees supported. Any desire to push resisted by breathing short, rapid breaths in and out until the momentary urge passes. Relaxation maintained between and *during* contractions.

13

Birth: Second-Stage Labor

Once the second stage begins a woman not only gives the appearance of, but often expresses, great relief. She is now able to help. Her backache disappears, things are making progress, and soon, in an hour or two, as she should be told, her baby will be born if she works with a will.

EARLY SECOND-STAGE LABOR

When the second stage is established the routine of labor changes. The patient should not be allowed to push violently at first, but merely to hold her breath and exert a little pressure with each contraction, leaning forward and pressing down on the top of the uterus (fig. 54). It is a great mistake to wear a woman out with violent muscular effort in the beginning of the second stage of labor. The uterus will do its work perfectly well with a minimum of assistance.

Pushing with second-stage contractions requires physical effort; therefore it is obvious that relaxation during contractions must be discontinued. But as soon as a contraction has ended the mother should lean back comfortably against a raised back support, close her eyes, take one or two deep in-and-out breaths, and completely relax *between* contractions (fig. 55). These contractions may come every five or six minutes at first, but gradually at shorter intervals.

After ten or twelve contractions it will be observed that the woman becomes very drowsy between them. This state of inattention to surroundings is nature's way of preventing pain by keeping the mother relaxed. It is not, however, for the purpose of taking pain away, because very few women have any physical discomfort at this phase of the second stage. It is the means by which a woman's mind and body are completely rested, creating a condition in which the body can *recuperate with great rapidity between its violent efforts.* She is thereby prepared for each succeeding contraction without becoming exhausted. It is essential therefore that *absolute quiet* be maintained in the labor ward.* Inconsequent conversation between attendants, clumsy movements, heavy footsteps, and banging doors are unforgivable sins in the presence of a woman advanced in labor.

Subdued lighting is important as an aid to her relaxation. Many women sleep between contractions, while others remain quietly unresponsive to their surroundings. Sometimes it is difficult to make them understand what is said without speaking loudly into their ears. Since they will often respond more automatically to a command given by the husband, the doctor gives the instructions and the husband relays them to his wife.

The Husband

An obstetrician should not allow the isolation of a husband to be established by his alienation from the birth of his child. His concern and his place in this family matter should be sympathetically recognized and every effort made to bring him into close contact with the event. There is little advantage

* Dr. Dick-Read makes no mention of the removal of a woman to a separate room for the actual birth. This is an American custom. In most of the world it is an accepted practice to permit a mother to labor, deliver, and recover in the same bed without being moved from her room.—Ed.

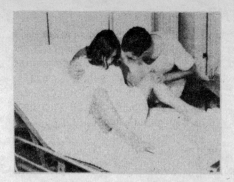

Fig. 54. Bearing down in labor room, early second stage, knees drawn up and widely apart, back rounded head bent forward.

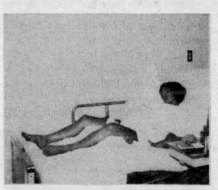

Fig. 55. Complete muscular relaxation in "reclining chair" position, between bearing-down efforts.

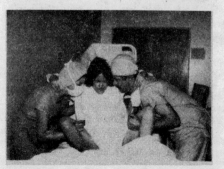

Fig. 56. Bearing down correctly, with husband and nurse assisting.

to be gained by making childbirth an incomparable delight to the woman if in so doing the husband is estranged and seeds of discord are sown in the home. Much trouble and sadness occurs from the isolation of the husband.*

Position

As soon as the second stage is under way and the mother is helping to push her baby through the birth canal, she should be placed in a semisitting position with her knees wide apart. Adopting this modified squatting posture gives the greatest freedom of muscular action to her, and also allows for the maximum size of the pelvic outlet to be obtained.

In order to achieve this position she should be propped up on a backrest to an angle of about 45 degrees. During a contraction she is to lean forward over the abdomen, with her knees drawn up beside her body, near her armpits. As she grips under her knees with her hands and pulls them outward and upward, her feet are to be supported either on the stirrups or by her attendants (fig. 56).

Other positions are adopted by the women of races whose lives habituate them to different customs. For instance, some of the Far Eastern peoples squat on their feet when their babies are delivered. Certain nomadic races kneel, giving birth to their babies very easily in that position. In some countries the horseshoe-shaped labor chair was in use until the beginning of the nineteenth century, and may well appear in modernized form; a good deal can be said in its favor.

---

* The husband will of course observe the customary aseptic techniques before accompanying his wife to the delivery room (figs. 57, 58). He will scrub, and wear appropriate operating room attire, including cap, mask and conductive shoes. He can help his wife become comfortable in the correct position on the delivery table, adjusting the backrest to her particular needs, and can help support her when she leans forward to push. He can repeat the doctors' instructions to her, remind her to take cleansing breaths after pushing, and thus become a valuable member of the birth team. In the drowsy state of second stage, a woman responds best to his familiar voice.

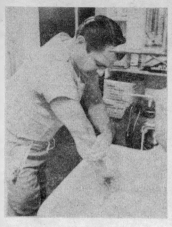

Fig. 57. Husband scrubbing before accompanying wife into birth room.

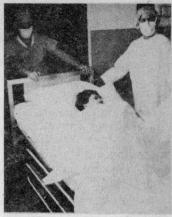

Fig. 58. Moving from labor room to birth room.

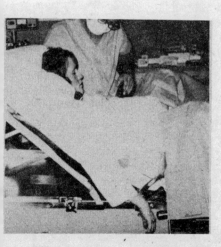

Fig. 59. Mother of twins totally relaxed between second-stage contractions.

WELL-ESTABLISHED SECOND-STAGE LABOR

Breathing

Once the pushing reflex is well established during the second stage of labor, respiration ceases while the woman leans over and bears down in an expulsive effort. At the same time the uterus is contracting firmly and the high quantity of carbon dioxide accumulating in the blood is shown by a change in the color of the woman's face as the contraction persists. She may become swarthy and cyanosed, which is a blue tint under the skin, for blood containing an excess of carbon dioxide is a dark blue-red color. Therefore, she must be trained during pregnancy to hold her breath, for by so doing she can learn to retain in her blood the slight increase of carbon dioxide without distress, and at the same time overcome the desire to let her breath go when it is advantageous to hold it.

That is why *after each expulsive contraction she is told to lean back against the backrest and take two or three controlled, full, in-and-out breaths,* thus replacing the oxygen used and clearing the lungs of carbon dioxide. Then she should completely relax and wait restfully for the next contraction in a state of peace (fig. 59).

Respiration between contractions is quiet breathing, that is, "sleep" breathing, the abdomen rising and falling slightly as the patient rests. The absence of muscle tension between contractions minimizes the need for oxygen and the formation of the waste products of tension. It also permits complete dilation of both the arteries and veins in the abdomen and pelvis, and enables a free intake of all the fuel necessary for the low state of metabolism between contractions.

Relaxation

One could not require, nor would it be possible to obtain, physical relaxation during expulsive contractions of the sec-

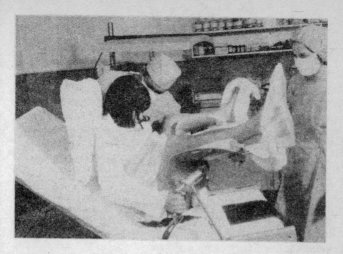

Fig. 60. Bearing down with second-stage contraction, back curved, head forward, knees wide and back toward shoulders, husband supporting shoulders.

Fig. 61. Complete relaxation against backrest between second-stage contractions, husband giving instructions.

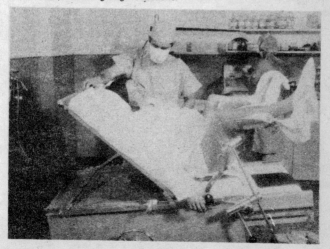

ond stage (fig. 60). The idea of nature here is that, the door being widely opened and the birth canal ready for the baby to pass through, the mother can assist the muscles of the uterus by pushing down vigorously. This requires real physical exertion, and since after each second-stage contraction the woman will be plainly out of breath, deep in-and-out breaths must be taken to quickly replace the oxygen used. Then, *between* the contractions complete relaxation is necessary, for relaxation is the most effective manner of quickly reconstituting muscle power (fig. 61).

It is usual for the membranes, the bag of waters in which the baby is contained, to have ruptured before this time. *A woman should always be reminded of the imminence of this event,* because many are alarmed by the sudden and unexpected flow of a large amount of water.

Anesthesia

There is very little, if any, discomfort in the average, properly conducted second stage of labor. During the first stage many women become bored, and a little tired of the feeling that nothing can be done. Thus a tremendous sense of relief very often fills a woman's mind as she realizes that not only can she help, but the greater effort she applies, within reason, the greater sense of comfort she will get. There is no pain with a good honest second-stage expulsive effort until the first awareness of dilatation of the perineum is felt. I am not, of course, speaking of abnormal cases, such as those in which large masses of piles come down as the head stretches the anterior wall of the rectum, but of the normal, unimpeded case in which no pathological condition is present at all.

No woman should be allowed to suffer pain in labor, and every method discovered by science should be used to prevent it. If there is true pain, anesthetics and analgesics should be exhibited at once, but the absence of severe discomfort contraindicates its use. *It is as great a crime to leave a woman alone in her agony and deny her relief from her suffering as it is to insist upon dulling the consciousness of a natural mother who desires above all things to be aware of the final reward of her efforts. Each of these two unforgivable errors is constantly committed.*

There should always be an anesthetic or analgesic apparatus at hand during labor, and if necessary the patient should be instructed in its use. Women adequately trained for natural childbirth very rarely desire anesthesia and frequently refuse its use. Women who have not had the advantage of preparing themselves to give birth may have considerable pain, which they are causing themselves; therefore analgesia and anesthesia should be used. It must be recognized, however, that 95 percent of these deprived women could have had natural labors if they had been properly prepared.

When there is a *definite abnormality,* such as disproportion or a malpresentation or one of those rare complications which must be diagnosed and treated by an experienced obstetrician, drugs and anesthetics should be adequately applied under his instructions as quickly as possible. *That is one of the greatest benefits anesthesia has brought to humanity, and when a woman suffers the pain of abnormality in childbirth it should never be withheld.*

The administration of anesthetics and analgesics should have definite indication in obstetrics as it has in every other branch of medicine or surgery. Pain is the most frequent justification; it does not matter whether the pain is secondary to fear or whether it is primarily physical. Natural childbirth mothers have no fear and therefore little discomfort. Because the discomfort is minimal few, if any, of these prepared women demand relief.

When the head gets down onto the muscles that form the floor of the pelvis, a woman often finds it difficult to relax the outlet, because she gets a sense of the passageway opening up, a new sensation to every first-time mother. If she is alarmed by this sensation and endeavors to resist as the head arrives within an inch of the outlet, contracting her pelvic floor and squeezing the vulva and rectum tightly, she runs a very good chance of having not only acute pain but also, by increasing resistant tension, a torn perineum.

At this time a definite wave of fear comes over most women, caused by this feeling of opening up below, and an uncontrollable desire to *escape*. It is important not to yield too quickly to the assumption that the woman is in pain, for this threat to her self-control is not difficult to overcome. She must be strongly reassured that she will not "burst," that the opening will not hurt as it stretches further; she must be told how to overcome the discomfort. At the next contraction she is to *concentrate and push as firmly as she can*. As soon as she exerts this *maximum* pressure, the pelvic floor becomes distended and the head rapidly passes down to the vulva without further discomfort.

CROWNING

When the head is visible and no longer slips back between contractions, what is called *crowning* has occurred. As the vulva dilates to about two inches in diameter the outlet can be felt stretching, a sensation that has been described as one of burning or bursting.

It is important that a woman *relax completely* at this time, letting her jaw fall slack and *breathing with her mouth open*. The muscles of the perineum relax as her face and mouth relax. She should be told that the sensation of bursting is a myth. The head will not tear the perineum if she is *completely relaxed*, all her muscles slack and her facial muscles relaxed, and if she breathes softly in and out through her *open mouth*. It is astonishing how large a baby will then pass through what appears to be a small vulva without any tear to the perineum at all. If, between the final second-stage contractions, after the head is adequately crowned, the attendant can persuade a woman to remain relaxed in this way, the complete absence of difficulty with which the head can be produced is surprising. I am sure that a large number of torn perineums are due to the effort of the woman to resist the oncoming head by violently contracting the muscles at the outlet. If her husband sees her close her mouth, or set it in a grim line, he should immediately remind her to relax her face and breathe through her open mouth.

As soon as the head has crowned, *all efforts to bear down should be stopped*. During contractions the uterus itself will slowly urge the child forward while the woman fully relaxes, opens her mouth, and breathes in and out quickly, to keep from pushing. In this way the vulva is gradually distended without discomfort. It must be distended gradually without any violence, for tears of the skin and even of the muscles are frequently produced unnecessarily because a woman is erroneously encouraged to bear down at this time.

BIRTH

As the head is born, it must be supported by the attendant and turned up over the pubis of the mother. Once the baby's head is born there is often a pause (fig. 62). It may cry before the shoulders arrive. With the next contraction, which again must be completely controlled by the attendant to keep the baby from moving too quickly, the baby's body emerges (fig. 63). He may ask the mother to refrain from pushing during contractions, or he may have the mother bear down very gently if the uterus requires a little assistance from the mother.

When a baby arrives under these conditions the woman, being conscious and not filled with anesthetic, often realizes that her baby has been born only after she hears it cry. A child passes through a relaxed vulva with almost complete absence of sensation to the mother. There is no doubt that with relaxation of the vulva there is also a temporary natural anesthesia of its sensory nerves.

The case of a young woman whom I attended is an example of this. As her second stage of labor began, I instructed her in how to bear down, and asked her gently to increase her efforts. Then I sent for the medical students to come observe. They seemed unable to believe that she had passed so smilingly and so comfortably through the first stage. After a few more honest contractions, the rectum bulged. Soon the head appeared, and she looked at me inquiringly and said, "Can I really stretch enough? It feels as if something must give way." I pointed out to her that this was the invariable sensation of a conscious woman, but that it was only a temporary sensation, for as the head was born it turned away from the point where she was feeling the pressure. She accepted my assurance confidently, and in three or four more contractions a large baby's head was born easily and painlessly into my hands. I told her that her baby's head had arrived and that it was a lovely child. She was unwilling to believe that I was not encouraging her by making her think the head had come when it had not, so I pointed out to her that she could feel the child's head against her thigh and also see it if she looked. She was incredulous as she looked down and saw her child.

I asked her to bear down gently so that the rest of the child could be born. She said, "Tell me at once if it is a boy. We are longing for a boy." And so I was able to lift up to her a crying, beautiful baby boy of eight pounds one ounce, as we soon discovered upon weighing him. Her joy was indeed a picture to behold. There was no question of pain, she had been instructed how to use the inhalant but had refused, assuring us that there was nothing in this experience but the most unqualified delight. At first she was too excited to speak as she took the child in her hands, but then she said, "I must look carefully—it is difficult to believe I have a boy. It is wonderful!" And as she laughed and fondled her child, tears of joy rolled down her cheeks.

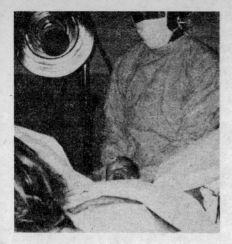

Fig. 62. Baby's head is born, supported upward by attending physician.

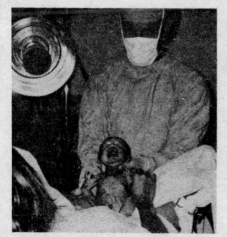

Fig. 63. Baby's body is born, supported upward, over the pubic bone and toward the mother, by attending physician.

Summary of Second-Stage Labor*

I. Early Second-Stage Labor

1. Expulsive reflex not strong. Backache ceases.
2. Temporary revival of personality and determination.
3. Semisitting position on birth table, backrest at 45° angle. Breath holding during contractions followed by one or two deep breaths. "Sleep" breathing and relaxation between contractions. Leaning forward to push, arms out at right angles, knees drawn back toward shoulders. Leaning back to rest.

II. Well-Established Second-Stage Labor

1. Head progressing down birth canal to pelvic cavity. Expulsive effort stronger. No discomfort but hard work.
2. Woman's true self evident. Sometimes discretion and discrimination is "low." Increased drowsiness between contractions. Sudden impatience and desire to escape as head reaches pelvic floor.
3. To overcome discomfort, take a deep breath, hold it, and push as firmly as possible. A partial expulsive effort may seem uncomfortable, a complete expulsive effort overcomes the discomfort.

III. Birth

1. Stretching and thinning of the perineum. Crowning, and burning feeling around the vulva temporarily, disappearing as stretching increases.
2. Exasperation as the burning is felt, discretion low, but response to the encouragement of attendants. As head is born, drowsiness replaced by mental alertness and incredulity. Weariness vanishes.
3. Perineum to be kept fully relaxed. No bearing down as the head or shoulders emerge, but rapid in-and-out breathing to keep from pushing.

* Key: (1) Physical symptoms; (2) emotional symptoms; (3) position and aids to comfort

14

Immediate Newborn Period:
Third-Stage Labor

In natural childbirth, once the baby is born, there is no need for relaxation. Here we get the beautiful *tension* of satisfaction. The sympathetic nervous system sweeps in with all its joys and its pleasing emotions, and so there is no desire for relaxation. The strain and weariness of muscular effort are swept from the mother's memory by the sound and sight of her newborn child, and this stimulates the uterus into the action of the third stage.

When the child is first born it is my custom to lift him up for the mother to see (figs. 64, 65), then lay him flat on the bed between his mother's thighs and wait until pulsation of the cord has ceased before severing it. Sometimes it may be four or five minutes before pulsation fades, during which time the baby is covered with warm towels.

If there has been a small nick of skin which the obstetrician considers will heal better with one or two stitches, these can be inserted while the perineum is still numb, with a minimum of discomfort to the woman and without any anesthetic. The woman is asked to relax while they are being inserted. I use a semicircular needle of an inch, or an inch and a quarter in its greatest diameter, passing the point of the needle quickly through the skin at right angles to the surface both in and out.

This must be done at once, however, because the natural

anesthesia of the vulva disappears in a very few minutes. If it is delayed for a quarter of an hour or more, then some local anesthetic, such as 1 percent novocaine, should be injected into the area through which the ligature is passed. These stitches are not tied until the placenta has arrived, and it is interesting to note that the tying, if not very gently done, is likely to prove much more uncomfortable than the insertion. This relative natural anesthesia of the perineum persisting in the early part of the third stage of labor is worthy of note, for it permits immediate suture, if needed. It is probably true also that lacerated surfaces brought into apposition before coagulation has occurred heal more quickly and more firmly than those which remain open before they are repaired. If an episiotomy is performed and a more extensive repair is required, the routine procedure of the attendant obstetrician will be adopted.

As soon as the cord is severed, the child is wrapped in warmed towels and given to his mother to hold. Some have an immediate desire to put the baby to breast. This contact stimulates, by direct reflex, strong contractions and retractions of the uterus, thus hastening separation of the placenta and the closing of the blood vessels in the part of the uterus to which it was attached.

This may be confirmed if one's hand is placed lightly on the abdomen as the baby is put to the mother's breast. Thus one of the most important benefits of the physical contact of the newborn with its mother is this rapid separation of the afterbirth, and the absence of any excessive hemorrhage. Those of us who are aware of the results of the mismanagement of the third stage of labor can adequately assess the importance of this phenomenon.

After the mother has held her baby for a few minutes, he is placed in a warm crib beside her. She is given a hot or cold drink with plenty of sugar, to replenish her energy and the loss of fluid in her system. Many women have violent *shivering attacks*, at about this time, which are alarming if not ex-

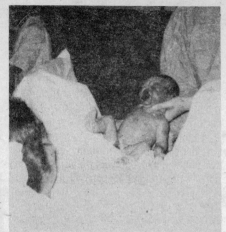

Fig. 64. Attending physician holds baby up for mother to see.

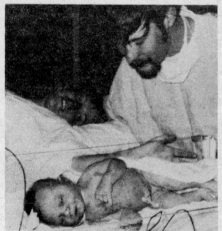

Fig. 65. Proud parents admiring newborn.

plained. Shivering is the natural method of replacing some of the body heat lost when the waters, the baby, and finally the placenta leave the mother's body, and is equivalent to shivering when we feel cold, the producing of maximum warmth with minimum exertion. The mother should be helped to become comfortably warm again. (Shivering experienced earlier in labor is a nervous reaction to emotional states, causing cold sensations and excessive muscular tension. It rarely occurs in a trained, relaxed woman, unless the room is too cold or her covers insufficient for warmth.)

It should not be overlooked that many women believe the delivery of the afterbirth to be an event of considerable severity and discomfort. Therefore the care of a woman's mind during this twenty minutes or so continues to be important.

She need not relax, but may be asked to bear down gently with these painless, miniature second-stage type contractions. Not infrequently a mother will expel the afterbirth without any assistance from the physician, and with a minimum of blood loss. This is possible because of the absence of either exhaustion or shock in a natural birth.

The placenta is a spongy, soft organ that varies in size with the size and weight of the child. Usually oval or circular in shape, it measures from six inches to nine inches wide and about three-fourths of an inch deep at the center, thinning off at the edges. The average weight is about one pound. It shapes itself very easily to the contour of the birth canal and is passed without difficulty.

Years ago it was unheard of that a woman should wish to see the afterbirth. Today nearly every mother who watches her baby born asks me to show her the placenta. (A few women have no desire to look at it.) This I do if she requests it (figs. 66, 67), pointing out the bag in which the infant, now lying peacefully in her arms or by her side, developed and became a perfect little human being (fig. 68). I show her the cord and its attachments, and the manner in which substances are

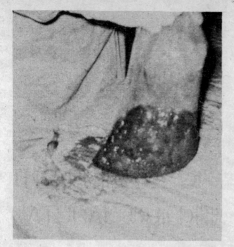

Fig. 66. Physician showing parents the placenta in the membranes.

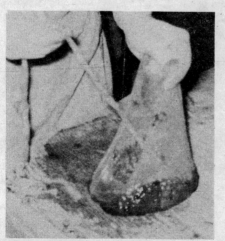

Fig. 67. Physician showing parents the membranes in which the baby lay, and the cord attached to the placenta.

filtered from the maternal blood to build the body, mind, and nature of her child. The amazing powers of selecting and rejecting substances that the placenta has for the fetus at its different stages of growth is remarkable. Its capacity for selecting the correct food in balanced quantities and refusing to admit much, though not all, that might be harmful, makes the intelligent mind appreciate the incalculable genius of creation in all its phases and designs.

"Madam," I tell my patient, "when man can make one of these, he will have reached the footstool of the Creator. As I hold this discarded mass in my hand, I am humbled by the limitations of science." Such references create respect and help us visualize childbirth in its correct perspective. By speaking of the placenta in these terms, the importance of judicious diet and the influence of harmful chemicals that may pass into the baby's blood can be more fully appreciated.

After the placenta is expelled, the nurse then swabs the vulva and perineum carefully with an anesthetic and a sterile napkin is adjusted to receive what is known as the *lochia*. So labor ends, and the woman, accompanied by her husband, is returned to her bed (fig. 69), where she is given a cup of tea, orange juice, or other nourishment and made comfortable to rest from her exertions. The newborn baby should remain with his mother.

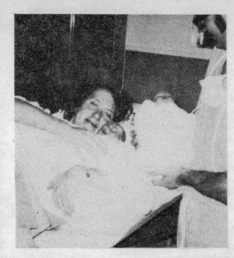

Fig. 68. Twins!

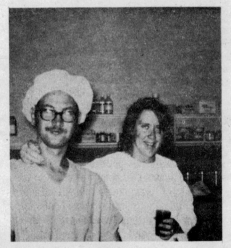

Fig. 69. Walking to room with husband after giving birth to twins, orange juice in hand.

INSTRUCTIONS ON THE IMMEDIATE
ROUTINE CARE OF THE NEWBORN*

1. The baby is kept horizontal at about the level of the placenta until cord pulsations have ceased.
    a. During this time, first nasal then pharyngeal aspiration is accomplished.
    b. The nurse will remind the attending physician at both sixty seconds and five minutes for Apgar ratings.
    c. It is to be noted that the baby's head is not to be lower than the feet (to prevent excess intracranial pressure), nor is the baby to be held for any significant length of time above or below the level of the placenta until after the cessation of cord pulsation.
    d. The notable exceptions to the above rules would be in the premature infant or in the Rh or ABO sensitization, when early clamping of the cord is indicated.
    e. In all mothers who are Rh-negative, and/or previously sensitized, a cord blood specimen, including Coombs, Rh, and type is to be taken. If the mother is known to be already sensitized, further specimens of oxalated and whole blood obtained for other study is indicated, such as bilirubin and hemoglobin determination. If a mother who is Rh-negative has an Rh-positive baby, the mother then becomes a candidate for Rho Gam injection.

2. As soon as the cord has stopped pulsating and has been clamped and severed, the baby is immediately transferred to a prewarmed IMI warmer or similar type birth room warmer, and skin thermostat applied.

3. Identification of infant is performed in the birth room and checked by both the nurse and the physician.

4. 1% silver nitrate is placed in each eye.

* See also *Standards and Recommendations for Hospital Care of Newborn Infants* (American Academy of Pediatrics, 1966).

5. Vitamin K_1 is given I.M. to each newborn baby, in the birth room when possible.

6. If the mother has been prepared to start early nursing, she may do so on the delivery table by moving the hood of the IMI warmer over herself and keeping the skin thermostat attached to the baby, to control and register the temperature of the baby and maintain newborn body warmth. With the exception of a problem in the newborn, the newborn is to be placed as close to the mother as possible for as long as possible before being transferred to the nursery.

7. The baby is not to be removed from the birth room until his condition is considered normal or the attending physician so orders.

8. The only cleansing of the baby is to be the cleaning off of blood and/or meconium with lukewarm water. At times, it may take a small amount of baby oil to clean adherent areas of meconium. All vernix caseosa is to remain on the baby. In order to keep the baby close to the mother as long as possible, it is preferred that the baby not be returned to the nursery until the mother has been returned to her postpartum bed, at which time the baby should be returned to the mother for rooming-in. The exceptions to this are when the mother is recovering from an anesthetic, or she does not wish the baby, or the doctor requests that the baby not be taken back to the mother at that time.

9. All mothers on a childbirth training program and listed as early nursing mothers should have their baby brought to them as soon as possible after the mother has returned to her postpartum bed, and remain with the mother as much as possible during the first twenty-four hours of life.

10. Whenever possible during this first twenty-four hours the husband should be permitted to be with his wife and to hold their baby. He should first have pHisoHex or equivalent scrub of his hands and wear gown and mask during this period. No other visitors are permitted when the baby is with his mother.

15

Natural Childbirth in Emergency

There are times when we all have to face unexpected emergency, and it is our reaction to it that is often more important than the sudden unexpected occurrence or situation with which we are confronted.

Women all over the world are, and may continue to be, caught in the emergency of unexpected labor—if only because they are alone at home or in the country or, as I have seen several times, in a public place or vehicle. Labor is not a frightening incident in the life of a woman if she has learned what goes on and how her body produces the child when it is ready to leave its mother's womb.

What can a woman do when and if in circumstances of unexpected emergency her labor begins, with no competent person to help her, and perhaps only herself to help her child safely into the world? If she has no knowledge of her own natural processes and how to assist and not hinder their performance, she creates many difficulties and much discomfort to herself, and perhaps also for her child. A known and well-proven scientific fact is that nothing disturbs the course of natural labor more than fear. Fear is caused and intensified by ignorance. The first need, then, is for the woman in such circumstances to be prepared in advance by knowledge and understanding of how to give birth to her child.

When the baby is ready to be born it lies comfortably in the uterus or womb with its *head downward,* for it is usual and best for babies to dive, not step, into the world. The baby announces its coming arrival in three ways—by a *show* of mucus or blood from the outlet of the birth canal, by a *leaking* of water from the uterus, or by *rhythmical contractions*, which increase in frequency and in strength.

The first two of these warnings, in the absence of the strong contractions of the uterus, usually give plenty of time to prepare for the baby's arrival. But under the stress of accident or the threat of death-dealing danger, as in time of war, the intense defensive reaction to paralyzing fear is almost complete relaxation and inactivity of the muscles that control the passage of the baby from the womb. Under these circumstances labor is often what we term "precipitate," and the baby arrives with very little discomfort or difficulty to the mother. Terror-caused paralysis of the muscles of the pelvic floor, allowing spontaneous evacuation of the bowel and urinary bladder, is well known, and at the end of pregnancy the same reaction to terror may occur with the uterus. This unusual state is the reverse of the fear-tension-pain syndrome.

When the intensity of fear diminishes and brings conscious realization of being in labor, women resist the effort of expulsion and thereby create a state of tension by opposing the muscles that are contracting to push the baby out. This is the reaction of emotional stress. *There is a very real difference between the emergency of precipitate labor due to external stress*, with the primitive defense reaction to violent and imminent destruction, *and the labor of a woman in fear of labor itself*. The defensive reaction in cases of external fright is one of emotional and physical paralysis, but in the fear of labor alone it is one of emotional and physical resistance to the work of the uterus. I have seen in trenches, on shell-swept plains, and in the rubble of bombed cities women in such emotional terror that they have lost all voluntary control, and have compared them with women in perfectly safe surroundings, frightened by the process of labor itself. These women suffer even though under the care of well-meaning attendants, whose tender ministrations and sympathetic manner reveal that they expect their patient to be in pain, and thus add to her tension and discomfort.

The most important thing to remember, then, is that it is *fear* of pain that produces all the severe and unbearable suffering of labor. In an emergency, a *calm* woman who remains in control of her actions will have little discomfort as she awaits the progression of the natural events about which she has learned.

During labor a woman should pass urine from time to time, in order to keep her urinary bladder empty. This should be done in a squatting position at any reasonable place, according to the dilemma in which she may find herself.

Then, wherever she is, in a wayside ditch or a ruin-covered cellar, in a stranger's house, a caravan, or tent, she should find a place to *sit down and lean her back against*—wall, bank, or any available support. She should pull up her knees and rest her buttocks on a folded coat, a bunch of leaves, or anything that will lift her slightly off the ground. She should *not lie down on her side or her back, but sit* as near as possible in a squatting position, taking the weight of her body upon her buttocks. If left alone in labor, she may escape one of the greatest causes of trouble, which is interference by those around who, being kind but misinformed, feel they must *do* something for her. The safest medical attendant in such an emergency is nature, by whom woman has been marvelously equipped for this purpose. The baby is not to be interfered with by its mother's mind or a volunteer assistant's hand. Just courage and patience are required, and faith in God, if she is a believer, to produce a healthy baby and be a happy mother.

As the woman sits and waits patiently for the baby, she will soon feel a desire to push down. At first the effort to push must be very gentle. She should only take a deep breath and hold it, without pushing. There may be some backache, but it will soon pass. If there is no one there to rub her back she must relax and try to put it out of her mind, for the backache will soon disappear. When the desire to bear down becomes too strong to resist, she may begin to push firmly, but not too hard, and without expecting immediate results. If it is her first baby, it may take one and a half to two hours of expulsive effort before the baby appears. Sometimes two or three deep breaths, in and out, may be taken during one contraction, if it is too long for one breath alone. Breathe in, hold and push, breathe out and in, hold and push.

As the contraction fades she will relax sleepily, first taking two deep in and out breaths, then quietly resting until the next effort begins. Her drowsiness may be so deep that her mind is concentrated only on the one task of producing her child. I have seen women during air raids who, although by nature nervous people, were not disturbed by the noise or the flashes of bombs that rocked the walls about us. On one occasion, being disconcerted myself by the volume and proximity of missiles, I was slow to notice the onset of my twenty-two-year-old patient's next contraction. She said testily, "Another push, doctor. Come on, don't worry about the noise!"

Just before the head can be seen some women have a strong desire to "escape" the impending birth. When this occurs the woman should remember to ignore the feeling and *push firmly* for the next two or at the most three contractions. Such concentrated expulsive efforts to help the contraction will quickly overcome the temporary discomfort and desire to escape. Shortly after that the hair on the baby's head will show at the outlet. If there is a looking glass handy, so the mother can see her baby, it will help her take an active interest in helping him arrive. She will then concentrate upon the baby and his arrival and forget thoughts of her own well-being. The second or expulsive stage of labor need not be painful if the mother is in the correct squatting position, keeping her outlet relaxed and pushing properly with the contractions, though it may be hard work for the birth of a first baby. This stage is to be a conscious, controlled, and painless repetition of pushing to urge the baby forward as he moves through the natural twists and turns, flexions and extensions of the head that prevent damage to both mother and baby.

As the head starts to distend the vulva, a feeling of burning of the labia or lips of the outlet may alarm her. She must realize that it will quickly disappear *if* she does not squeeze up against it. The outlet must be relaxed and allowed to bulge as it will. But she *must not bear down* any more. Instead, she should breathe short breaths in and out, letting the abdominal muscles stay relaxed, allowing the uterus itself to urge the child slowly forward in a relatively painless birth of the head.

At this time she will have lost her drowsiness, and will be able to adjust her position, leaning back at an angle of 45 degrees—about halfway between flat and upright. With contractions she should pull her knees up and, with her hands, hold them wide open and at right angles to her body, with her feet resting on whatever support is handy.

As the baby emerges into the world face downward, the woman should lean over and put one hand on the area between the anus and the vaginal opening, so that the forehead and face of the child pass gently into her waiting hand. She can thus support her baby's head as it arrives, directing it *upward* toward her abdomen. Under no circumstances should she pull the baby out straight before her! She must remember to *help the baby upward and over the bone of the front of the pelvis,* using her second hand to support the baby's body as it emerges. Lifting the baby upward helps prevent tearing of the outlet.

If she is alone or with inexperienced people, she must not become excited or hurried. Slowness, quietness, and gentleness are the qualities of a good delivery. The crying baby is then to be laid flat on the ground, his head still supported in her hand, until the cord that joins the infant to her ceases to pulsate or throb. It will shrink and become pale and limp. By this time the placenta or afterbirth may have separated from the womb and be in the vaginal canal.

As soon as the cord has stopped pulsating and is long enough for the woman to lift the child without any pull on the cord, she should put the child to breast, raising the child gently with one hand under his head and the other under his hips. Cradling him so that he lies level along her arm she should allow him to grasp the nipple. If he will not take it as most do, she should gently rub his mouth and nose against the nipple, to stimulate her uterus.

Soon contractions will begin again, and the second stage of labor is then repeated, in a diminutive form, for the birth of the placenta, the third stage. If the afterbirth does not come of its own accord, the mother can keep the baby supported on one arm and place her hand on her abdomen above the uterus, which will be felt as a coconut-sized lump reaching just above the navel. If she presses gently on the abdomen with the palm of her hand, and then gives one or two sharp coughs, the afterbirth may come out easily.

In emergency labor the cord should not be cut until after the afterbirth comes away. Until then the baby is kept warm in its mother's clothing, either on the ground beside her or in her arms, preferably held to the breast. When the afterbirth has been expelled, it is to be wrapped up with the baby until experienced medical help is available.

Whatever clothing is available may be used for the baby and for the mother. As little as possible should be put over the birth canal outlet, which must not be touched with unwashed hands if this can be avoided, although emergency labor seldom results in infection.

Most women, after the labor is completed, are able to walk with their babies to a place where clothing and cleanliness may be obtained, and perhaps medical aid and advice.

The *dignity and control of childbirth* can be maintained even in circumstances incredibly different from our accepted standards. I have attended women in many strange places and circumstances and know that this is true. A woman must remember that faith is not only an ethical and emotional acquisition. It is also a state of mind, which creates within the body physical harmony in the activities of living that maintain the highest standard of health and resistance to disease.

16

Care of the Newborn

A newborn baby remains part of its mother just as much after birth as it was while *in utero*. Indeed, the added association of personality and behavior brings them even closer together. When a baby is born it is equipped by nature with the means of survival in relation to its mother.

In the absence of experience it does not interpret incidents in the adventure of living with adult understanding. Its physical demands are for food, warmth, and rest. Its awareness to things and people about it develops rapidly, however, and within a few hours of birth it seeks security in the widest sense. In the early days of a baby's life security implies the provision of the essentials for survival and protection from outside injurious influences. *For that security a newborn baby turns to its mother.*

BODY CONTACT

When a child is born the mother should hold it and fondle it immediately. Some mothers have the desire to put the baby to the breast. This initial skin-to-skin contact of warmth (figs. 70, 71, 72) between the mother and her child has a most salutary influence upon the progress and behavior of them both. After the mother returns to her bed, the baby is placed in a crib beside her. Knowing her child is there, she does not worry about it. She feels that her child is secure. Whenever she desires she can put the baby to her breast. For not only do breasts have the supreme function of lactation, they are also the ultimate manifestation of the mother-child relationship. As surely as the umbilical cord sustains the vital unity of the mother with her intrauterine fetus, so the nipple retains that mystic union with the child that is no longer within her. In those peaceful moments the infant floods its mother's mind in meditation, which brings reality to her most cherished dreams. His restlessness is quieted and his awareness of others stimulated through this physical and affectionate contact. An older baby often pats and fondles the breasts as he nurses, and stops to smile at his mother. Through her breast they are unified in extrauterine life as closely as in the months of gestation.

After the baby has been put to the breast it is held and cuddled, becoming familiar with the mother's ways while she herself becomes familiar with his. When a mother fondles and cuddles her baby as it nestles and nuzzles against her breast and in her arms, she is unconsciously laying a foundation of that mutual confidence and companionship from which all that is best in human nature develops.

The baby is then replaced in the crib by her bedside. Infants treated in this way are peaceful and quiet and very rarely disturb their mothers by crying.

COLOSTRUM

When a child is put to the breast shortly after birth he gets no milk, but there is a substance known as *colostrum* that exudes from a well-prepared nipple. There is still much to be learned about this valuable, thick fluid. We know that it contains substances that produce within the infant immunities to certain bacteria that might cause diseases. It contains a certain amount of milk globules and cells containing fat, which are called *colostrum corpuscles,* but the actual value of these to the baby is not yet fully known. Colostrum seems to have a beneficial effect upon the baby's bowels, helping to expel the

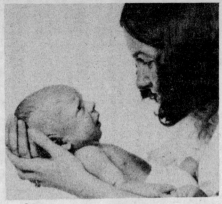

Fig. 70. Stimulation of infant through mother's hands.

meconium that is contained in the intestines of the newborn. It may be of help in breaking down the mucus in his throat when he nurses immediately after birth, by stimulating the swallowing reflex or causing him to cough before he can swallow. Colostrum may also provide enzymes for protein metabolism.

Colostrum is also of great use to the breast and nipple of the mother, for the suckling of the baby helps to stimulate the activity of the glands by which the milk is secreted. By the third day or less after the baby has been put to the breast, these milk glands become enlarged, filling the ducts leading from the breast to the nipple, of which there are about twenty. Since the baby has drawn away the thick colostrum from these ducts, the milk flow is much more quickly and easily established without engorgement, for *where the infant feeds there will be food*.

Nature provides the newborn infant with a considerable amount of fat. During the day or two before the milk is secreted in the breast, this fat in his own system is absorbed as his own natural nutrition. It is largely this provision of food within itself that accounts for his loss of weight until the mother's milk supply is established. I certainly do not advise

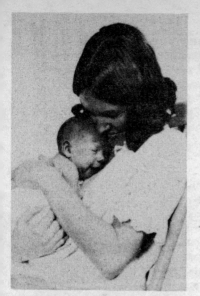

Fig. 71. Newborn maternal closeness.

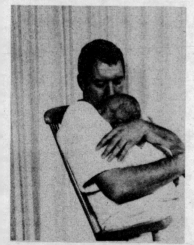

Fig. 72. Skin-to-skin with Daddy, too!

giving the baby any prescription before the natural food is available. It has enough nourishment in its own body to live comfortably until the milk supply is adequately stimulated. Not infrequently its desire to take the breast is decreased if it has supplementary or "pity" feeds, and this delays further the establishment of his mother's milk supply in an easily accessible flow.

FEEDING ON DEMAND

A child does not wish to nurse continuously. At first, when hungry, he will swallow as rapidly as possible, but he must rest. Although he does not relinquish his hold on the nipple he will stop taking milk for a short time. If he appears to be drifting into sleep, a gentle touch on the upper lip with the mother's finger will restimulate his sucking reflex.

Although it is not strictly accurate to say that the infant sucks the milk from the breast, we will use this term for the sake of simplicity. In reality, he presses the milk out by closing his mouth on the nipple with a squeezing action. The only real sucking is the action of the baby's tongue in lifting the nipple up to his palate.

An infant takes nearly all his food in the first four or five minutes, and if he becomes lazy he should be taken off the breast. This can be done without discomfort to the mother by lightly compressing the baby's nostrils so that he opens his mouth to breathe.

A newborn baby requires feeding again as soon as its last meal has been digested. One will take a large amount, and four or five hours pass before he feels he wants more and cries to gain the mother's attention to his hunger. Others may take smaller amounts, or have a more rapid digestion, and will cry after three hours or even less. The demand in a baby's voice is recognizable from all other cries, and a mother quickly learns the difference between the cry of hunger, the cry of colic, the grumble of an uncomfortable diaper, or the irregular bursts of a cry due to pain. Mothers must learn to recognize the normal conversational cries of their children by close association from the time of birth.

Demand feeding has many advantages. It is obviously wrong to force a baby to take food into a stomach that is not demanding it, and, although many will do so, they are more predisposed to colic or spitting up than those who only accept a meal for which their stomach is ready.

Much crying in a frustrated baby is undoubtedly a greater evil than has been recognized in the past.* Violent crying deprives a child's brain of the full quota of oxygen that he would have in a restful state. Many babies cry very violently when they are annoyed by not having what their body obviously demands, and these fits of irritation can definitely do harm, not only to the child's personality, but also to his physical and mental development. The baby, and the baby only, feels when he is ready for nourishment, and a mother, feeding on demand, soon knows to within a few minutes the digestive cycle of her child.

BABY'S PERFECT FOOD

Mother's milk has certain qualities that cannot be exactly duplicated. It has been created specifically for the human baby's own digestive system. It develops within the child an immunity against certain diseases, infections, and tooth decay. In families that suffer from such allergic diseases as asthma, eczema or hives, infants who are entirely breastfed for the earlier months of their lives are less prone to develop these conditions.

Breastfeeding is easier for the mother, for the baby's milk is always fresh, clean, easily available, and at the correct temperature. It is also both economical and labor saving, for there is no need to waste time sterilizing bottles and preparing

* Margaret A. Ribble, *The Rights of Infants,* rev. ed. (New York: Columbia University Press, 1965).

food, or buying expensive prepackaged formula in bottles. It contains all the essential elements of food for the baby.

ROOMING-IN

The profound importance to the baby of the first forty-eight hours of its neonatal life does not receive the emphasis many of us wish it had. For my own part I extend that thought to the development of the mother in the first forty-eight hours of motherhood. A newborn baby should remain with the mother during this extremely important period, where she can constantly see him and attend to him if necessary, even from the first day.

Forty-five or fifty years ago nurseries for all newborn babies were hailed as one of the latest advances in maternity wards. Up until that time it was usual to have the babies in cots either attached to or standing beside the mother's bed. The change proved to be a most unfortunate divergence from what was then termed the "old-fashioned" principle of leaving the babies with their mothers. It arose because of the increased use of heavy anesthesia for the mother, who was then in no condition even to be aware of the presence of the child and might cause him harm before she awakened to consciousness. The babies also needed much more constant medical supervision because of their own sedated state and associated problems.

But in recent years several important factors have brought about a change, so that in many up-to-date hospitals rooming-in has been reestablished.* One of these factors is a recognition of the importance of the mother-child relationship and the emotional development of the baby during the first few days of

* *Standards for Obstetric-Gynecologic Hospital Services* (Chicago: The American College of Obstetricians and Gynecologists, 1969), pp. 14 f., 44 f.; *Standards and Recommendations for Hospital Care of Newborn Infants* (Evanston, Ill.: American Academy of Pediatrics, 1964), pp. 30–33, 77.

his life. A mother who has been alert and cooperative during the birth presents no danger to the newborn left under her watchful eye.

Unless stringent protective measures are constantly employed, devastating epidemic infections in hospital nurseries still threaten to occur, for these infections now resist the previously effective antibiotics. Infants kept with their own mothers escape the risk of infant-to-infant skin, intestinal, and respiratory infections.

The results of a long and intricate investigation of rooming-in by Harvey Carey of Auckland University have been published, along with a number of similar studies. He found that the mother was the safest person to handle the baby, his research demonstrating that the nursing staff could be a source of danger in spreading the lesions of the staphylococcus, even though uninfected themselves. Rooming-in means that as far as possible no one but the mother handles the baby. The additional great advantage is that the baby receives individual attention, is fed when necessary, and is made comfortable when required. Researches show that babies put on weight better under rooming-in and that the mother is more confident in handling her baby, even though she now leaves the hospital only a few days after the birth. And of course under these conditions breastfeeding also has a much better chance of being successful.

Editors' Addendum

INFANT CARE IN THE NURSERY*

1. For a nursing mother, the "normal" baby is to be given no supplements, either milk or water, unless requested by the attending physician and/or the mother of the baby. If during the night
   in the first twenty-four hours a nursing baby appears fussy
   and the mother is asleep, the mother is to be awakened to
   nurse her baby, unless the mother states or gives other instructions.
2. If the baby and mother are discharged home in the first twenty-
   four hours and the PKU test has not been performed, the
   mother must be given instructions to return to the laboratory
   the next day with the infant for this test.
3. Personnel wash their hands before and after handling each infant. Newborn infants are to be under unremitting observation
   for the presence of cyanosis, hemorrhage, jaundice, dyspnea,
   vomiting, dehydration and/or abnormal activity.
4. The first stool and urine is noted and recorded. An antiseptic
   is applied to the umbilical cord. Infant's temperature is measured on admission and every four hours until stabilized, and
   then once daily.
5. Each infant is weighed once daily.
6. On discharge, the nursery nurse discusses with the mother
   any questions or problems concerning the immediate home
   care of the baby and checks to be sure the mother has an appointment back to her attending physician for the follow-up
   care of the baby.
7. All placentas are to be tagged and saved for the first twenty-
   four hours. If at the end of this time there has been no request
   to send the placenta to the pathology laboratory, the placenta
   is disposed of in the usual manner.
8. The following list is to be considered a newborn critical list and
   requires pediatric consultation:
   a. Respirations above 60.

* See also Haire, Doris, *Implementing Family-Centered Maternity Care with a
Central Nursery:* (CEA of New Jersey, 1968).

b. Persistent *cyanosis*.
c. Repeated vomiting first 48 hours.
d. Loss of more than 10 percent birthweight.
e. Absence of *meconium* in first bowel movement.
f. Abdominal distention.
g. Rectal temperature over 101° Fahrenheit.
h. Birthweight under four pounds eight ounces.
i. Viable infant with severe malformation.
j. Rh sensitization.
k. Jaundice in first twenty-four hours.

SUGGESTED ROOMING-IN PROCEDURES*

Keeping the newborn baby as close to the mother as long as possible on the first and second days of life is advantageous both to the mother and the baby, psychologically and physically. Nursing personnel should be trained to encourage and assist in accomplishing this type program, as efficiently as possible within the facilities available.

1. Immediately following birth and in the birth room, the baby is to be first placed in the warmer, which should be placed right next to the mother. As soon as the temperature has stabilized in the baby, the mother is encouraged to hold the baby and touch him, having previously cleansed her hands (as has the husband), and the new father is also encouraged to touch his baby or hold him.
2. If the mother desires to nurse on the birth table, this can be accomplished. Moving the hood of the warmer over the mother assures the warmth of the baby.
3. A scale should be in the birth room so the baby need not be taken to the nursery to be weighed, or his data recorded.
4. The baby in the warmer is to stay in the birth room as long as possible while the mother is being prepared to return to her ward bed.
5. The baby can then be taken to the nursery for any additional care, but as soon as it is convenient for the nursery staff, hope-

* See also *Standards and Recommendations for Hospital Care of Newborn Infants* (American Academy of Pediatrics, 1966), for both nursery procedures and guidance in rooming-in in American hospitals.

fully within the first hour, the baby will be returned to the mother and to the bassinette at her bedside. Many times the baby bypasses the nursery, going with his mother directly from the birth room to her postpartum room.

6. When there are no other patients in the room, it seems advisable for the baby to stay with the mother as much as possible and as long as she requests his presence.

7. When the baby is in the room with the mother, the only visitors permitted will be the husband, who must be properly gowned, capped and masked. The infant's mother and father are the only two people in the world with whom he is bacteriologically compatible.

8. If other visitors are to visit the postpartum patient who has a rooming-in baby, the baby must be returned to the nursery while the visitors are present.

9. It is an important part of the staff's responsibility to take time whenever possible to help educate the new mother with as much information as possible for newborn baby care at home.

17

The New Mother

After the natural birth of a child a healthy woman need not remain in bed for more than two or three days. No mother should become bedridden after childbirth. Unless there is any definite contraindication, which the medical attendant will judge, she can be out of bed for short periods of time on the day her baby is born. On the second day she can be up a little more. Any feeling of tiredness is the signal that she has been up long enough, and she should rest as soon as she feels the need. The upright position and the exercises she does after the baby is born have many advantages.

The immediate adoption of good posture is important. So many women walk about after labor as if they had been seriously ill for a month; we see them in maternity hospitals after an uncomplicated birth stooping, hanging onto someone's arm, and staggering rather than walking. This postnatal assumption of illness is, in most cases, a psychological demand for activity, and an entirely uncalled-for condition in a healthy woman who has been properly cared for. She should be a happy, upright, easy-moving person glowing with the bloom of health, and with the expression of happiness on her face that is the prerogative of young mothers.

A certain amount of sensible discretion must be used when the mother arrives home with her new baby, and her husband or other helpers should take over her regular household chores for a week or ten days so she can devote her full attention to her baby without becoming weary or discouraged. At the end of six weeks she should revisit her physician.

AFTERPAINS

Women who have had more than one baby may have painful contractions of the uterus for the first day or two after the baby is born. Sometimes these are very slight, occurring especially when the baby is put to the breast. This is due to the reflex stimulation of the uterus from the breast, which makes it contract tightly during nursing, and assists in the rapid restoration of the uterus to its nonpregnant state.

Relaxation does not always relieve the pain, for it may spring from a different cause than in labor. If these contractions are severe enough to hurt, it probably means that there is a small blood clot or piece of membrane that has not yet come away from the uterine cavity. Many women resign themselves to these afterpains, which is wrong. If this discomfort arises they should say so immediately, for there is no reason why they should not be relieved of it very quickly. A mild pain reliever such as one quarter grain of codeine followed by two tablets of aspirin four hours later usually works like a charm, and the discomfort probably will not recur.

LOCHIA

For two weeks or even longer after labor, a discharge persists from the genital canal. This discharge, or *lochia,* is largely composed of the debris of the uterine and vaginal walls as they cast off those membranes and tissues which were of service during pregnancy and birth. It consists largely of thin blood with a few small clots and, in three or four days, turns a brownish color. Apart from frequent cleansing and the wearing of sanitary napkins, this should occasion no more inconvenience than rather prolonged menstruation.

CARE OF THE NIPPLES

The nipples must be kept soft and elastic. They should be cleansed with warm water only, for even soap has a drying effect. The application of chemicals with the intention of making them hard and strong does more harm than good and predisposes to cracking and sore places. The nipples should be made to stand out so that nursing is easy for the baby; this can be done by proper care during the last weeks of pregnancy, as described earlier (page 150).* Sore nipples should be exposed to the air for fifteen minutes after nursing. A cream such as Nivea is soothing.

If milk has to be expressed from the breast after nursing has been established, the expelling movement is the same as that used in preparation of the nipple. The left hand used for the right breast and the right hand for the left breast, the base of the brown area should be pressed gently between the thumb and forefinger. The breasts should be relieved in this way of a little milk whenever they become uncomfortably full and it is not time to nurse the baby, to prevent painful engorgement. Gradually the amount of milk produced will adjust to the amount the baby requires.

BREASTFEEDING

Every mother should feed her baby at the breast. The advantages to the baby are often mentioned, but it is equally important to the mother's health and emotional well-being. It consolidates the mother-child relationship from the earliest hours of birth. The breastfeeding mother is conscious of a

* A variety of breast shields are available that are helpful in overcoming such problems as inverted nipples, weak suckling as in a premature infant, or sore nipples. These problems should be under the physician's care and advice.

satisfying sense of achievement when her baby is at the breast. The close contact and physical stimulus of the baby's suckling bring nearer to her mind the reality of motherhood, its joys, and its responsibilities. We must not overlook the importance of the daydreams of a nursing mother. Not infrequently a new outlook upon life is developed that brings a serenity of mind, enhancing for all time the patience and self-control so necessary in the upbringing and training of children.

Nursing the child not only assists the uterus and birth canal in returning to their normal shape and size, but it also releases into the mother's bloodstream chemicals that have a tranquilizing effect upon her, once breastfeeding is well established. Before that time, consciously relaxing will help the breast "let down" the milk. The problem in breastfeeding is not the supply, but the "giving" of the milk. A tense mother inhibits the "let-down" reflex of her milk, so that both she and the baby become frustrated. When she has learned to relax well enough to allow the milk to flow as the baby nurses, the stimulation to her system will result in still further calmness and pleasure.

A mother breastfeeding her baby must be in a comfortable position so that she can relax well, and avoid any strain on her back and shoulder muscles. Many women sit hunched up with their heads dropping forward to watch the baby anxiously, only to find that in a short time their backs are aching from the neck to the waist. It is best to sit in a high-backed chair with a pillow across the knees and the baby lying on the pillow, its head level with the nipples. The mother puts one arm around the child and lets its head rest on her forearm. With the other hand she gently depresses the breast from under the baby's nose to give him a free airway.

If she prefers to lie in bed, the baby can lie beside her. This is not only comfortable but enables the baby to take the nipple into his mouth without dragging on the breast.

It should be remembered that if an infant is fed from below, with the nipple pulled downward into his mouth, after three or four months the shape of the breast may be irreparably damaged. Thus, if a mother wants to keep her attractive physical shape, the correct position for nursing is important.

Let me offer this solace to the woman who would, but cannot, feed her baby at the breast. She will find this disappointment can lead to a deep and cherished bond that turns the water of weaning into the wine of spiritual communion. A gypsy mother, whose breasts had been incurably mutilated by the flames of an exploding stove, was feeding her fifth baby from a bottle. She had breastfed the four beautiful children who ran to greet me. They were clean, friendly, and lovable in their picturesque, highly colored clothes and gilded earrings. I sat in the spotless caravan and told her how grieved I was to have to suppress her milk flow. "Don't worry, doctor," she told me. "It's all the same if you put your heart into the bottle."

If a mother must bottle-feed her baby, let her give him the milk herself, with warmth, love, and security, snuggled to her heart in the silent serenity of mutual satisfaction. It is well to let the baby snuggle "skin-to-skin" against her breast as he nurses from the bottle. Then little will be lost and much will be recovered.

ROOMING-IN

Many mothers suffer silent acute anxiety for the welfare of their babies during the first three or four days of life if the baby is in some place apart. But if it remains in the room with her, she will see the nurse change the baby's diapers and oil its skin, for newborn babies are not bathed with water and soap for the first few days. She will learn what his different cries mean and will gain confidence in her ability to care for her child, under the supervision of the nursing staff. This closeness to the infant, so that he can be fed on demand any time of the day or night, stimulates early and efficient breastfeeding, often before the mother leaves the hospital.

It is not correct to say that the presence of a baby is disturbing to a mother and does not enable her to have sufficient rest. The baby that is "roomed-in" with his mother is very rarely restless, and the mother who wishes to have her baby with her is almost invariably at peace with herself and the world.

DIET

The same principles of good diet apply during breast-feeding as during pregnancy. The nursing mother should continue to take two pints of milk a day, and drink more water than before the baby was born. Apart from that, she should eat sensibly, simply, and discreetly, recognizing the essential constituents of food and including them in sufficient, but not excessive, amounts to maintain good health and provide for the development of the baby. She should look upon meals as important and pleasant pauses in the daily round, eat slowly, enjoying the natural flavors of food, for quality is of more pleasure than quantity, and should stop before feeling full. She should be restful and relaxed in comfort and conversation, stop before feeling full, and should spend fifteen minutes in quiet reading or rest before returning to the duties of the day. This aids digestion and prevents the signs and symptoms of avoidable indigestion.

POSTNATAL EXERCISES.

The objects of postnatal exercises are:
1. To promote efficient circulation of the blood.
2. To maintain the habit of full and controlled breathing learned during the prenatal training.
3. To regain good posture and carriage.
4. To aid the absorption and natural distribution of fat stored in and on the body during pregnancy.
5. To restore the firmness and muscle tone of the abdominal and pelvic muscles.
The average mother does not have much time for exercises

and relaxation, especially if she has one or two other children to care for. She will be less tired, however, and more efficient if she organizes her daily routine so that a quarter of an hour is spent on these few exercises, followed by fifteen to thirty minutes of deep relaxation.

Breathing

Deep, full breathing should be begun on the second day. It is enough to take *six full, controlled breaths three times during the day*.

Firming the Pelvic Floor

It is extremely important that the muscles and tissues of the pelvis, which have been stretched and considerably loosened during childbirth, should be restored to their normal tone and strength. Many of the discomforts that follow childbirth are due to the absence of this care. This exercise should be done on the second day after the arrival of the baby, and continued for the rest of the mother's life. It is the same exercise as exercise 5 in the prenatal instructions.

Tightly squeeze together the muscles of the vulva and vagina, much more firmly than the effort required when there is a desire to urinate at an inconvenient moment. This "squeezing up" need not be associated in any way with movements of the thighs or buttocks. After tightening these muscles, hold them tight for a moment when the tension is greatest, and then relax them slowly. This has the effect of drawing up the pelvic floor, tightening the ring around and within the vaginal orifice, and closing firmly the small tube through which urine is passed. This should be done *twelve times, two or three times a day*.

Firming the Abdominal Muscles

On the third day after the arrival of the baby, after taking a few full, deep breaths, lying on the back, raise the left knee up to the chest, with the knee bent. Straighten the leg and lower it slowly onto the bed. Repeat with the right leg. Do this with each leg once or twice the first day, gradually increasing to *five or six times once a day*.

Firming the Breasts

This is the same as prenatal exercise 4. Grip each arm firmly behind the wrist and raise the arms to the level of the shoulders. Push the skin of the forearm up while tightening the arm muscles and the muscles of the chest, lifting the breasts. Release the tension slowly, so the breasts do not drop suddenly. Repeat *ten times, once a day*. It is especially important to continue this exercise during weaning, to keep the muscle support of the breasts in good tone.

Pelvic Rock*

This is the same as prenatal exercise 1. On hands and knees, let the back sag. Slowly raise the back, at the same time squeezing together the muscles of the buttocks, pelvic area, and upper legs.

Conclusion

After completing the exercises, a period of relaxation should follow, lying on the abdomen with the legs extended, or in the lateral side position as in pregnancy and labor. These positions take the weight of the still bulky uterus off the pelvic floor and help to prevent it from falling backward and down toward the pelvis as it returns to normal size.

I advise women to exaggerate their posture for the first few days, pulling the abdomen well in and the hips under, and

* The arms must be kept extended during this exercise, with the elbows straight, so that the chest is not lower than the hips. The "knee-chest" position sometimes prescribed for postpartum patients is to be avoided, as it causes air to be sucked into the vagina, and may create an air embolism in the bloodstream.

"standing tall," with shoulders back and head and chin up. Breathe in such a manner that the chest expands and fills the hollows below the collarbones. This slight exaggeration of posture enables rapid reabsorption to take place in the softened connective tissue around the pelvic joints and lower spine, with the minimum risk of discomfort from backache.

Relaxation must be persisted in, for it is of great advantage in successful breastfeeding. If the mother has opportunity for relaxation as she nurses her baby, does her breathing and other exercises, and persists throughout her life in the habitual performance of the pelvic tensing and relaxing, she will be laying the foundation of good health and happiness for herself, as well as efficient breastfeeding of her newborn infant.

Part III

THE PIONEER OF
NATURAL CHILDBIRTH

These chapters have been compiled from the many personal experiences about which Grantly Dick-Read wrote, scattered through his books and letters. They give us an understanding of the man as a person that few of his contemporaries had.

During his life he was an enigma to many people. He was a farseeing man who looked beyond the immediate. He observed details in the natural world around him that escaped the attention of others. He looked back through the centuries in search of wisdom and forward into the future of the human race.

As the years passed, his goal in life focused increasingly on one essential purpose—to make this world a better place in which to live, through happier mothers and homes. As he grew older he became increasingly outspoken in his views, in contrast to the timidity of his earlier years. The fact that he was right did not increase his popularity among his colleagues!

Yet it was not arrogance that drove him on, but an inner anguish over so much needless suffering that he had found clues for overcoming. It was the anguish similar to that of another prophet, who cried, "There is a fire burning my bones, and I cannot keep silent!"

18

Early Impressions

In my library there are thirty-seven volumes, each leather bound and stamped in gold, *Mother's Letters, from 1915 to 1941*. These manuscripts of indescribable beauty are not to an only son, for I was born in 1890 as the sixth of seven children. In these letters, schooldays and Cambridge, the London Hospital, World War I, are all recalled and reviewed in terms of sympathy and understanding, admonition and advice. Betrothal, marriage, and parenthood are discussed with me in words of which Madame de Sévigné might well have been proud. Year after year this fount of mother love poured its influence into my life and still, at eighty-eight, this grand old lady filled me with pride when I read her views on things of today, written in the light of long years of quiet observation and deduction.

There is no logical reason to presume that the influence of one mother is exceptional. It is my belief that I quote an example only from many thousands, and there would be many more with each generation if this great source of power were fostered and nourished by the obstetric physicians. The science of obstetrics must be recognized as an invaluable adjunct to the health and happiness of humanity. From earliest childhood, since as far back as my memory reaches, I have devoted nearly all my interest, and most of my energies, to this cause.

When I was a small boy, I delighted in hearing my sister play "The March of the Gladiators." Many evenings before my bedtime she would sit at the piano and play it to me, until "old Ellen" came to take me up to bed. One night I sat by her, listening and supremely happy, when three revolver shots rang out from the woods at the bottom of the drive. Then I heard that "old Ellen" had been shot dead by the soldier she had been going to marry.

For the rest of my life, one phrase in that tune, if ever I am forced to hear it, brings back to me the chill of horror, the agony of fear, and the inconsolable anguish that I suffered that night. "The March of the Gladiators," by association, ceased to bring me pleasure, but was a conditioned stimulus for violent emotional disturbance—so much so that, ten years later, when I was in medical school at Cambridge and it floated across the campus to my room during lunch, I suddenly felt sick and had to leave the table, only realizing afterwards that it was a reaction to an almost forgotten emotional state. This experience later helped me to appreciate the negative emotional reactions of a woman to any mention of childbirth, if she had unhappy memories concerning it.

As a child I was very happy and fortunate to spend at least six months of the year at our Norfolk home, which was a farm, where I became acquainted with nature and enjoyed it far more, I regret to say, than I enjoyed the society of my older brothers and sisters. I got to know my animals, the cows, the pigs, and the horses. I sat with my bitches when they had their puppies, and caressed Topsy when she had her kittens, those natural things children do under the happy circumstances of such an upbringing. I spent much of my time on my own because I believed so unquestionably in the miracles of nature—they were all mysteries to me of absorbing interest. I sought the loneliness of silent places where only naturalists really find companionship.

On one occasion during my obstetric practice in later years, a nursing student remarked to me: "We have only had normal cases lately, but Mr. X is coming in later on this afternoon to put on forceps. The woman has been in labor two and a half days—we think she is an occipito posterior. It should be quite interesting."

"Ah, splendid," I replied to this lady, who though a student was a potential mother of tomorrow, "very interesting. I expect the woman is getting interested by now!"

Of course it is exciting to see the abnormal, and necessary for training, but must the normal and natural be considered dull? It is only in these cases that any beauty can be found in obstetrics. The simple, straightforward performances are the perfect initiation into motherhood; surely here is the field for observation. Each constituent of the ordinary is so extraordinary when understood. It is so in nature, in every sphere, one of its great fascinations. It is more thrilling to watch an avalanche crash in a cloud of snow to the bottom of a ravine, to hear the roar of its thunderous progress and witness the devastation in its path, than to lie on the edge of a Norfolk marsh. Yes, more thrilling—until you have looked quietly and closely into the reeds.

Here as a boy, prone on the grass, I observed the peaceful beauty of nature as its constituents gradually appeared. Silver fish lit up the shallow water, great swallowtail butterflies flitted decoratively from ragged robin to wild flower; small cotton tufts revealed the newly hatched cocoon; each wee spider was a thrill as it set out on its great adventure. I heard the moorhen call and hurry her fluffy offspring past my observation post as a bittern* boomed in the distance.

At every turn of the eye the simplest form of nature is found to be full of excitement and fresh beauty to the quiet, respectful observer. As we look more closely, the treasure house opens fresh doors of wonder until we become absorbed in the perfection of simplicity and the magnificence of the ordinary. I have continued to do this so often during my life that the intrusion in these marshes during the past several years of foreign bodies in smelly motorboats is equivalent to

* A medium-sized heron notable for the booming sounds it utters.

disease attacking the peacefulness of natural beauty. The thought of these disturbers brings resentment; they are not interesting. They upset the natural order, and are unheedful of the beauty around them.

In all observation of a natural state, the more concentrated and penetrating it becomes, so much the more is found to observe, to understand, and over which to marvel. Many people think the Norfolk marshes dull. They abhor the silence, so they bring radios and recorders* and regale the voices of nature with ragtime. These are the same people who love to be on the Jungfraujoch with me and count the roars of avalanches and say, "Stupendous!" while I say, "Dead ends falling off dead beginnings." These are the type of people who also find normal labor dull, but who are thrilled with a forceps operation, a postpartum hemorrhage, or a face presentation. If only they would look closely into uncomplicated labor, observing every change in the mind and body of their patient, how much they would find of absorbing interest, and how all-important the harmony of nature would become!

One day in 1907 I made my first observation upon the pains of childbirth. There were a number of cottages on the Norfolk farm, and I had discovered that when a woman in one of the cottages had her baby, it was an anxious day of woe and sadness. The maids climbed up at our windows to see when the doctor galloped past our house on his horse. My mother went quietly down the drive to the cottage with a basket on her arm in which was a chicken or jelly or something she was taking to Maria, Mary Anne, Robina, or one of the others.

I questioned my mother about this, and she told me that it was a dreadful thing to have a baby. This didn't make sense to me, for as number six of seven children born in eight and a half years, I thought my mother looked awfully well to have gone through seven really dreadful experiences in such a short time! But, owing to the peculiar nature of my extremely pious

* Wooden flutes.

and religious upbringing and my observations on the marshes, I turned to her and said something that was probably the stepping-stone that changed the course of my whole life. "That's not true, Mother! It must be man who is making the mistake, not the God of nature in Whom you have taught me to believe!"

After an awkward moment she said to me, not unkindly, "I think you must realize that these are things you should not discuss. You are much too young to understand. But in time, perhaps, you will realize what a serious thing it is for a woman to have a baby."

For years her answer troubled me, and prompted me to keep my thinking on the subject to myself, but inwardly the direction of my thought had been determined. I had learned by this time that the Creator uses neither the words nor the methods of human beings to obtain results more magnificent than our greatest scientists can ever aspire to. It is an essential law of nature that all species should be reproduced in the safest and easiest manner possible. Two of nature's greatest laws are the law of reproduction and that of the maintenance of the species. If either fails, we all fail.

Sir Thomas Browne's statue stands in the marketplace of my own home town. It was there he lived and wrote the famous *Religio Medici* in the seventeenth century. From the time I was a boy one of his most famous statements has remained in my mind: "Nature does nothing in vain." I have learned nothing new from the work and writings of man. Man's discoveries, innovations, creations, and cleverness are only nature opening a little wider the window through which all knowledge will, in time, be found. Nature separates the apple from the tree. We must learn to work in harmony with the law of nature if life on earth is to survive.

In the following year, 1908, I started my medical career with these impressions already forming in my mind. But my sense of discovery and adventure soon brought me face to face with inflexibility. My chiefs were more rigid and less approachable than any senior staff is today. Their noses were so long, it seemed to me, that when one looked down his at the junior who was inquiring, he became an indistinct object that could not be clearly focused. His questions were an even more distant blur upon the horizon of the great man's dignity. The answer I received in the classroom was, "My dear boy, we are trying to teach you, and before asking questions you don't understand, I suggest . . . etc., etc."

Fortunately, because of my love for sports, I soon learned to appreciate the reality of blunted noses against my boxing gloves. Some of the owners of these previously haughty noses became my lifelong friends. Strangely enough, it was here by the ringside, on the playing field, on the football field, the tennis court, or golf links that my chiefs, off duty, approached their juniors without restraint. Here I learned that they were men of great accomplishment and human understanding. They were people who could laugh at themselves more readily than at their colleagues, and whose hands were always outstretched to receive the grasp of a man who needed guidance and help. A little later on I began to realize that long noses were only lifted as a means of self-protection, protruded when difficult situations or even more difficult questions threatened the proprieties of orthodoxy.

It was my good fortune during the years of my training to have been under the able teaching of Professors Shipley* and Gardiner,† Langley,‡ and Anderson§ at Cambridge. I reveled in the study of zoology, biology, and physiology because of my hobby of natural history. The notions and ideas upon the birth of the young of any phylum, class, or order that I saw or studied filled me with wonder and curiosity. It was not in-

---

* Arthur Everett Shipley, a famous biologist, zoologist, and naturalist.
† Charles Fox Gardiner, known for his work on the use of natural therapeutic agents in the prevention and cure of tuberculosis.
‡ John Baxter Langley, *Via Medica* (London: Hardwick, 1867).
§ Sir Thomas McCall Anderson, *Lectures on Clinical Medicine* (London: The Macmillan Company, 1877); see also John Baxter Langley and Sir Thomas McCall Anderson, *Journal of Physiology*, 1893–94.

herent discernment that drew me to this research, but a resentment that the law of nature should be held responsible for such injustice to women.

I was also privileged in having such men as Rivers* and M. D. W. Jeffereys as my professors for my courses in anthropology. In the years 1908 and 1909 I often sat with one or two of my friends on the floor of Professor Rivers' rooms at Cambridge, drinking tea and eating cookies with him, while listening to much that was fascinating, interesting, and almost terrifying to us undergraduates, as he related the experiences he had had in his life of pioneering work in social anthropology. And Professor Jeffereys had spent thirty years of his life as a government official in East Africa before retiring to a university appointment as Senior Lecturer in Anthropology. From these men and others I learned that we must not draw deductions from small premises!

In 1910, while still at Cambridge, I spent considerable time in collecting varieties of color associations and the visual patterns of numerals. This was especially interesting to me as I have, among other peculiarities, a certain form of color blindness. Later I persuaded some of my musical friends to record the forms and colors connected with sound. We found that, with practice, definite types of color pattern were consistently associated with the characteristic works of different musicians. Here, in musical works, we discovered that the mind of the creative genius not only conveyed clear and unmistakable pictures to us by sensuous auditory paths, but imprinted them on our memories as well. When these pictures were reproduced in mental imagery behind closed eyes, they aroused again in our minds the musical patterns, airs, and harmonies that they represented. Dvořák has painted the simple pathos of the Negro slave; Tchaikovsky has unveiled the panorama of tragedy and woe; Handel has opened our eyes to a great

* William Halse R. Rivers (1864–1922), author of *History of Melanesian Society*, 2 vols. (1914); specialist in experimental medical psychology.

celestial choir massed upon white clouds beneath the azure dome of heaven, flinging its song of praise across the amphitheater of illimitable space. Thus I found that sights, sounds, and associations, real and imaginary, imprinted themselves upon the human mind, molding and influencing its present reactions to past experiences.

These observations later raised in my mind the question concerning what mental image might be within the mind of a woman in labor, and how this might influence her actions at that time. But I still kept such thoughts and impressions to myself, unable to find anyone with whom I felt free to share. Once I mentioned this in a letter home, and my mother replied: "I know that you are lonely; it is possible that you will be for many years. But we are close together in spirit and you are never alone, for God is with us both."

During my four years as a medical student at Cambridge, on only one occasion did I gather courage to ask specifically about pain in childbirth. I was watching one of the experiments by Professor Langley, in his study of the sympathetic nervous system. In this instance the nerves to a cat's uterus were being stimulated with nicotine, and I asked, "Is it possible that these sympathetic nerves have some bearing upon pain in the uterus during childbirth in a human being?" Professor Langley looked up sharply, and then, after a moment's pause, said, very quietly and very slowly, "Yes—yes, that is indeed possible." That is all that was ever said on the subject.

In 1912 my internship began at the London Hospital. It is situated in the heart of the East End slums in an area called Whitechapel, where fifteen hundred to two thousand patients passed through the outpatient department every day. It was an exciting and a busy time for me. On the surgical side I felt that I was dealing with real science, and on the physician's side with humanity, which interested me even more. But nothing so far turned my interest so close to excitement as gynecology and obstetrics. When I first arrived I had not yet seen for myself what childbirth was really like, but felt that at last I was on the threshold of discoveries that would help answer the troubling questions in my heart and mind concerning it.

Among the women I attended at Whitechapel there was one in 1913 whose casual remark had a far-reaching influence on me. The whole picture made an indelible impression upon my mind, although at the time I had no idea that it was the seed that would eventually alter the course of my life.

I had plowed through mud and rain on my bicycle between two and three in the morning down Whitechapel Road, turning right and left, and innumerable rights and lefts, before I came to a low hovel by the railway arches. Having groped and stumbled my way up a dark staircase, I opened the door of a room about ten feet square. There was a pool of water lying on the floor. The window was broken; rain was pouring in; the bed had no proper covering and was kept up at one end by a sugar box. My patient lay covered only with sacks and an old black skirt. The room was lit by one candle stuck in the top of a beer bottle on the mantel shelf. A neighbor had brought in a jug of water and a basin; I had to provide my own soap and towel. In spite of this setting—which even at that time, near the turn of the century, was a disgrace to any civilized country—I soon became conscious of a quiet kindliness in the atmosphere.

In due course the baby was born. There was no fuss or noise. Everything seemed to have been carried out according to an ordered plan. There was only one slight dissension; I tried to persuade my patient to let me put the mask over her face and give her some chloroform when the head appeared and the dilatation of the outlet was obvious. She, however, resented the suggestion, and firmly but kindly refused to take this help. It was the first time in my short experience that I had ever been refused when offering chloroform. As I looked at her, I saw an expression on her face that showed she hoped she hadn't hurt my feelings by refusing the offer.

As I was about to leave some time later, I asked her why it

was she would not use the mask. She did not answer at once, but looked from the old woman who had been assisting to the window through which was bursting the first light of dawn. Then, shyly, she turned to me and said, "It didn't hurt. It wasn't meant to, was it, Doctor?"

For weeks and months afterward, as I sat with women in labor, women who appeared to be in the terror and agony of childbirth, that sentence came drumming back into my ears: "It wasn't meant to, was it, Doctor?"

That young woman doesn't know what a tremendous fund of comfort and happiness her casual but purely honest cockney remark has made to the women of the world. So it is from the seeds dropped unknowingly and in unexpected places that the greatest trees may grow.

Not long after successfully completing my final medical examinations at the London Hospital, I was called into military service, as World War I was raging. Dejected, I wrote home that "I had hoped my life would be in the reproduction of the human race. I don't want to be called on now to attend to those who are mutilated, and watch them die!" But England was at war, and, like countless other young men, I had no choice but to serve my country. I was attached as a doctor to an ambulance unit, and soon sent overseas to Gallipoli.

I do not lightly recall my most hideous hour; it was in August 1915, shortly after we had landed at Suvla Bay. My watch upon the beach began at 2:00 A.M. On the edge of the mud of Salt Lake, crystal-coated and faintly glistening in the brilliant starlight of a moonless sky, was my first-aid station. Some three hundred badly wounded men were lying shivering in the cold night air; the fierce heat of the day had fled with the fading light, and in a few hours men's breath was frozen on their beards. To those who were in pain I gave the maximum dose of morphia; rifles and bayonets used as splints required adjusting; tourniquets had to be released and reapplied. Water was scarce, but some could ill afford to be left without their share of our meager supply. The monotony of this round was depressing, for there were no ships' boats to take the wounded off the beach. From time to time, Death seemed to reach down from the empty spaces and seize this man or that, and, on each round I made, a carcass lay where but a short time past I had heard courageous words of patience and gratitude.

I sat to rest upon a mound of sand from which I could hear any call from my stricken flock, and wondered if the living knew that their silent neighbors had passed on. It became so still that only the breathing of the sleepers could be heard, and suddenly I became aware of utter loneliness. I thought afterward that some instinctive warning brought that strange desire to fly. In fact, such an impulse was unthinkable, but in theory at least I was reacting to an undefined fear. I had not many moments to wait for the explanation: from only a mile across the bare lake, on Chocolate Hill, a rifle was fired, rending the stillness so unexpectedly that I started and became alert. It was followed by a sound of war that still rings in my memory, more terrifying than the bombs of World War II that are bursting near by as I pen these lines, falling close enough to rock the lamp on my table.

It was the sound of a bayonet charge; the lights leaped from beyond the hill; the shrill yells of madness and bloodlust mingled with the wild whoops and screams of victor and vanquished. A few revolver shots, and soon the lights died down. The stillness was a thousand times more intense after that mad quarter of an hour. I knew our line was feebly held by tired and battle-strained troops. I peered into the distant blackness, wondering who had won. Had the Turks broken through, and should I see the gleam of steel and the fire of mad eyes looming up from the darkness?

I would have given anything within my power to have had a trusted companion with me, even if only to ask him who he thought had won. But I was alone, and that sickening doubt wore down my vitality. I stumbled, tired and frozen, around my patients; my hand shook as I held the water bottle to their lips; my eyes turned unwillingly, but half expectantly, to the black mile that stretched to Chocolate Hill. My mind ran riot, and I suffered agonies of apprehension and fear. Not long after, dawn broke in gray and purple lines across the hills. The doctor who was to relieve me came with the first rays of the sun, and he asked me about the night. I gave him my report, and he looked at me and said, "You look worn out. What's wrong?" He was an old Cambridge friend of mine, and my answer was: "I have never known before how frightful loneliness can be."

The landing on the sixth of August several days earlier, with its hail of fire over our heads, had been the reality of slaughter, but it was not so fearsome as that lonely night on which I died a hundred deaths. Later on I was in many battles —on the Somme, at Ypres, Arras, Amiens, and Cambrai; Bourlon Wood, Farbus, Flecquiere Wood, Fampoux and a dozen others where there was ample reason to be afraid—but I never suffered so acutely in any of these as when I learned that night what loneliness can mean.

Perhaps that is the reason why I shudder when I pass the door of those wards where women lie alone, enduring the first stage of labor with no understanding of what is taking place, fearfully imagining what greater agonies may await them.

One day while still at Gallipoli, a shell burst over me and I was seriously injured. Some time later I regained consciousness enough to discover that I was on a hospital ship, a converted cattle boat, bound for Malta. There I was taken, along with the other wounded survivors, to the Blue Sisters Convent for medical care. As I sit with women in labor, I not infrequently remember those dark days in 1915 when I arrived there, blind in one eye and with clouded vision in the other, almost completely paralyzed below the waist, weakened by dysentery, my pulse at thirty, and with a raging fever. The surgeon would have removed my injured eye if he had not been so pressed with caring for those he thought more likely to survive. As the weeks slowly passed I longed to live, yet at the same time wished that I could escape from life.

I recall the horror of those sympathetic visitors who brought me flowers I could not see; told me to cheer up, I should soon be home. "Remember how lucky you are to be alive," was their parting comfort. It made my whole body burn with agonizing tension; my head throbbed and uncontrollable twitchings came into my legs; my spine felt as if it were torn in two at its fractured vertebra. I perspired, and had I been able would have yelled in a wild mixture of pain and fury.

One of the sisters came in after they had gone and saw me alone in my trouble. I had been given a room to myself. She was a tall, stern-looking woman of some fifty years whose features I could not clearly define. She took my hand in hers and stood silently beside me. After a time she knelt beside my bed, and in broken English said: "I will stay with you. We will be peaceful, you in your way and I in mine."

Can I ever forget the miracle of that understanding? My back relaxed and ceased to torture me; the uncontrollable spasms left my legs; my clouded eye seemed to clear, and before I sank into my first long sleep for weeks I saw her head bowed and her eyes closed as she sought in her own way the peace that swept over me.

We may all have our own way of bringing peace to women in labor, but it is in the end a balm of restfulness to a tired mind—a mind that has no energy to withstand the irritations that intensify its discomforts.

I finally recovered enough to be sent home to England for further rehabilitation, fifty-six pounds lighter than my usual hundred and ninety pounds. Determined not to remain a lifelong cripple, I cooperated fully with the hospital program of heat and massage to restore feeling to my legs. Grimly I exercised my useless legs day after day and week after week, until gradually coordination began to return.

Because of the great shortage of doctors on the battle front, I was sent back to active duty in foreign lands soon after regaining the use of my limbs. This time I was attached to a cavalry unit. One of the things that occupied my mind during quieter hours was the weighing of the reactions of the men around me to danger. I described my reactions in long letters home:

I am not pretending to like shells nor to pose as a fearless fire-eater. I know well enough how I loathe it all. The excitement for me is the fight between body and mind. Instinctively I should run away, fly to cover although the shell is nowhere near. But of course one doesn't. I have that instinct more or less under control. Then comes the fight to stand still, to continue dressing a wounded man; not to start or jump but to continue talking, eating, writing.

People will confound and muddle the terms "fearless," "brave," "heroic," "gallant." The fearless man cannot be brave, he has no physical fear (and there are such). He has no battle of the mind versus body. He can be heroic or gallant—but never brave. The only brave man, to my mind, is the one who is afraid. That sounds like a paradox. But the man who cannot breathe because of fright, who is pallid, whose legs shake and whose voice quivers, who feels death at his very throat, at whom each shell is personally aimed, but who yet forces his legs up the embankment, who sees men fall back dead and wounded, who forces words of encouragement through his teeth and leads the first wave over; that is the man.

He is the man who has all the glory for me. He is the best fighter, fighting as no other man can, because suddenly the bonds of fear become loosened and the whole tense physical strain relaxes into an overwhelming reaction.

It is no honor to be fearless; it is a gift. To be brave is more than glorious. If I won honors or died, I could wish for nothing less than for it to be said of me, "He went fearlessly into his duty." That is no praise! It is but making light of an arduous duty. Let it be said of me: "He was afraid, but went because it was his duty." Then honor is earned.

I am afraid. I have not won so far because I have not yet had a severe test compared to many. I am not brave, and that does not apply only to war. There are many things at home around which the same conflict rages. What I want you to do for me is to send me the thoughts to win on. And if I am not here to write, you will know that I have won. . . .

But I learned more on the battlefield than just from observations of myself and the men around me. It was during this time that I witnessed several women having their babies in the most natural and apparently painless manner. But I also saw those who suffered pain and to whom the birth of their child was an experience horrible to remember, and weighed in my mind what it was that made such a difference. I learned more that was to be of service to me in obstetrics than I would ever have learned had I remained safely in England.

On one occasion a young woman approached the trench and asked for a doctor. The soldiers brought her to me, as she was obviously very pregnant. I had sacks hung up at the end of the dugout and placed her on a stretcher there, while the orderlies on the other side of the improvised screen continued dressing the wounded men who were being brought in. I examined her and found her well advanced in labor. She seemed to be having no discomfort at all. Soon the baby appeared and all was well. She seemed bolivious to the noise of war all around us, sat up on the stretcher, laughed, and took the child in her hands at once.

Four British soldiers came to carry her gently away on the stretcher, rather than the usual two. I could not forget the look of joy on her face as she was carried off with her new baby. She probably would have walked away had the soldiers permitted her to do so. If this is childbirth, I thought, how can childbirth be compared, as it is, with the pains and agonies and hopelessness I see among the wounded men who are brought down to this very same place where this child was born?

One day I had been off the base playing polo, and on my way back to camp came across a Flemish woman leaning against a bank in the field where she appeared to have been working. I tethered my horse and walked over to her to see if anything was wrong, telling her both in French and in English that I was a doctor. She spoke only Flemish, but indicated with gestures that she was bearing a child. She did not in any way appear to resent my intrusion. With the recurrence of the contractions, which appeared to me to be out of all proportion in their strength to those of the average European woman, her face became set, not with pain or fear, but with an almost stern sense of expectancy. I sat down and smoked a pipe and waited, knowing enough of this people's customs to realize that no interference would be welcome.

Within a short time a child arrived. It is possible that during the last ten minutes her expectation almost became apprehension. The child appeared when she was in a half-sitting position. She smiled almost immediately. I felt then that my presence was unnoticed. For some minutes the child lay on the ground and cried, and then she took it in her hands. After a time its yells were all that could be demanded of a newly born baby, and I observed that the cord was already like a thin white string. She took this in her fingers, about six inches from the umbilicus, and neatly severed it—whether by tearing or with her long nail I could not see. She wrapped her baby in the cloth that was around her own shoulders and then looked at me and laughed. It may possibly have been five minutes later when contractions recurred, and with minimum effort the afterbirth arrived, certainly with minimum hemorrhage, for there was none that I could see.

I left her then, hastening into the village on horseback to see if any of her people would come to help her home. They appeared unconcerned and shrugged their shoulders, so I galloped back to where I had left her. I met her walking back to the village, carrying her baby.

The spirit of joy, the spirit of happiness and pride at the arrival and sound of the child, appealed to me. I had never seen a cord so rapidly anemic. The separation of the placenta and its expulsion all appeared to be carried out under the influence of the joy that the mother was experiencing. For the first time it entered my mind that this joy was not for nothing, and that this perfect physiological process could not be an accidental occurrence. My visions of postpartum hemorrhage, blue babies that would not breathe, uteri that would not contract, and placentas that would not separate, all seemed entirely foreign to this exhibition of labor, conducted more efficiently than I had ever visualized in my most ambitious moments. Elation, wonder, tenderness, and the pride of creation appeared to combine in a great storm of pleasing emotions, and under their influence the birth of a child had been perfected.

During the war I was transferred from my unit to the Indian Cavalry Corps, as deputy assistant director of Medical Services. One of the black-bearded Indian officers noticed one day how tired and jumpy I was after having cared for the wounded under fire and losing several men. He approached me and politely asked if he might demonstrate how he and so many of his people overcame tiredness. He explained in great detail how to achieve complete muscular relaxation. Afterwards, on many occasions I recovered from the stress of my duties by relaxing completely on the little broken-down sofa in my quarters, breathing deeply and quietly as he had taught me.

As the end of the war approached I gave many thoughts to my future, and wrote home how I felt about it:

I am not suited to be a general practitioner. My object is not to become popular. It would be madness for such a man to settle down in suburbia. It is far better for him that he should aim at a position where the work matters more than the pay he receives, where the service to which he is called is not constantly and obviously in view, where he is not overloaded with the various social and domestic impediments which have spoiled the work of more than half of our good men in the provinces.

. . . Some months ago I was thinking about things, just sitting quietly with my feet on the table, trying and managing to pick holes in myself. Then I turned and picked up a *New Testament* and read, for no reason at all, *James*. I just seemed to drop on to it and came upon some rather startling phrases when you remember the trend of my thinking. I know that service and not self-aggrandisement is the only life one is justified in living. I *know* it. That is the great subconscious influence governing and guiding the whole trend of my thought, and then I read it as if I had been arguing with James himself: "To him that knoweth to do good and doeth it not, to him it is a sin." That is plain enough, is it not?

Again I was injured near the front—playing football! Some of the men and I were enjoying a bit of recreation on a stretch of open land just beyond reach of the German shells. I was returned to England with a broken leg, shattered by a swift kick in the shin from one of the men who had been aiming at the ball. But I recovered before the Armistice was signed in France. I was reassigned as a brain surgeon in a hospital at Le Havre, meticulously taking shrapnel out of wounded heads.

When eventually the war ended in 1918 I returned to the London Hospital as the senior resident obstetrician, overjoyed to be back in obstetrics. I got out all my old papers and research notes on childbirth and began going over my developing theories again. Here in the hospital I found the same contrast occurring that I had seen on the continent of Europe. Most women seemed to suffer greatly, but here and there I met the calm woman who neither wished for anesthetic nor appeared to have any unbearable discomfort.

It was very difficult to explain why one should suffer and another be free, apparently, from pain. There did not seem to be much difference in the actual labors; they both had to work equally hard; the time factor was not markedly different one from the other. Perhaps those who had suffered had slightly longer labors on an average than those who had less discomfort. In those days we did not know the mechanism of pain as well as we do today, and a good deal was overlooked that certainly would not have passed unnoticed in the light of our present teaching. It slowly dawned on me, however, that it was the peacefulness of the relatively painless labor that distinguished it most clearly from the others. There was a calm, it seemed almost faith, in the normal and natural outcome of childbirth.

So gradually my mind was influenced by these observations to investigate the part played by the emotions in the natural function of reproduction. Was the nature of the labor responsible for the emotional state of the woman, or was the emotional state of the woman to a large extent responsible for the nature of her labor? Which was primary and which secondary? Could it be that fear of impending pain actually set in motion those factors that caused pain?

Fear is not necessarily abnormal; it is a natural protective state. In the presence of danger, fear engendered by knowledge is the stimulus that prompts escape according to that which threatens. For example, we slow down, if we are wise, when passing through dangerous crossroads. There is, however, an exaggerated state of caution. As students at the university we heard many stories about the "height of precaution," like the decrepit old gentleman who always wore the armor of a first-class wicket-keeper when he went out to play croquet.

In childbirth, fear and the anticipation of pain give rise to natural protective tensions in the body. Unfortunately, the natural muscular tension produced by fear also influences the muscles that close the womb and thus delay the progress of the labor and create pain. What I was witnessing in the labor wards of the hospital convinced me of the truth that this aspect of childbirth held. The Whitechapel question still came back to me: "It doesn't hurt. It wasn't meant to, was it, Doctor?"

Now at last I knew that I had found an answer, and that answer was "No. It was not meant to hurt."

19

Prophet Without Honor

It was my good fortune to serve as house physician under Sir Henry Head* for a time after my return to the London Hospital. He is one of the great pioneer neurologists whose writings have helped form the framework for the later rise of the branch of science known as psychosomatic medicine. He demonstrated that somatic or physical changes may occur as the direct result of psychological states. I had the privilege of many conversations with him. These were always a source of great pleasure, because of his enthusiasm not only for his specialty but for the art of living. This stimulated most interesting discussions filled with observations upon his wide experience of human relationships.

Knowing my interest in gynecology and obstetrics, he turned my attention on a number of occasions to the mind of woman and its activities under different circumstances. The obstetric orthodoxy of the day required the mother to be drugged into unconsciousness during labor and birth to spare her from "suffering." Nothing is more to be abhorred. The forceps deliveries of normal babies—blue and flabby babies who will not cry, babies drugged and anesthetized, were common pictures in current practice.

As senior resident obstetrician I began probing deeply into

* Sir Henry Head, *Studies in Neurology* (London: Oxford Medical Publications, 1920) and *Henry Head Centenary*, ed. K. W. Cross *et al.* (New York: St. Martin's Press, Inc., 1961).

my patients' backgrounds, hoping for more clues, observing their state of mind. I sat for long hours at their bedsides in labor, seeking to ascertain the strength of the relationship of fear and tension to pain. In every spare moment I searched through every textbook that might provide a clue. I could not relax until I was satisfied that I had found an answer.

And then, in 1919, when I was nearly thirty years old, I gathered together my conclusions from my copious notes into a manuscript painstakingly written out in longhand, hoping eventually to have it published. I had had no one with whom I could share my views freely, but finally I gained courage to present it to my three obstetric professors for their evaluation. They were kind men, and accepted the manuscript graciously.

For some time there was no response. But finally I was called in to meet with them and given their decision. "Look here, old chap," the spokesman of the three said quietly. "The truth is we think you really ought to learn something about obstetrics before you start writing on the subject."

Deep in my heart I had known that this would be their reaction. Although my thesis still contained a great deal of orthodoxy that I had not yet discovered could be discarded, it still represented a major change from current obstetric thinking. "All right. I'll learn," I told them. Returning to my room I buried the manuscript and notes deep into my trunk and went for a long walk alone through the gray, dismal back streets of the East End slums. I never brought up the subject again while at the London Hospital.

When the time came for permanent appointments to the hospital staff to be made, I was passed over, much to the astonishment of my fellow classmates. This meant I had to leave my loved work in obstetrics and go into general practice after all.

Soon after entering general practice, in partnership with an elderly physician in a small town away from London, I married, and in due time our first child arrived. I was not permitted to be present, and was found, when informed of the child's birth, reading the daily paper, apparently calmly—except that the paper was upside down! This, I regret to say, was true, for every obstetric abnormality I had ever seen was, to my knowledge, occurring upstairs.

A few years later, in May 1926, I entered into a clinic practice with three other doctors so that I could devote my time completely to obstetrics. The idea of specialists working together from a single clinic was such a new concept in medical circles that what we had done was not well received. A wave of resentment among the doctors who heard of our action set in, and one of them reported us to the ethical committee of the local division of the British Medical Association. They investigated us, but eventually ruled in our favor.

Now at last I could concentrate fully on my specialty, continuing to apply my theories to my patients, perfecting my methods both from their comments and from my own observations. On one occasion I had spent three hours with a girl of nineteen, and just at the beginning of the second stage of labor she assured me that everything was fine. She had learned how to conduct herself and her labor, and everything was going extremely well when her mother tiptoed into the room. Wearing an agonized expression on her face, she went to the other side of the bed and took her daughter's hand. She stood there during the next contraction, and then, with tears rolling down her cheeks, whispered, "Darling, if only I could bear some of your agony for you!" Fortunately, by that time my patient had transferred her confidence to me, because she smiled at her mother and said, "Yes, it must be painful for you to watch. Now please go." I added in a stage whisper, "Yes, please go."

I shall never forget the harassed, agonized expression on the face of another nineteen-year-old girl whose doctor had sent for me. The labor had been slow, and the mother-in-law—a perfect example of one of the major pests of parturition—rushed dramatically into the driveway and flung open the door of my car before the chauffeur could leap from his seat. She tugged my arm and cried, "Come, oh come quickly. They are killing my daughter. Save her! Save her!" I ceased to be popular when I looked down upon her and asked with a smile, "From whom?"

The scene upstairs was one of tribulation and turmoil. The girl, uncovered from the waist downward, was biting a towel that had been stuffed into her mouth. When I entered the room the towel was taken from her mouth, and she flung a tired arm across the bed to me and said, "For God's sake give me peace!"

There was nothing abnormal in her labor except its conduct. Each contraction had been a signal for loud shouts of "Push, shove, pull, hang on!" Pressure on the abdomen alternated with the raising of the left buttock to see if the child was appearing. Nurse, doctor, and even mother-in-law gazed at the inoffensive outlet in an agony of anticipation. But the cervix was not fully dilated. It was suggested that they were all very tired; I advised a large brew of tea—downstairs, away—and a cup of tea for the patient and myself upstairs, weak and warm. In one hour a normal second stage had produced a healthy baby. A few whiffs of gas just at crowning time, for she was still very alarmed, and peace reigned. The pitiable request of that girl, tortured by the turmoil of her parturition, "For God's sake give me peace!" embedded itself in my mind and left an indelible impression of the power of calmness and confidence.

It had become obvious to me long before this that the first place to strike in eliminating pain was at the cause of tension. An aphorism was already imprinted on my mind: "Tense woman—tense cervix." All obstetricians know the effect of a tense cervix: pain, resistance at the outlet and the innumerable complications of a prolonged labor, with probably an operative finale. I believed the cause of tension to be fear. Restoring a measure of confidence to this badly frightened young woman had released tension enough to produce the baby without difficulty within a short period of time.

However, the fear of childbirth originated from so many

sources and from such high places that the whole scheme of society would have to be altered if the attack were made at the source! It was equally obvious to me that those who had suffered were very unlikely to refrain from saying so, and even less likely to preach that their suffering was unnecessary. It was also rather difficult to go around saying that the Bible and the Prayer Book did not really mean what they said on the subject! The Prayer Book had not been altered since 1662, and contained a special service known as "The Churching of Women":

Forasmuch as it hath pleased Almighty God of his Goodness to give you safe deliverance, and hath preserved you in the great danger of childbirth; you shall therefore give hearty thanks unto God and say . . . "The snares of death compassed me round about and the pains of hell gat hold upon me. I found trouble and heaviness, and I called upon the name of the Lord . . . I was in misery and he helped me. . . . Thou has delivered my soul from death."

Oh, Almighty God, we give Thee humble thanks for that Thou hast vouchsafed to deliver this woman, Thy servant, from the great pain and peril of childbirth.

And finally, I came to the conclusion that it would not be much fun to shake a theory in the face of my contemporaries in the attempt to persuade them that all our greatest obstetricians were wrong, and on no account should anyone believe what they were saying! It appeared to me to be rather like a flyweight squaring up in the corner to not one, but a dozen professional heavyweights.

It will be seen that the correct line of procedure was not obvious. On the other hand, I must own to a profound affection for my theory, and that, combined with a modicum of quiet pigheadedness that always stimulates a Norfolk man to discount odds, prompted me to get on with it without further "quavery mavery." Thus I began making an effort to educate women in the facts of childbirth during their pregnancy, in addition to striving to calm their fears during the labor itself. I soon received encouragement, for many women instinctively felt the truth and disbelieved in the necessity for suffering.

At first this did not appear to be enough, for too often, as soon as labor began, the exaggerated receptivity of the mind to all forms of stimulus, both physical and psychical, swept aside their good intentions. Some method had to be found to overcome this main weapon of the enemy, which was muscular tension.

So the practice of physical relaxation that I had learned from the Indian officer during the war was introduced. I had my patients learn to relax well, applying it during the last four or five months of pregnancy for health reasons. Again in labor they were to relax all muscle tension. It was found that when the muscles were flaccid the mind remained at rest. More gratifying than anything was that the interpretations of the sensations experienced during labor were not invariably that of pain.

Relying almost entirely on this simple, Oriental method of muscular relaxation, in a short time I was more astonished than my patients. In the absence of turmoil, anguish, and misunderstanding, many of the phenomena of labor appeared in their true light. After not more than two years the results of the application of these procedures had not only established my own belief but—what was more important—the large majority of the women whose labors had been conducted in accordance with them had an entirely new attitude toward childbirth.

It was during this period that I began including the husbands in prenatal education, encouraging them to learn and to be with their wives during labor and birth. Our clinic practice was prospering, and my file of case histories growing. Each time I returned from attending a birth I carefully recorded all details of the case, the woman's attitude, and my own handling of the labor and birth, including my mistakes.

By 1929 evidences and experiences in homes and hospitals satisfied me and a large number of patients that the effort to learn and follow the untarnished physiological pattern of normal childbirth was acceptable to nine out of ten women who knew there was such a procedure. I began preparing a book on childbirth, working from my 1919 manuscript and compiling material from the massive library of case histories that I had been building. I did most of my writing at night. Now for the first time since my mother's rebuff to my boyish question during my teen years, I ventured to bring up the subject to her again by letter:

My work has led me to a line of thought which I believe will become of tremendous importance to all women one day. It is to the end that motherhood in the normal case is not a painful and terrifying proceeding but one which is without pain and beautiful beyond all other experiences.

Since the work has developed, a large number of women have testified to the truth of the teaching. Without any anesthetic and with no pain or discomfort they have learned the joy of natural motherhood. To have had children has been their greatest happiness and the act of childbirth has been the most wonderful experience of their lives.

Now you will agree that is a work which may justifiably enthuse any man. It is a service which it is more than a privilege to render. If motherhood can become a painless joy, how great a change in the whole nation. That is my ambition . . .

But behind my enthusiasm is the drag—opposition to my greatest usefulness. Again my old enemy, professional jealousy, is working slowly to take away from me what might make me so worthwhile to others. But this time I say: "NO! It is too big to give up." It is my only justification for being alive at all.

And so I go on firmly, quietly, certainly. Perhaps in the end the Prayer Book will be altered . . . and there will just be a simple thanksgiving that a woman has, by God's grace, been admitted to the joy and wonder of motherhood and all the marvels of child-birth—God's greatest miracle.

You will keep this confidential to just us, won't you? It has been so nice to write this; so grand to have you still there, so many years after my leaving home, to pour out my whims and my grouses, my ideals and ambitions, knowing that you will understand and sympathize.

By 1930 my manuscript was completed, and I chose as a title the words *Natural Childbirth*. Before submitting it to a publisher I first showed it to one of my personal friends, Dr. John Fairbairn, who was at that time one of Britain's finest obstetricians. He returned it to me later, thanked me for letting him see it, but then added, "Look here, my boy" (He still called me "my boy," even though I was over forty!), "you aren't really going to publish this, are you?" I told him that I hoped to.

He said soberly, "It will ruin your practice, you know. Ruin it!" I asked him why, and he replied, *"Because it's true,* my boy. It's true. But it's a truth which will not be accepted by our profession. If you can stand having that sort of trouble, go on, but if not, then my advice is that you should give it up." He patted my arm, and left.

In the months that followed I submitted the manuscript to one publisher after another, all of whom rejected it, some without comment, some with formal "regrets." Finally, two years later, William Heinemann (Medical Books), Ltd., accepted it for publication with certain reservations, upon recommendation of Dr. Johnston Abraham, a well-known London surgeon who was one of their directors. A letter from them in October 1932 stated:

We have now received the report from our reader on your manuscript and while he considers it an extremely interesting work, full of valuable ideas, he does not think, owing to the fact that you have no definite obstetrical appointment and are comparatively unknown, that it would have any commercial value for a large sale.

If you like, we will be pleased to publish it at your expense with the proviso that as soon as we have sold a sufficient number of copies to cover our cost, the money will be returned to you and a royalty paid on subsequent sales. We shall only print 1,000 copies to start with and probably 500 will have to be sold before the cost is covered. If this idea appeals to you, will you be good enough to let me know and we will send you an estimate for same.

It was nine months before the book was ready for publication, but in 1933 *Natural Childbirth* was published, and not only did the subject become controversial but the author "a controversial figure"! At first the book was received with gentle kindliness, more like sympathy, by my colleagues in obstetrics. The first reviews were surprisingly favorable. When my friends heard what I had found off the beaten track, they listened politely—much too politely for my comfort.

After the initial fairly favorable response, the reaction set in. My clinic partners dissolved our relationship, bringing against me charges of unprofessional conduct. For a year my professional life hung in the balance. I could not legally practice until the charges were resolved. Ten months later the court cleared me of every charge for lack of evidence, and I was free to open a practice on my own.

But it was difficult to find patients. At first I did not understand why, until someone informed me that I had been anonymously reported to the General Medical Council for advocating cruelty to women! Husbands called me on the phone to cancel appointments for their wives. Pregnant women hurried past my door like scalded cats. But in spite of it all I was satisfied to be nobody with something special, rather than somebody with nothing.

On the advice of friends, I applied for a Chair of Obstetrics that was vacant at one of the universities. My application was rejected. During this difficult period my health became affected. The old war injuries in my back and legs caused increasing pain and paralysis. I was able to get around with difficulty by using walking canes, but could only manipulate stairs to reach my patients by dragging up on hands and knees.

But encouragements as well as discouragements began coming. Eventually my practice began to grow again, prospering far more than it had in group practice. I maintained a second office on Harley Street in London during part of each week.

I began receiving an increasing number of invitations to lecture on obstetrics. In 1933, before the Ninth British Congress of Obstetrics and Gynecology I read a paper that I called "Prophylaxis of Fear," using that name to explain how to prevent the pain of uncomplicated childbirth. I was invited to address religious gatherings as well as medical groups, in which talks I laid stress upon the family and the importance of the husband's role. Among the addresses I made were to two conferences of Catholic priests in 1936, one in March on "Psychological Aspects of Maternal Welfare," and one in July on "Maternal Happiness," explaining the importance of the husband for a woman's good childbirth experience.

I was invited to contribute a chapter in Professor Francis James Browne's textbook, *Antenatal and Postnatal Care*,* which was published in 1935. Apart from my own book, this was the first time that either the practice of relaxation during childbirth, or the thesis relating to the cause of pain, "The Fear-Tension-Pain Syndrome," had ever been published and widely circulated in the medical world.

From America a letter of encouragement came from Joseph De Lee, Emeritus Professor of Obstetrics at the University of Chicago, dated June 29, 1936:

I thank you for the book (*Natural Childbirth*) which you have kindly autographed.

I had already been reading the book, having obtained one of the first copies that came from the press. I agree with you to a very great extent on the thesis which you have therein set forth.

It may interest you to know that I loaned your book to Dr. Paul de Kruif, who made rather extensive references in some articles that he wrote for the *Ladies' Home Journal*.

I will incorporate some of these ideas in the next edition of my book on obstetrics,† which will probably be finished some time in 1938.

With best regards . . .

These encouragements made me eager to complete a more comprehensive book on the subject. Dr. Johnston Abraham

---

* London: J. & A. Churchill Ltd., 1935.

† Joseph B. De Lee, *The Principles and Practice of Obstetrics*, 7th ed. (Philadelphia: W. B. Saunders Company, 1938), pp. 339–340.

assured me that Heinemann would publish it, and Dr. Browne kindly offered to read the proofs.

When De Lee's book came out in 1938 he wrote: "It will take several thousand generations before we can train women back to the state which Grantly Dick-Read speaks of as 'Natural Childbirth.'" Because of his comment, it seemed best to prepare my new book as a teaching book addressed to women, and once again I spent long nights poring over my notes, and writing. I am sure that, had this great obstetrician lived, he would have modified his opinion concerning the ability of women to learn, for he set up an experiment using a hundred of his former students to examine the procedures. At the end of the experiment he announced the principles as sound and wrote asking if I could hurry along the completion of the new book. A few weeks later he died without having seen it.

My growing practice and lecture opportunities made progress on the book slow, but I learned from these as well. I was lecturing one time in a large county center. There were a number of medical personnel present, as well as two or three hundred practicing midwives who listened appreciatively to my observations. The matron, whose brilliant career at a London maternity hospital justified her appointment to a large county maternity organization, rose to speak. She spoke with simplicity and a charm of manner that accentuated the sincerity of her revelation:

"I feel it is the moment to disclose a secret. For a long time after I became matron I failed to understand why so many women asked to be looked after by the nurses and not by the medical men who attend the hospital. I was constantly embarrassed by the situations which arose, and finally decided to inquire why the request was so frequently and so urgently made. The reply I had was astonishing: 'Because the doctors all make us have chloroform whether we want it or not, and the nurses don't.'"

The matron in another maternity home told me, "The more

I see of this natural childbirth, the more I am persuaded that education is what really matters." I asked her frankly if there was any obvious difference in the conduct of labor in my cases from those of other obstetricians who also practiced there. She said, "Yes, in your technique, but the outstanding difference is in the women. They seem to know their job before they start. They understand why relaxation helps and why it prevents pain in labor. . . ."

Two brilliant and progressive headmistresses of large girls' schools in England became persuaded that the teaching of elementary biology and anatomy should be extended, in the higher classes at school, to human structure and reproductive function. It was believed that confidence in discussion would make it easier for girls to have a balanced acceptance of womanhood upon leaving school. But before introducing the subject they felt it necessary to obtain the opinions of the parents of the three hundred girls in one of the schools, as a guide to what the reaction would be in all the others. The response was prompt and dogmatic. If, under the guise of biology and physiology, the parents said, their daughters were to be introduced to the subject of sex and reproduction while still in school, they would be removed immediately!

The tremendous need for such training was brought home very closely to me when one of my own daughters, at the age of seventeen, made these remarks in her weekly letter home: "Jenny's mother is going to have another baby; she is terribly upset about it and awfully worried because her mother told her it was absolute hell. Isn't it too frightful for her?"

It was near the end of the term, so I did not reply in any controversial manner, but neither did I waste any time at the beginning of the holidays in introducing my daughter to the opinions of those who not only entirely disagree with Jenny's mother, but who would have liked to tell her of the infinite harm this effort to gain the sympathy of her daughter had done. To my own child this was an example of the hearsay with which sooner or later all girls become familiar, even in those schools where it is not a frequent subject of conversation among the girls themselves.

One problem that frequently confronted my patients was the unhappiness of the other women in labor. One of my patients was very comfortable and progressing well toward second stage when the loud cries and moans of a woman in labor from a neighboring ward floated through to the peaceful room in which we were situated. My patient hastily grasped my hand, looked appealingly at me, and said, "How unnecessary it is that she should suffer. Can't you go and help?" I said that I was indeed grieved, but it was no business of mine to interfere uninvited with other cases. I assured her that the chances were the cries were not of suffering, but of fear, and under the influence of narcotic drugs. About an hour later, from the ward on the other side, groans obvious to me to be those of a woman in real pain came loudly across the passage. In a few minutes we heard clearly the crescendo of her screams for help. This was extremely disturbing to my patient, who said, "Surely that is not another?"

I explained to her that a perfectly competent doctor was attending her, because I had gone out to see whether she was asking for help that could be given by me. This went on for an unhappy quarter of an hour and I was afraid it would disrupt the harmony of my own patient's labor. But she proceeded quietly, saying, "I am not having any pain, why should they?" Some time later her baby was born perfectly.

Two women medical students were present at her labor. They had asked to see how natural childbirth was conducted. I was as much interested in the expressions upon their faces as I was in the normal, peaceful birth that I was conducting. Their mouths opened, and, in silence, their eyes opened wider and wider. They looked at the woman as though she were mad or demented; they failed to understand that she was speaking the truth. They had, each of them, seen and conducted many labors, but did not realize the importance of certain simple phenomena of labor that can only appear under these conditions. As I came away after the birth, one of them commented,

"It's perfectly simple to have a baby like that. If that is what obstetrics means, there is nothing in it." I replied, "Exactly. Obstetricians are essential to deal with the abnormal—they should not complicate the normal."

When I stopped by to see my patient later, she asked about the two other women whose babies had been born that same night. I told her in plain words that all was well with them, but did not tell her that one of the women had been deeply anesthetized for an hour and a half, her child extracted by forceps, and a large tear of her perineum repaired. The other one had had her perineum repaired later in the night. I kept for myself all thoughts, and merely left her with the knowledge that they were two mothers with two babies.

All this did not endear me to some of my colleagues! There were those who encouraged and helped, but there were others who not only disagreed, but continued to make a number of untrue accusations. The most frequent and most damaging of these continued to be that I did not allow anesthesia or anything else to relieve pain. This accusation was brought to my notice by a doctor whose wife wanted me to attend her. He had read a book in the medical library that stated that I would not give anesthesia. I knew at once the book to which he referred. It was popular with medical students because it was short and easy to read. The author never corrected the statement, although he knew full well that it was a deliberate falsehood. My teaching on this has always been clear: (1) no woman should be allowed to suffer; (2) analgesia must always be available for the woman to use if she needs it; (3) analgesia is to be administered according to the clinical indication and the judgment of the attending physician.

One lady wrote and told me my name should be struck off the medical register; such inhumanity was unbelievable in our enlightened age. Society whispered that I sat and watched women writhe in agony. A doctor who had intended to invite me to attend his wife wrote and explained that he did not think I was quite good enough as an obstetrician.

Another startling accusation was that there was some kind

of mystic quality I possessed that made the good results possible, but of course other physicians were not so endowed and could thus be excused from even trying to achieve the same results. Others dismissed the results as a kind of personal hypnotism. Frankly, when I saw myself in the mirror mornings, I hesitated, for one brief moment, before even considering this distinction!

I had considered hypnotism in my early research, along with anesthesia and every other means of relieving suffering, but had dismissed the thought of learning to use it. Why hypnotize when education and understanding give better results? Hypnotism only hides the phenomena of normal labor behind the ephemeral curtain of disassociated consciousness.

It is true that I possessed one personal quality that helped make the good results possible. But it is a quality I share with tens of thousands of other doctors the world over. It is said by psychologists that in the subconscious mind of woman there are but two types of men—those who injure and abstract from her and those who protect and give to her. The first of these is the materialization of cruelty, and the second the personification of kindness.

There is no more definite division of men than that which is found among the attendants upon women in labor. For, without any question, some by their presence alone stimulate the normal neuromuscular activities of parturition, and others, in spite of the utmost sympathy, appear to cause delay and suffering. In short, there are "motor men" and "inhibitory men" in obstetrics.

An example of the sympathetic yet inhibitory physician is a medical man I once overheard try to encourage his patient. "Ha, ha. Cheer up, old girl. You've got to go through hell, but I'll go anywhere with you, so keep smiling. Ha, ha!" Then there are others who inhibit because they are prompted by the impulses necessary for the perfection of the work *they* have to do during parturition.

Fortunately there are many others who are truly activated by motives of kindness and human understanding, willing to assist the woman in her work of giving birth and to let her be the "star" of the show. These I characterize as "motor men." One of the many accusations made against me was that I was a "motor man," but this I did not mind.

One thing I would never do was to induce labor unnecessarily or hurry things along for my own convenience. We still hear of normal cases having the membranes ruptured early or the labor induced in some other way, so the physician can get the case over in time to do this or that. We still hear of anesthesia and forceps being employed to assist in the maintenance of a social program, and even for the purely selfish motive that it is the quickest method. Obstetricians are sometimes busy men, but there is no reason why busy men should not be good obstetricians! I have frequently been told, "But my dear so-and-so, I simply do not have time to do all this. There are other things to attend to, and other things to be done."

For three years in succession my summer holiday was planned for three weeks, giving ten days clear at each end from any booked dates for births. Each year from ten to fifteen days of that three weeks had to be sacrificed to infants who insisted upon remaining *in utero*. It is not surprising that my family had a poor opinion of obstetrics as a hobby! To invite friends to dine was to precipitate a labor during dinner, and to fulfill a long-standing promise of a family evening at the theater was practically impossible. The special days of the school term when the children looked forward to a visit from their "baby doctor" father were frequently days of disappointment.

Late in the summer of 1939 I had finally been able to take my family for a short two-week holiday at the beach. On the last Sunday, we were all in church when the pastor made the announcement that war had been declared on Germany just a few minutes before. We hurried back to our home, which was only twenty-five miles from London, only to find it filled with evacuees. Our first air-raid warning came quite soon after, and, in the absence of any proper shelters, the women and children hurried to the cellars in which we have the boilers and furnaces. I stayed upstairs to make tea for the "party," feeling that bomb splinters upstairs were preferable, should they arrive, to a nightgown party in the cellars with females and boys.

My practice on Harley Street in London was gone. My big car had to be put away for lack of fuel, though two small cars were still available for my local practice. During the Christmas holidays that year war and peace were strangely mingled. I sat in my study after an air-raid warning was over one day. Suddenly the irregular zoom of an airplane, quite low and coming toward the house, attracted my attention. I listened and, as I did so, there was a loud, shrieking rush of a heavy bomb seemingly howling past my window.

Within a few yards of the house I found myself at the raised edge of a crater sixty to seventy feet wide and about twenty feet deep. The cottages near were blasted to a ruined, dusty mass of rubble. All of us, including a nurse who was staying with us, worked like Trojans to find some traces of life. By pushing my arm in the rubble I came upon a small hand. It had a pulse, firmly and surely beating.

Hurriedly working my way up the arm I gave directions to the others to clear away the debris from the face to which the hand belonged. Soon the mouth was free, and then the head and shoulders. A little more clearing and I pulled the child out by the shoulders. He was a boy of about twelve, who soon recovered consciousness and was taken away by the nurse.

I delved again and found another hand and arm—but this time, no pulse. The body was quickly pulled out of the wreckage. Together we worked rapidly until all were accounted for, some dead, some surviving.

That evening my daughters gave a previously planned party for about twenty couples. The evening went well. We had no near bombs that night, and at 3:00 A.M. the last guest went out into the darkness, cheerful, war free, and contented. So life and death lived side by side.

Inwardly I had decided to burn my new manuscript. I was

fifty years old, and although my teachings had become known throughout Europe and in America, they were still unacceptable to the majority of medical men in my own country. Besides, no one knew when this dreadful war would end. I gathered up the chapters that were finished, and the notes, and stuck them into a far corner of the library.

Babies keep coming in wartime, too. A doctor's wife had come to the maternity home in labor. As her baby was born, the labor ward was shaken by the concussion of guns and shells; the first cry of the baby was in concert with hordes of German airplanes going over the maternity wards. I looked at the maternity supervisor and we wondered what might happen next. The blitz was at its height, but the mother, who had been very nervous of these things, took her small child in her hands and played with it with all the utter carelessness of joy that only this occasion witnesses. It was an extremely pretty picture.

But as I stood and watched these two, still the German hordes went over our heads; the roar and thrum of their engines, the crash of guns, the bursting of shells, and from time to time the bursting of their bombs seemed to make the picture of peacefulness in that labor ward unreal, ephemeral, or a figment of the imagination. It was the permanent record of humanity at its best, and overhead were the emblems of humanity in its most primitive barbarity.

I think perhaps I shall never forget this series of events. In the immediate presence of childbirth there was no thought of fear within any mind in that labor ward. Our work was the privilege of those who assist in laying the foundations of a fuller life, and our thoughts were far beyond the activities of those who seek to destroy. When I went out, having put on my tin hat and placed my gas mask beside me in the car, and drove the three miles home through the blitz that was harassing the countryside, I was possessed of a sense of elation that here indeed is the true calling of an obstetrician.

20

Man Without a Country

There were bombs and many deaths in those days. It may have been despondency or frustrating incredulity that men, so gloriously born, could be such fools that made me lose all faith in purposeful writing. But my wife Jessica rescued my original manuscript from being consigned to the flames. She found it, unfinished, discarded in the corner of my library. She placed it before me on my table, asked me some rather pointed questions about myself, and finished by saying, "Don't you realize? That is what women have been wanting for centuries!" So, thanks to her encouragement, the book was finished.

In 1942 William Heinemann, Ltd., published *The Revelation of Childbirth*. It was a more complete book upon the principles and practice of natural childbirth than the one I had published nearly ten years before, its thesis tested and perfected during the decade between. It was followed in 1943 by the publication of *Motherhood in the Post-War-World*.

The early reviews of *The Revelation of Childbirth* were not discouraging. The British medical journal, *The Lancet*, spoke of it as "this rather 'Through the Looking-Glass plan,' " but ended by saying, "The book is simple, kindly and often brilliant."

The reviewer in the *British Medical Journal* said:

This book accuses the medical profession in general and the consulting obstetrician in particular of gross mismanagement of all cases of normal pregnancy and labor. . . . In spite of all this, no one can doubt Dr. Read's sincerity and the book contains a message to all who work in the field of midwifery—namely, that the physical condition is considered at the expense of the psychological and that neglect of the latter frequently converts what would have been a normal physiological function into a pathological process.

The *Journal of the American Medical Association* advocated that "this small volume should be read by every obstetrician and every student in the physiology of reproduction."

But some of my colleagues, for whose academic attainments I have great respect, argued: "You assume too much. This is not proved—this is not strictly scientific. We disagree with your neurology and your psychiatry is misleading, therefore you must be wrong."

My reply has been, with all humility: "Yes, of course," and I have returned to the labor ward to be greeted by happy women with their newborn babies in their arms: "How right you are, doctor, it is so much easier that way." Frankly, if there is a whole series of academic flaws in my argument, I cannot be too seriously concerned, for its practical application shows clearly that "it works" with considerable success. My thesis was evolved from observations made by the bedside, not in the laboratory.

Reviews continued to pour in from all over the world, nearly all of them favorable. Natural childbirth became the topic of many lively discussions from Canada to Australia. Requests for translation rights began to come in from several foreign countries and were granted. A request came from Harper's in New York to publish the book in the United States, and it was thus that in 1944 *The Revelation of Childbirth* was published in the States, under the title *Childbirth Without Fear.**

* *Childbirth Without Fear* was published by the staple trade department of Harper & Bros., which was under the direction of George W. Jones for about twenty-six years. The book sold slowly at first, but by the early 1950s had reached a sale of 100,000 copies.
When the sales of a book reached this figure, it was the custom at

At first the book followed a course in the United States similar to the original publication of *Natural Childbirth* in England eleven years previously. It brought new thoughts from an unknown pen and introduced theories upon the pain of labor that appeared at first sight to challenge the validity of much that was considered basic orthodoxy. It did not die, however, but survived in spite of small support from the obstetric field. It was neither obstetric nor academic perspicacity that gave it security, but women, from whom letters began arriving in increasing numbers, thanking me for making possible the beautiful births of their babies, and often relating by contrast previous unpleasant childbirth experiences. Many thousands of similar letters have swelled my files as the years passed.

As the war came to an end, invitations to lecture in other countries increased. Among the invitations was one from the United States that arrived at Christmas time, 1946. The president and board of directors of the Maternity Center Association issued a large number of tickets for a meeting at the Academy of Medicine in New York: "Dr. Grantly Dick-Read of London, England, . . . comes to this country to discuss for the first time on this side of the Atlantic his concepts of natural childbirth. . . ."

Over twenty-five hundred medical personnel were present,

Harper's to have a copy hand bound in leather for the proud author. Grantly Dick-Read was in South Africa at the time, and he and Mr. Jones had not yet met. Mr. Jones had the book leatherbound as was the custom, and shipped to South Africa, "expecting the letter of burbling gratitude authors usually send on such occasions. I was deflated but also amused by Dick's reply, 'Thank you for the handsomely bound book. However, I wish to point out that there are 3½ million babies born every year in the U.S., and I think you have merely scratched the surface.' " When the doctor returned to England he and Mr. Jones became firm friends, and remained so until Dr. Dick-Read's death in 1959.

By the mid-1960s the book had reached a sale of 275,000 hardbound copies in the United States, and a million copies throughout the world. It has been translated into many other languages. —Ed.

an opportunity greater than I had ever had in my own country. The kind reception and interest in the United States overwhelmed me, although not all agreed with my beliefs.

While still in New York I was invited to attend a meeting of the senior obstetric specialists in the city. They gathered once every two weeks to discuss problem cases or current difficulties. I had gone as a spectator, but after the first case had been reviewed the moderator turned to the hundred and twenty or more medical men and women and said, "And now, since we have him here, we'll use him, and he can spend the rest of this session telling us all about his teaching and explaining to us how it works." I need hardly say that before such an illustrious audience, to be thrown unprepared into an hour and a half's lecture and discussion might well have been an ordeal. But again, there was the same spirit of friendliness in our differences of opinion, and we had many reasons for good laughter.

Toward the end of the afternoon a brilliant psychiatrist and scholar, who stood well over six feet, suddenly strode to the foot of the platform and addressed the moderator in a furious voice: "What sort of nonsense is this? Are we supposed to believe his ideas?" He turned on me. "Tell me, sir, could I pass a coconut through my anus without pain?" There was a pause while we all collected our wits. He pressed his question: "Well, Doctor, what have you to say to that?"

Fortunately, the gods visited me hurriedly and fairly. I apologized politely that I was unable to give him a definite reply. "Because," I added, "I am not familiar with the orifice!" His anger turned to friendliness, and the perspiration dried off his forehead in the good humor that followed.

I found that some senior gynecologists who teach abnormal obstetrics disagreed with prenatal instruction of women. "It is better for us if they don't know anything about childbirth, and anyway, it is our job, not theirs," I heard more than one say. That is the war I have referred to of *man against woman*. There existed a demand that women be kept in ignorance of the truth of childbirth, so that they would be unquestionably submissive to the recommendations and demands of the orthodox obstetric profession. The women did not know that this submission might expose them to routine interference and physical injury, without any clinical indication that could justify such assaults upon their bodies.

I was proudly told by a gynecologist, before a gathering of colleagues at another meeting, that 75 percent of his women were delivered with instruments. The labors of 85 to 90 percent of his patients were surgically or medically induced to have their babies at a time convenient to all concerned. He said also that no woman was allowed to be either sensitive to the sensations of labor or conscious when her baby was born. "No human being," he exclaimed vehemently, "should be allowed to suffer this appalling agony." All women having their first babies were operated upon by having the outlet of the birth canal cut open to make it wider, and he did not advise women to breastfeed their babies. It was an unnecessary call upon their time and it made them tired; social and domestic routine was disturbed and formula feeding gave better results.

He refused to listen to argument or discussion. "I have used my methods for twenty-five years," he said, "and I see no reason to alter my ideas."

I asked him if he was interested in cerebral palsy. He was not—it was the pediatrician's business. Had he read the results of the recent wide-scale investigation and the report that medical authorities believe that over 70 percent of these disabled children had been crippled by interference at birth? He replied that there was undoubtedly a lot of bad obstetrics, but what could be done about it? I pointed out that there were thirty thousand new cases in the United States every year, making a total of one and a quarter million—did he not think that the natural or physiological method might be worth a trial in this fight against the tragedy of so many maimed babies?

He replied that with all respect he must tell me that there

was no such thing as natural childbirth. It had ceased to be a physiological function; culture had seen to that, and civilization must be blamed for the diseases it brings with it.

Did he know that 10 percent of all the children of low-grade mental development were in their sad plight because of meddlesome midwifery? He found the evidence difficult to accept and preferred to leave the cerebral trauma children, epileptics, and the results of birth oxygen starvation to the experts. He was an obstetrician.

Had not the obstetrician a great responsibility to the nation as well as to the parents and homes? "Yes, certainly, most important," he said. And so the conversation finished.

Only twelve weeks after returning from the United States I gave a course of lectures at the Clinique Tarnier in Paris, in May 1947, at the invitation of the late Professors Brindeau and Lanteujoul. I mention this to demonstrate that the general acceptance of this work resulted in a large number of invitations and requests to lecture. I lectured in French. It was at these lectures that the late Dr. Ferdinand Lamaze of Paris first became aware of natural childbirth or, as it was later termed by him, "painless childbirth."

During the years since 1933, the year my first book appeared, I had lectured upon this obstetric teaching in seventy-one different universities and maternity organizations in the British Isles and at forty-two universities and maternity organizations in different countries on three continents.

On a visit to a certain country in Europe I was shown, rather proudly, a first-stage ward where there were nine patients. When I went in with the professor who was conducting me around, I realized that there was no nurse present. We walked among the patients and I noticed that three of the nine were already in second stage. They all thought their neighbors were suffering the most intense agony, and when kindly spoken to they nearly all expressed sympathy with others. Only one demanded sympathy for herself because of her own personal discomfort. This distressing scene impressed me with the fact that prenatal care was at fault more than labor. Had these women understood labor, learned and practiced what to do, and been helped by trained attendants, it would have been so different.

Reports were becoming public by this time of several controlled series of births carried out under the natural childbirth procedures, from as far distant countries as the United States in 1946, by Blackwell Sawyer of New Jersey, and Durban, South Africa, in 1947, by the Department of Anesthesia, Addington Hospital.

In 1947 I published *The Birth of a Child* and began compiling material for *Introduction to Motherhood*. At this time the National Health Service was about to be introduced in Britain, so I went to inquire of Sir William Gilliatt, president of the Royal College of Obstetricians and Gynecologists, whether there might not be opportunity to be accepted as a member under the new arrangements. I asked for an assignment to carry out controlled studies in Britain itself, such as those being conducted in other places. He was very charming in manner but offered no hope, and hinted broadly that I should consider leaving the country! On my return home, I wrote him a long letter:

. . . In the absence of any official investigation or indeed recognition of this doctrine by your College, I must ask you to accept my statements as accurate, full of evidence which surrounds me here in my library as I write to you. From all over the world there is a vast fund of evidence that this approach to childbirth has brought safety and happiness to thousands of women. . . .

A frequent request from doctors, matrons and sisters of maternity establishments is: "Where can I come and study these methods?" Doctors in China, America (many), South Africa, Australia, Sweden, Holland and France have all expressed the desire to visit a hospital in England to learn and witness this work. . . . Books upon this subject are bought and read by thousands in the British Isles and America. They are translated or extracted in ten languages at least, probably more by now. Few editions of medical, obstetric or nursing journals are published without some favorable reference to the benefits of the "new approach to childbirth." . . .

To me this work is no longer an obstetric practice only, but a mission—no longer a pursuit, but a calling. I am not holy or pious, but I sincerely believe that time has shown clearly that the only justification for my personal existence, now that my family is grown up, is to give up everything to spread this gospel of safe and happy childbirth. I mean everything—my practice and, if need be, my home. I cannot sacrifice wealth as I have not attained it beyond providing for my wife and the future of my children. I want to teach and demonstrate and have a platform where all who wish may listen and learn and, in due course, perfect the technique of which I have evolved the elementary principles. . . .

I must set my course for the future. I hope to have ten years or more of life given to me in active work. I want to use it to good purpose. Can you therefore tell me, in order to assist me in deciding on my disposal: Is there a place for me in this country where practical teaching and demonstration may be given to those who accept these tenets? Do you still consider that my best course is to leave the country and try somewhere else? . . . I know this thing has got to come—and in the near future. The demand for it is growing like a rolling snowball across the face of the earth. Do you wish it to come from within or without?

By November 26 word came that my request was being considered, and on January 25, 1948, I received word that an eighteen-bed unit at Isleworth was to be placed under my clinical care. It had two labor wards and facilities for a prenatal department. The hospital would provide two obstetric nurses, and one or two of the medical residents who would be trained to carry out my teachings.

It seemed too good to be true! And it was. I discovered that the unit was separate from the main hospital, and had been damaged in the war. The eighteen beds were rickety and old. One of the only two toilets in the unit was out of order. In the room where the babies would be changed and bathed, the washbasin was broken and the baby's tub of cracked enamel was covered with a plain wooden board, on which were piled the dressings that were to go into the sterilizer. Shelves in the walls around were stuffed with an assortment of cups and saucers, bedpans, and spare rolls of toilet paper. Paint and plaster were peeling off the walls, and some of the windows were broken and boarded over. The labor wards were tiny, with bare wooden floors. In one of them the only ventilation was through a small window fan, set in a window that would not open. Instruments would have to be boiled in an enamel basin on the kitchen stove.

I inquired if the place could be repaired and brought up to date. The answer was no. I invited the maternity supervisor of a large hospital to take a look at the place the Royal College had offered, in which doctors from all over the country and world would come to witness demonstrations of my teaching. Her reaction was the same as mine. It was impossible.

I was nearly sixty years old. My health was breaking under the strain of opposition. The old World War I injuries were again causing searing headaches and problems with my back and legs. My world seemed shattered around me. Where could I go? What should I do?

Then I remembered what my mother had written me many years before: "Put your hand in the Hand of God. I have done so in all my troubles and have never failed to find comfort and help." I followed her advice, got down on my knees, and prayed.

Editors' Addendum

A new possibility presented itself to Dr. Dick-Read when a group of South Africans proposed building a magnificent hospital for women just outside Johannesburg, and invited him to come take full charge of the obstetric section as soon as it opened. On March 27, 1948, he made a preliminary visit to South Africa, prior to another lecture tour of several countries, with the promise to return to the position in the fall.

But it was not to be! His teaching had caught the attention of the press, and this nearly caused the end of his practicing career. On June 28, 1948, the following article appeared in the London *Daily Mirror:*

I understand that Princess Elizabeth is preparing, by careful study of the nature of childbirth and by doing muscular exercises, to have her baby without an anesthetic. The Princess has told friends her belief that pain in childbirth can be greatly reduced if a woman has a calm understanding of exactly what is happening when her baby is born. . . .

In all these matters she will, of course, be advised by her obstetrician, Sir William Gilliatt. But I am told that Sir William is not a great believer in natural childbirth. And the Princess will be giving a lead and encouragement to millions of women who fear confinement because they believe it must necessarily be accompanied by dreadful pain.

This "natural childbirth" system was first advocated in modern times by Dr. Grantly Dick Read.* Though it is accepted by many doctors all over the world, an early book on it nearly put him out of practice. . . .

Princess Elizabeth has read Dr. Read's book. When it first came out it was almost impossible to sell it. Now it has been translated into five languages, is a best seller in America and is selling at the rate of thousands of copies a month.

Dr. Dick Read is a tall, jovial man with a Cambridge degree, a Harley Street practice and a private clinic in Surrey. . . .

Once that story appeared, the rumor of Princess Elizabeth's proposed natural delivery swept the world. The French newspapers came out with bold headlines such as this: ENGLAND IS DIVIDED INTO TWO CAMPS—FOR OR AGAINST PAIN. In Australia the *Melbourne Sun* reported:

Princess Elizabeth, who is known for her enquiring mind and logical approach to life, has taken an intelligent interest in motherhood. . . . Although it is reported that she is doing regular muscle exercises hoping that she will be able to have her baby without anesthetics, bushy-eyed, sixty-year-old Sir William (Gilliatt) says that he thinks it most unlikely. . . . But the Princess has read *Revelation of Childbirth* by Dr. Dick Read, first advocator of "natural" childbirth. This book sells over a thousand copies a month in England, has been translated into five languages and is a best seller in America.

* The English do not hyphenate compound names. Because Americans did not realize that "Dick" was part of the surname, American editors began using the hyphen in American editions.

Some news reports even rumored that Dr. Dick-Read was replacing Sir William Gilliatt as the Princess' obstetrician! Yet at the time the articles appeared he didn't even know she was expecting, or that she had ever heard of his books. The news preceded him to South Africa, where the Natal *Daily News* said:

South African women, accustomed to having things done for them, will not take too kindly to the advice of Dr. Dick Read, whose theory of painless childbirth has created tremendous interest in the United States. But perhaps the fact that Princess Elizabeth is having her baby the "Dick Read way" may give a fillip to a revolutionary concept of childbirth which, paradoxically, is as old as woman herself.

Other headlines in South Africa appeared, such as the one in the Johannesburg *Sunday Times* on October 31, 1948:

JOHANNESBURG TO BE NEW WORLD CENTRE OF PAINLESS CHILDBIRTH

Johannesburg is to become the world centre of "painless childbirth." Dr. Grantly Dick Read, the famous British obstetrician who has taken terror out of childbirth for women all over the world, plans to move his entire organization from London to Hurlingham, a suburb of Johannesburg. A South African architect has visited Dr. Read in London and discussed with him his plans for the proposed hospital. . . . The building of the hospital in South Africa will mean that students of the new system of obstetrics will have to come to So. Africa for training.

Dr. Read visited Johannesburg in April of this year and demonstrated to doctors and women that normal childbirth can be free from pain. . . .

Thus it was that news items, many of them inaccurate in a number of details, caused him far more harm than anyone could have deliberately planned. The day he left England, December 19, 1948, millions of Britons read the untrue headlines of the *Sunday Pictorial:* DOCTOR QUITS IN DISGUST.

The news flashed around the world, in varied and distorted ways, and thus, predictably, on March 26, 1949, the London *Evening News* carried another item:

HARLEY STREET MAN BANNED IN SOUTH AFRICA

British obstetrician, Dr. Grantly Dick Read, who took fear out of childbirth for women all over the world has been refused registration by the South African Medical and Dental Council.

The council took its decision in committee and later confirmed it in open session. Officials of the Council refused to comment on the decision. . . .

The charges against him by the council were that he had solicited "advertisement" from the lay press, and thus was not a "person of good character," and was unsuitable for registration as a practicing physician in South Africa. Dr. Dick-Read hired a lawyer to prepare an appeal. While the legal argument raged he was without income and forbidden to practice, though scores of women wrote or besieged him by telephone begging him to attend their confinements. Scouts were even sent to spy on his home, in case he might be accepting patients secretly!

Finally the Medical Council held a special session to hear the appeal, given by A. J. Israel, one of South Africa's most brilliant lawyers:

According to the evidence before you, Dr. Read is a man whose work is well known. . . . Whether his methods and teachings are correct or not, it is not for me or you to say. This application is not concerned with that aspect. It therefore seems that an unnecessary attempt is being made to prejudice him when one sees that members of this Council wish to indicate that here is a man who is nobody and has done nothing. The type of question put by a member at the meeting of the Executive Committee indicates this. It is wrong to have put that type of question, to belittle a man and his work. It has nothing to do with an application for simple registration. . . .

We have put in letters and evidence from famous obstetricians and gynecologists and other medical practitioners who have written and read papers on his work. . . . I handed in today letters from the Lord Chancellor of England and from Dr. Thoms, head of the obstetrical department of Yale University; letters from the School of Medicine at Boston; letters from Canada and other places where Dr. Read's work and lectures are known and appreciated and he is treated with consideration because obviously his work is recognized as of some value to the profession.

But here, without any necessity, it is suggested that his lectures and work are, in effect, so bad that an application for him to practice is treated with contempt.

. . . Mr. Chairman, I think I am putting the case fairly when I say that, at the Executive Committee, Dr. Read laid himself open to examination and not only to examination but severe cross-examination of himself, where there was no right or even necessity to hold an enquiry. But nevertheless, he answered every question put to him candidly and he must have dispelled any impression that he is not a "person of good character."

Following the appeal, the nineteen members of the council took a vote. One abstained, and eighteen voted against permitting Dr. Dick-Read to be registered!

Only one recourse was left—an appeal to the Supreme Court of South Africa for a judgment. Three separate hearings were held, and on June 23, 1949, the Supreme Court ruled that he was to be issued a certificate of registration without further delay.

In the meantime, the plans to build the new hospital had long since been abandoned. But once he was entitled to practice in South Africa, a small but beautifully equipped maternity hospital, the Marymount, run by nuns of a Dominican order, invited him to come, promising to cooperate fully with his teaching. He had not been there many weeks before he said to them, "In another eighteen months it will not be a question of keeping the beds full, but of building to provide double the number, so that we can cope with all the demands for our services." His prediction was correct.

21

The Women of Africa

My wife immediately organized a series of prenatal classes for expectant mothers. The classes were held once every two weeks for women who could attend. Usually ten was the maximum number taken in any one class, which started about the eighteenth week of pregnancy. It was fascinating to watch the difference between these organized classes conducted by my wife and my early efforts of trying to teach women myself. The clumsiness and misunderstanding of men—I don't mean to derogate my sex—but the advantage of women being taught by women is that they understand the mysteries of a woman's mind, as man cannot.

The women were taught many things at these classes, including all the principles of postnatal care from the day the baby was born. It was soon found that these classes became gatherings of friendly women, even though they were very mixed in terms of social position or deprivation. They had a common interest and a common desire to learn the truth and apply it.

I slipped into the prenatal classes one day while the women were relaxing, to see if I could discover to what extent the relaxed women showed any sign of residual tension. The room was darkened and quiet; I entered without any unnecessary noise, the instructress greeted me, and although speaking quietly she used her normal voice. I walked around the women, some of whom were in the left lateral and some in the right lateral position. They had been relaxing for about ten to fifteen minutes. I sat in a chair and watched them individually, and although several had obvious evidence of incomplete relaxation, which was not unreasonable since they had only attended four classes, I was astonished at the sleepiness of all these women, who were not actually asleep. As I sat there in the peace of the room it came to my mind how easily anyone who was not initiated might have presumed that these women were being subjected to some form of hypnosis. When given instruction they reacted slowly but accurately, and it reminded me of the dictum of Edmund Jacobson, referring to relaxation: "No university subject and no patient ever considered it a suggested, hypnoidal or trance state, or anything but a perfectly natural condition. It is only the person who has merely read a description who might question this point." I talked for a short time with the instructress and left the room. I learned afterward that only two of the class had known of my visit.

What was the result of this preparation of women? The result has been that all over the world today the tenets that emerged from that relatively small school are the basic foundation for the organization of prenatal care of women in universities, teaching colleges, and maternity homes. They are not yet as common as I would wish, but that time will come.

The actual time I practiced in Johannesburg was just under four years. In that cosmopolitan community all sorts and conditions of people came under my care. I saw about six hundred babies into the world, of almost every European nationality under the sun. For simple enjoyment it was too many, but for the privilege of attending different types it was unique—English, American, Belgian, Czechoslovak, French, Latvian, Norwegian, Italian, Spanish, Greek, Yugoslavian, German, Armenian, and Jewish women who had lived in or been born in Russia, Poland, Bulgaria, and Austria. I mention this at length because the physical and psychological characteristics of these people differed considerably. The mental background of the refugees, those who had been in concentration camps, differed from any I had previously met. Some had witnessed the indescribable horrors of slaughter and torture, and others had seen friends and parents walk away from them forever, to be deported to a distant country or to death in the gas chamber.

There were also the women of old Boer stock, physically fit and strong, mentally imperturbable, without fear or frustration. These were women of families of the gold rush whose grandparents had farmed the grasslands, and whose cattle had grazed upon pastures with millions and millions of dollars' worth of gold beneath their feet. These people demanded my books and translated them into Afrikaans.

Here indeed was a heaven-sent opportunity to observe the influence of the new approach to childbirth; call it natural, educated, or physiological, what you will, the result was the same. Physically, in the mass, all women are the same—good, bad, and indifferent anatomical structure. Disproportions between fetus and the maternal pelvis occurred much as they do in England and probably all over the world. But psychologically the picture was different and, in my opinion, more difficult: I attended women with neuroses, psychoneuroses, hysteria, and anxiety states, with real terrors of death and conflicts at diverse psychic levels and intensities. Some had emotional struggles and the mental suffering of ambivalence —for and against children, husbands, marriage, motherhood, homes, social life, and sexual desires. All these came to learn to the best of their ability, at the magnificent prenatal school organized and superintended by my wife.

Of all these, except for those few who required, through disease or disproportion, some operative interference, 96 to 97 percent, of their own free will, refused the analgesia within their reach, preferring to be fully conscious and watch the birth of their babies.

It was possible during these years to make a sixteen-millimeter sound and color film of three natural births, as well as a sound recording.* It was not possible to pick and choose "ideal" cases, but when the cameraman was hired, the film was made of the next women who came in to have their babies.

But I still had one lifelong dream unfulfilled, that of investigating the childbirth customs of the people who lived closest to nature and furthest from both the advantages and disadvantages of modern science. For weeks and months my wife and I talked about such a project. There were still villages where tribes of Africans were living, in the jungles and on the mountains, in the swamps and on the sand-swept plains, where white men seldom go and never stay. We decided to go and see for ourselves what the customs of these people were.

For over forty years I had held the beliefs of my medical colleagues as suspect, feeling that they were misinterpreting the laws of nature. I felt that they had used modern scientific methods, not only to hide the pain of childbirth, but also to hide their own failure to understand its cause. I had satisfied myself that the physiological and anatomical apparatus the Creator had evolved for childbearing women was a magnificent manifestation of Divine genius. No further observations were necessary to uphold the belief in my contentions. But the years were telling on me. Night work took toll of my vitality, and tiredness such as I had never known brought home to me the fact that many of my contemporaries had already reached retiring age from hospitals and medical schools.

So the plans were made, and we sold home and practice, had a mobile home built on a bus chassis, and set off into the unknown, hoping to visit not just a few tribes but a hundred, two hundred if possible, to learn of normal childbirth in its natural environment. We wanted to prove or disprove the reports we had heard of the horrors of childbirth among the unwesternized people, the sufferings of women, and the enormously high rate of neonatal deaths. In our hearts we would not believe these stories without a closer examination of the facts.

* See Appendix.

During our journey through Africa we found doctors, priests, and others keenly interested in helping this project with personal experiences of their life among the African tribes. They brought Africans in to add their information on tribal lore and custom, and interpreted for me. It was generally agreed that childbirth had earned a bad name because of the relatively few complicated cases that were seen by medical people, who never saw the normal. And, further, I discovered that difficult labor cases were only brought in after a long wait in the villages, so that women who could have been successfully treated without any danger were much worse when finally brought in than those with similar complications among Europeans. This was due either to the distances involved, or to the ignorance and delay caused by the witch doctors.

One of my first visits was to the Moffatt Mission, where Dr. Manson from Scotland was in charge. He was certainly typical of the best of the doctor missionaries we came across. It was a strange coincidence to find that I was no stranger to him, although I must say I did not remember him myself. He had been present at my lectures in Scotland during the days when I lectured at the university there, bringing to the attention of the students the physiological approach to childbirth. He told me a lot about childbirth among these people. He was a keen obstetrician, and made me realize how much we had to learn.

From there we went a short distance north and called on a Canadian doctor at the Seventh-Day Adventist Mission Hospital, Dr. Jack Hay. When I told him my name he said, "This is nothing short of a miracle! My wife has had three babies, and studied your books very carefully with each one. She had not the slightest trouble or difficulty. In fact, she was so enthusiastic about the method that she started prenatal classes for the African women." After a year she found the numbers to have increased so much that seven hundred women attended in that one year. And it was the old women who usually insisted on the girls coming to learn.

I learned that the law of the jungle has two main branches. The Africans told me of the manner of the *maintenance* of individuals and their tribes, their systems and organizations, religions, food and drink, victories and defeats, drought, flood, fire, and disease. But they always expressed surprise that a white man should want to know the other branch of jungle law: the *reproduction* of the people, the marriage customs, and the girlhood of the women who bore children to reinforce the manpower of the tribe.

For this information I had to speak to the women, old and past the years of shyness and reticence, those who were chosen to guide and care for mothers when their babies were born. "Why do you want to know?" they asked me, and I said, "Do you not want to hear the ways of white women?" It was an exchange of confidences freely given, and I believe most of these ancient midwives with whom I talked were honest in their replies, for so many answers to my questions were the same, although from different tribes who lived thousands of miles apart, and spoke totally different languages.

But even if they did not tell the truth it was only to be kind. Dear old Bwalya Kalunda, whose interpreter was a lady of a Protestant mission, replied to me in her own language, although she spoke reasonably good English. "Bwalya Kalunda," I said, "how many children have you had?" Miss X translated that she had had twelve.

"Was it easy to have babies?" The question was put to her very sternly as if to say, "You know the answer to this one." In English the old lady replied in a monotone, "For my sin I suffer the torture of damn."

But, choosing her moment, she gave me a naughty wink. I understood and said, "Bwalya Kalunda, you like having babies?" She smiled, and through Miss X she said, "I love it, and did not want to stop!" Miss X told me Bwalya Kalunda was an ardent Christian. My obvious rejoinder was, "A grand old lady, and very loyal!"

She was one of so many with whom we talked. The young women were difficult to talk to, for most of them are coy and proud of their feminine assets, a fairly general trait throughout the world. They are taught it is a woman's business to be attractive to a male and on her best behavior before strangers.

But when we talked to the old dames, those who had been "through the mill," had seen life and looked after others, I found them not only charming and polite, but quiet, kindly women and surprisingly knowledgeable. They spoke of the one great experience, motherhood, not only of having their own children and all it meant to them, but of the young women they looked after. They told me, freely, so much that I came to the conclusion that the white man has a lot to learn from the black man, who should receive our greatest respect.

Until people have been to Africa they are inclined to think of jungle women as subhuman types. This is entirely wrong! Within the edicts of their own laws and customs they are dignified, and many of them are beautiful people. They are essentially feminine, and there seemed to us to be very little difference between "woman" whether she is European, Asiatic or African. The African women desire to be attractive, and spend a large part of their time beautifying themselves, particularly their hair. This is done in many different styles among the various tribes.

Black African women are people of amazing character. First and foremost we were impressed by their beauty, and when I say beauty I mean it. It isn't necessarily that they have the same outline of features you would expect to see in a London street or in New York, but they carry with them a personality that is astonishing. As we passed them sitting in groups at the edge of the forests, we stopped and laughed with them often, making signs and getting in touch with them in the different ways we had learned, because none of them spoke any language we understood. We got along well in the towns with our French and English, but in the jungle had to go back to the old primitive method of enjoying each other's company by signs, hands, eyes, and smiles. And there is nothing that gets one further with the African woman than a smile.

Among the majority of the tribes we visited the women in

the villages were looked after by the older women in the families, not necessarily relatives but old people especially chosen for this purpose. Very few African women attended a hospital for birth unless there was some definite complication and delay during labor. The more urbanized Africans who lived in the town brought their wives into the hospital, and we were told that they had more discomfort and made more noise than the village women at home.

While customs differed, the following procedures were the most common: The babies are born with the mother squatting on the floor, leaning against the side of the hut. Usually there is someone behind to support them during the later stages of labor, when the midwife takes up her position in front. The village labor is conducted in silence. There appears to be very little discomfort though sometimes considerable hard work on the part of the mother.

The woman who is attended in the village is never left alone. Most of them are well instructed in the course of labor by old women in whom they have complete confidence. And while their errors are tragedies, for they do not have the knowledge or ability to treat the 4 or 5 percent of irregularities that occur, their customs do not allow the acts and interferences that account for over 60 percent of maternal morbidity in the white man's countries. There will always be abnormalities in all forms of reproduction throughout the realms of nature, but the complications of pathological childbirth are few compared with the man-made troubles that emerge in civilized countries, when there is failure to understand the simple physiological mechanism and its demands. A mission doctor reported that 18 percent of his patients had abnormal labors *after* admission to the hospital. This I am willing to believe, but I found no evidence to support such a high percentage of abnormal labors in the villages.

A British provincial commissioner told me of one experience he had had when he was carrying an African man and wife on his boat. The wife began labor during the journey, so he stopped. She went into the bush and the husband waited nearby. In a relatively short time the woman emerged with her baby and the journey resumed.

We learned the profound respect that every tribe and village has for the afterbirth, and the manner of its extrusion from the birth canal. They do not interfere with nature's work, and allow no child to be separated from this wonderful structure, which gave it soul and body while it grew within the mother's womb, until it has been born and lies beside the child. Then, and only then, may the cord be cut and the offspring given to its mother to embrace. In many tribes, no one is allowed to touch the placenta, or afterbirth. It is taken away by the woman in attendance and buried. There are many superstitions concerning it, and its burial constitutes an important rite in the birth of a child.

The major cause of difficulty among the nationals, apart from anatomical disproportion or malpresentation, is that often the aged midwives insist on the mother pushing down hard from the beginning and using all her strength. This has resulted in many unnecessary troubles. Prolapse of the uterus occurs, and sometimes the pressure, before the cervix is properly opened, produces swelling and edema of the outlet, which actually impedes the progress of the oncoming child. I saw a number of fistulas from the vagina into either or both bladder and rectum, rupture of the uterus, and servere exhaustion and shock. When labor is prolonged, the woman might be accused of adultery, adding mental suffering to her physical difficulty. These were the chief complications of labor, and although compared with the normal cases they were only a small number, even these troubles could have been prevented, for the African can also learn from us.

The Africans are intelligent people, but it must be remembered they have a different culture from ours. Their way of life is that which one could expect from those who live nearest to nature, the nature from which they come and upon which they survive. In this journey of ours we found that the simple biological law of all life has stood immutable since the creation of the first living soul, and in a word it is—survival!

As we traveled through strange places among people whose manners and customs were new to us, we were conscious of the power of this fundamental principle. We found it everywhere; human beings, animals, insects, the trees of the great forests and the creatures of the rivers and lakes survive in a ruthless war one against the other, but man in many ways has a higher intelligence than other living creatures, and from the earliest records of his existence we have reason to believe that he has been aware of an all-powerful influence that rules over his destiny.

At one place we had come upon a deserted, hidden temple. It was an awe-inspiring spectacle for me, for when one has lived for over sixty years one seeks some association with our own experience, and recalls analogies from memories past. What can any sensible human being say when he sees, thrown on the canvas of today, the genius of a people long lost in an oblivion that has destroyed their entity, and the brilliance of whose work is secreted beneath a shroud of rampant vegetation? All archeologists must feel the futility of our existence in terms of man's estimate of success.

It must be accepted that greatness up to a certain standard is attained by acquisition, discovery, and organizing ability, but we very rarely hear anyone say "thank you" to the powers that placed the substance there and gave man the faculties to utilize it for the development of the human race.

I can only say there are some things the black man knows that would be of tremendous benefit to us, though other things are best left where they are, gradually dying out in the hidden places of the jungle. The African is a proud, spiritually minded but essentially practical man. He has for generations been brought up to use his physical prowess as well as his wits for the survival and the maintenance of his people.

In an international medical magazine recently I read: ". . . when modern science has said its last word, and the patient is still no better, we are not justified in saying that the case is necessarily hopeless. There are still spiritual values to be considered, and spiritual resources of prayer. . . ." We are swinging around once more to the practices of the African over the centuries, in his awareness of spiritual forces in the universe.

In the scorching brilliance of a cloudless sky and in the damp of forest darkness, when wild turmoil bent and frayed the treetops of the valley, and again in the stillness and peace of tropic night, we heard the echo of a Voice in harmony with every discord of the jungle world: "I am Alpha and Omega, the beginning and the ending, the first and the last."

Why is it that the enslavement of the body appeals more to our sympathies than the more destructive slavery of the spirit, which is the ruling force of survival in the modern civilized or cultured world? Soon this glorious array of bounties, which until recently was known as "Darkest Africa," will have been dissolved by the torrent of the white man's infiltration. I give it ten years—until the early 1960s—and then all will be commerce. The destructive hand of Western influence will take so much that is good and replace it with the crumbs that fall from the rich man's table.

Don't look too far ahead. It will give no pleasure and no reward. Go now, not to kill beasts or to find minerals, not to grow cotton, coffee, or bananas, but to open, while there is yet time, the windows of your own souls. Let in the light that floods the forest of the valleys and the hills, the light that is the law of the jungle, the law of nature, and the law of God.

And try to understand.

22

Some Misunderstandings

During my years in South Africa, experiments in natural childbirth procedures continued to be carried out in all parts of the globe and the results made public. Among the most notable of these was that conducted by Professors Thoms and Goodrich* at the Yale University School of Medicine in 1949, and in 1951 by Lawrence D. Roth of Rochester, New York. Since then each year there have been one or more records and publications of controlled experiments in the use of these principles.

Shortly after arriving in South Africa I completed writing *Introduction to Motherhood*. My books already published or in progress in several foreign languages were: *Mutter Verden ohne Vrees*, in Dutch; *Die naturlige Fødsels*, in Danish; *Mutter Werden ohne Schmerz*, in German; *Att Föda utan Fruktan*, in Swedish; *Rivelazioni sul Parto*, in Italian; and editions were also appearing in French, Spanish, Portuguese, Japanese, and Norwegian. It can safely be said that this teaching was known all over the Western world before my years in Africa began.

Painless deliveries have been of interest to Russian physicians for many years. In 1936 I read of the methods of painless childbirth in Russian papers; at that time it was spinal

---

* H. Thoms and F. W. Goodrich, Jr., "A Clinical Study of Natural Childbirth," *American Journal of Obstetrics and Gynecology* 56 (1948):875.

analgesia. In 1946 a Leningrad doctor reported on the use of Vitamin B₁. In 1945 Dr. Velvovsky of the Ukraine, who had been studying methods of painless childbirth, first using hypnosis and then trying a variety of other methods, reached for the Pavlovian physiology to assist him in obtaining his design. In 1948 the Russians carefully investigated the benefits of the natural childbirth approach, which was then known all over the world. These natural childbirth experiments found favor among them. They were quick to appreciate its benefits for the health of their nation, but omitted any reference to factors not purely mechanistic.

At the Fourth International Congress of Catholic Doctors on September 29, 1949, the Pope gave an address, outlining the principles and practice of childbirth without fear. He compared it to the procedure in certain hospitals where the mother was plunged into deep hypnosis, stating that this procedure resulted in emotional indifference to the child, and was thus not recommended, but that natural childbirth did not entail this danger. He went on to relate the recent Soviet researches in obstetrics along these same lines, but implied criticism of the Russians for their neglect of the spiritual aspects. He said:

The Englishman Grantly Dick Read has perfected a theory and technique which are analogous in a certain number of points; in his philosophical and metaphysical postulates, however, he differs substantially because his are not based, like theirs, on a materialistic concept.

The laws, the theory and the technique of natural childbirth, without pain, are undoubtedly valid, but they have been elaborated by scholars who, to a great extent, profess an ideology belonging to a materialistic culture.

By late 1949 and 1950 the Russian experiments in natural childbirth were successful enough for them to call a conference on this subject at Leningrad in 1951. It was sponsored by the Clinical Department of the U.S.S.R. Academy of Medical Science and the Scientific Council of the U.S.S.R. Ministry of

Public Health. Here Velvovsky, Platonov, and Nicolayev*
read papers on the results of a *new* method of obstetric pain
relief now being practiced in a number of institutions in
Moscow, Kharkov, and Leningrad. It is difficult to know why
this approach was called new, since it had been in English
textbooks and used in many countries for twenty years! It can
be said that this work was known practically all over the civilized world by 1951.

In September of that same year (1951), Dr. Pierre Vellay
of France wrote me a very kind letter, saying that both he and
Dr. Lamaze had considered it a privilege to read the last
edition of my book, *Childbirth Without Fear*. I remembered
Dr. Lamaze from my lectures at the Clinique Tarnier in Yaris
in 1947. Dr. Lamaze was now the resident accoucheur of the
Ironworkers Policlinic in Paris, and Vellay had been his
assistant for the previous three years. Dr. Vellay stated that he
appreciated the help my book might bring to pregnant women,
and requested the right to translate it into French.

I replied, thanking him very much for his letter but inform-
ing him that the work was already translated into French, and
that my publishers had informed me that it would appear on
the market shortly. However, in spite of all our efforts to get it
through, it was not until eighteen months later that the book
finally appeared on the French market. This was always a
mystery to us, but eventually my book *L'Accouchement sans
Douleur* was published.

Early in 1952, while still in South Africa, I received information from Switzerland and other countries that Russian
gynecologists had described a new approach to childbirth
called "psychoprophylaxis," based on the work of a Russian
named Ivan Pavlov. Those who sent the information stated
that there was a striking similarity of what they were claiming
to have discovered to what I had been writing, lecturing, and

* A. P. Nicolayev: "Les Bases Theoriques de la Psychoprophylaxio
de la doleur dans l'accouchement," revue de la *Nouvelle Medicine*, 1
(1953):61.

teaching for so long in so many parts of the world, even to the use of the term "psychoprophylaxis" in relation to childbirth, which I first used in 1933. So I visited the Consulate of the U.S.S.R. in Pretoria, South Africa, to discuss the matter.

The consul invited me to send copies of my book, in English and translated into German, to Dr. Lurye of Kiev. These were dispatched by diplomatic bag along with a friendly letter asking to exchange observations:

Dear Professor Lurye:

Medical friends who have written to me from Switzerland and England inform me that you are using a method of natural childbirth based, from some of its aspects, upon the work of the great Russian physiologist, Ivan Pavlov.

I feel therefore that you will be interested to read a book that I published in 1942, *Childbirth Without Fear,* which has sold just under a quarter of a million copies. It has been translated into eight different languages and has been enthusiastically received wherever it has been adopted. And my investigations upon this subject were carried out for twenty years before my first book, *Natural Childbirth,* was published in 1933.

I enclose an English copy and a German translation together with a small practical manual, *Introduction to Motherhood* that has been published in four countries. I have no doubt that most of your colleagues will be familiar with one or both of these languages.

It seems that there is still in this world one common denominator for all humanity—motherhood. Motherhood has occupied my attention for the last forty years of my professional life and this alone allows me the presumption of writing to you and sending you a work that may prove interesting to those about you.

I shall deem it a great honor if you will read these books and send me some literature published in Russia on modern obstetrics. Please accept as from one colleague in this great work to another my cordial greetings.

Yours sincerely.

I received neither thanks for the books nor acknowledgement of the letter, although it is certain that they arrived safely in Kiev, since they were dispatched through official diplomatic channels. When I inquired at the Russian Consulate they expressed surprise, but offered no explanation.

There is no doubt that those who heard the Russian exposition of their "new" work were struck first and foremost by the resemblance of the speeches at the 1951 Conference in Leningrad to previous published papers of my own, even to the measures adopted for the preparation of women for childbirth, which, in the earlier stages of my work had no relation whatever to Pavlovian conditioning. In fact, Pavlov's book on conditioning did not appear until nearly fifteen years (1928) after my own work had begun, at which time I incorporated his explanation of conditioned reflexes, with due credit, as descriptive of what takes place through mental imagery.

Two years later, in 1953, I read a Russian claim that my work had been inspired by Ivan Pavlov but had not been a success! The only successful system of natural childbirth, it was asserted had been evolved by Soviet scientists from the teachings of Ivan Pavlov.

In 1953 Dr. Lamaze, who had been in Russia for six months to study their methods, started widespread publicity from the Metallurgic Hospital in Paris, claiming that the work he was doing was Pavlovian psychoprophylactic method. Visitors to his hospital again recognized the similarity in almost every way to the teaching that had been carried on in America and Britain for many years.

The truth is that the psychoprophylaxis of fear and pain in childbirth had already been discovered, published, taught, and used for nearly twenty years before the Soviet doctors realized its value and began to examine its principles. The fear-tension-pain syndrome has been the foundation of psychoprophylaxis and has proved its value in countries all over the world. Many have made small changes to suit their people and their climate, but only one country has claimed it as their own.

It is no concern of mine whether this general principle is applied with a hundred different variations, neither can I be concerned with the academic arguments of neurologists or neurophysiologists upon the functions of the brain. There is no end to their opinions. It has been my privilege to work with some of the greatest neurophysiologists of the last fifty years, but I have only come to the conclusion that they are uncertain of all the applied doctrines concerning the reception, integration, and interpretation of the afferent stimuli to the brain and the efferent messages from the brain to the periphery of the body. I speak of *human beings,* not machines made from *cerebrocentric reflex arcs.*

So long as the fear-tension-pain syndrome is broken down by safe and simple teaching and training, our purpose is served. It is a fact that a series of events takes place that, if disturbed at any level, results in the abnormality of severe pain. I look upon the claim, therefore, of the Communists to be one of ideological rather than medical importance. My sphere is to reduce the pains of labor, to take fear from childbirth, and to bring untarnished love into the homes of the people. My concern is for the betterment of childbirth, parenthood, and marriage, for happy families within the framework of our society, regardless of individual race, religion, or political creed.

This was made clear in my original publication in 1933 and has not changed since. Hundreds of thousands of women of all nationalities have breathed gratitude for the comfort and happiness this teaching brought to them. In 1951 the Russian physicians accepted the advantages of this principle, after two or three years of testing it in practice, and in 1953 it was propagated by Frenchmen, to whom I give all honor for their determination.* In *Revue Nouvelle Médécine* A. Bourrel

---

* Dr. Dick-Read was sincere in his praise for their efforts to make childbirth a happier experience for women. His concern was for the women, not for himself. In the same generous spirit he would approve the efforts today of the Lamaze-Pavlov and psychoprophylaxis child-

writes of the "new" preparation of women, all the details of which had been used for years by others. Lamaze, Vellay, and Hersilie write on a technique of childbirth without pain that was an imitation so similar to that already published that in its initial stages visitors who observed it in practice saw nothing new. Angelergues, in seventeen hundred words, states that I don't know anything about childbirth, that I don't understand Pavlov's work, in fact that this man Read knows nothing about anything! He forgot to add, "That is why his work has revolutionized childbirth throughout the world, and also why the Communists have rescued him from the risk of his own ignorance."

But there is a serious aspect of this work as it is used in Russia. There are still great scientists who value, before all things, *truth*. This requires a freedom not always available. I am told that in the Soviet states a scientist must say and do what he is ordered to do by officials in high places. I also understand that there is another sort of scientific worker in the U.S.S.R., he who, in full knowledge of the truth, adheres to the universal principle of academic honesty and who, for his love of science, desires neither to deceive himself nor his colleagues. The true scientist will always exist, and he must be recognized as different from he whose work is primarily designed to support, by all available means, the ideology of Communism. If this is compatible with truth, I have no quarrel. But if ideology is upheld at the expense of truth, work loses at once its scientific value and the workers are degraded.

The claims of original production and possession of innovations are effective means of establishing the greatness of an ideology and its leaders only where ignorance and fear prevent contradiction. For instance, we believe that Signor Marconi was an Italian and that Shakespeare was an Englishman and that Columbus discovered America. When, however, we

birth groups in the United States, which have developed from this source. The need is so great that there is room for all who are truly interested in making childbirth a rewarding experience. —Ed.

learn that these men were Russians, we cease to be surprised that Pavlov, without realizing it, disclosed that psychoprophylaxis in childbirth is a means of relieving the pains of labor. Such nonsense is not taken seriously by educated people, and neither is it worthy of our attention. I have followed the writings of Pavlov for fifty years and, so far as it has been of value to physiology, I have admired it. But this hysterical effort to found a philosophy on his physiology is pathetic, particularly when much of his physiological concept is out of date.

But there is one basic principle of natural childbirth that Communism does not imitate, and in this way they differ entirely from my teaching. They treat childbirth and motherhood as a *materialistic* and *mechanistic* performance with no spiritual association. The miracle of reproduction is distorted to become a means of demonstrating the absence of God and the omnipotence of the Communist leaders. Their teaching stops abruptly at that point where the spiritual associations of parenthood play such an important part. The benefits of their teaching on childbirth will be limited by the atheism and materialism of their ideology.

My teaching is exactly the opposite. I believe in the law of nature and a God-force. I do not accept man's limited understanding as all powerful; in fact, I am very conscious of the small fraction of total knowledge that is within the comprehension of man. To me, childbirth is a sacred event and brings humanity nearest to the spiritual and metaphysical world around it. It is a moment of emergence of new life with unknown potentialities.

When I see a baby born to a happy, healthy mother and witness the superhuman radiance that carries her to a new world of mystery and possession, I say to myself, "What sort of an idiot thinks he can make anything of this life without the hand of God to guide him?"

So, finally, there is no clinical difference between my teaching of natural childbirth and that claimed by the Russians in the early 1950s because there was no "new" Russian method, but only a Communist adaptation of a twenty-year-old teaching, distorted for atheistic, ideological purposes. That is where we differ. They teach antispiritual parenthood and the doctrine of mechanistic materialism. I teach the sacredness of childbirth as a spiritual event, the spiritual power of a mother's love, and faith in the truth of the law of nature, which to me is one of the great laws of God.

Ninety percent of all civilized countries profess to some form of religious persuasion. Religious teaching calls for obedience to its codes, homage to the Creator, and loyalty to its spiritual and material purposes in the mother-child relationship. This factor knits in a common bond all the people of the world. I am not persuaded that the Communist ideology can destroy in so short a time the inborn devotion of a vast people to generations of religious faith. I believe that in time these naturally devout peoples who constitute the worker masses of the U.S.S.R. will turn once more to the fervent faith of their forefathers.

Professor A. P. Nicolayev ends his lecture with the words of a Soviet woman after her labor: "I have no fear, I am happy, thanks to Soviet knowledge, thanks to Soviet doctors, thanks to the great friend of knowledge, our own comrade, Stalin."

I end my lecture: "Childbirth is a sacred subject, and I cannot be concerned with any who use it as merchandise to exploit it for personal gain, whether it be for money, social prestige or political propaganda. I am neither the arbitor of your opinions nor partisan to your persuasions. I endeavor to raise before you the high level of loving homes and families through happy childbearing, for in the end it is the homes of the people that become the standard of a civilization."

23

American Tour

When I returned to London from Africa I no longer practiced medicine. I had passed the age when appointments on hospital staffs could be obtained, even had they been available. Under the present organization of the medical health services in the British Isles, an age is fixed for retirement of physicians, in order to make room for younger men.

During my years of practice and research in Africa it was not possible to accept lecture tours elsewhere, but on my return I began writing and lecturing again, in response to invitations throughout Europe. In the three years after my return from Africa I received a large number of invitations to speak in the United States again. So, at the beginning of October 1957, after completing a lecture tour in Germany, we again made our way to the United States.

I had been invited by the Academy of Psychosomatic Medicine to speak at their Fourth Annual Meeting in Chicago, October 17 to 19. This was a great occasion, for we learned in a short time what was taking place in the United States in regard to understanding the mind of women in childbirth, much of which had not been published in English medical journals.

Our host at the congress, Dr. William Kroger, who was secretary of this occasion, met us as we arrived. We soon had a taste of the hospitality that was to be heaped upon us for the next three and a half months. During those months I was entertained by seventy different groups in the large cities and towns of the United States, as well as in several cities in Canada.

It was nearly eleven years since I had been in the United States. Everywhere we discovered some organization flourishing for the education of women in natural childbirth. The interest extended to great universities as well. Preparation for childbirth has come to stay, and although it had still not been accepted by all the large hospitals, the demand of women for knowledge, and for more personal, humane care, is not to be denied. I had found the same rapidly improving conditions in Germany, Italy, France, the Scandinavian countries, Spain, Portugal, and the great countries of South America.

While here I was fortunate in having some extremely interesting conversations with the doctors of large hospitals. I remember one staff especially, where there were environmental differences in practice, but whose fundamental approach to childbirth was as near to the natural law as was possible under their present circumstances. I was taken into ward after ward and introduced to the ladies whose babies had recently arrived. I was greeted like an old friend and told without inhibition the details of their labors. My wife and I agreed it was a wonderful thing to happen to complete strangers.

One of our warmest memories is of our arrival in Seattle. It was, to say the least, unusual! Our seats were near the end of the train, so we were the last to follow the luggage cart down toward the station. These platforms are very long. After we had walked about a hundred yards toward the station we thought there must be some kind of school picnic, for a very large number of small children were waiting with some adults at the end of the platform. To our surprise, one of the ladies in charge walked toward us and stretched out her hand in greeting. She was the mother of four of the children. The other women were mothers of the other children.

Two very small girls carried a banner that said, "Welcome

to Seattle," with my name printed underneath. As we approached, they set up a cheerleaders' shout: "We are Dick-Read babies!" I found it very difficult to know quite what expression to wear, but the spontaneous one was an amused smile, which crept over my face. Then, very solemnly, two other charming little girls walked forward to my wife and presented her with a beautiful bouquet. Then we all gathered around and had a good look at each other, with a lot of laughter. I told them it was the nicest thing I had ever seen.

On another part of our journey, while in Dallas, Texas, my eyes could hardly take in all that I saw in the great Neiman Marcus store. Although appreciating the elegance and art that was so obviously and beautifully displayed, I found myself wondering how long I could live in comfort, without working, for the amount it would cost me to buy my wife just those things I felt sure she would enjoy wearing.

The morning went all too quickly. As we left, our taxi driver threw away three inches of a Havana cigar, which smelled excellent to me. Then he opened the box on the seat beside him and produced another one, a good six inches long, which he lit as though it were his duty rather than his pleasure. Again I began, in a very English way, to wonder how much it would cost me at home to buy a box of fifty of those cigars. Although I had given up smoking some time ago, I used to be a cigar smoker, and Havana cigars are really good. For a moment I dreamed and, in the clouds, so tender to my nostrils, worlds long forgotten formed. I sighed and my wife said, "Isn't it beautiful?" "Indeed it is," I replied. She referred to an expensive coat, and I to a smell!

We were in Las Vegas only a short time, fortunately, just long enough to see a little of its gaudy illuminations and mechanical decorations, and people standing for hours pulling handles. It seemed to be a place where nakedness was in great demand—postcards, boxes of chocolates, flags, toys, books, and even chocolate bars all seemed to come as close as possible to presenting a naked man or woman. I suppose it is reasonable that a doctor in his late sixties should look upon this approach to life as rather unnecessary and not a little boring, and we were not sorry to get back on the plane.

Another experience that left an unpleasant memory occurred as our hostess drove us through a beautiful mountain range. Although the trees on its slopes had no leaves on them, we could envision them covered with foliage all the way down to the river below. But there we saw vast booms of logs, like enormous water lilies on phantom lakes, gradually moving downstream, on their way to finish life in a pulp factory.

Since I was a small boy, I have never been pleased to see trees cut down, which may be associated with the respect I have always had for anything that lives. To see a tree falling to the ax seemed like murder to me, and I wondered how the pain it must have suffered was interpreted. I was told there was still enough wood to go on cutting more than man could need for a hundred years, by which time the new wood itself would have grown up to continue the supply, yet I could not help being reminded of an occasion when my wife and I were in East Africa. We had been down the Crocodile River, more sight-seeing than anything else, when we came upon two large trucks pulled up by the roadside. In a variety of uniforms and weird outfits, about a dozen or more young men were strolling along carrying rifles. We looked at the trucks and saw they were piled high with impala deer, beautiful little creatures that had apparently been herded up, driven together, then shot and carted off in that way. Little white tails, or beautiful antlers, hung over the end of the trucks. Somehow it was a shock to me that men could go out and kill hundreds on one safari and then take them back to be skinned, their flesh dried and sold. It isn't for one moment that I would suggest this wasn't reasonable, because life very largely lives upon life, and yet we need to be more careful not to entirely destroy our associations with all that is beautiful.

During one of my lectures I was asked to tell about my experiences while on safari in the Central Congo, Northern

Uganda, and other places where the white man has not yet exerted any influence upon the childbirth customs of the tribes. I gave a short outline of the information we had gleaned and, so far as possible, the factors common to the two hundred-odd tribes and subtribes we had visited. I tried to put these observations in terms of physiology, and the manner in which the birth function was carried out both emotionally and physically in terms of the religious and social rites of the various peoples. In terms of pagan religions, the laws of the gods saw childbirth as the greatest gift of woman, and her happiest accomplishment.

I drew attention to the fact that I was not discussing the abnormalities that arose in 2, 3, or 4 percent of the women—which women died unless they were rushed to some European hospital maybe a hundred, two hundred, or three hundred miles through the jungle—but was giving my observations upon normal and uncomplicated labor, which represented well over 90 percent of all births. This we had seen when we were given the privilege of studying the analogy of the white races and the black in the minds and hearts of women. In Africa we often witnessed the natural law of reproduction with its love and its magnificence.

I was surprised when a man who was not even on the staff of the hospital where I was speaking stood up, looking very angry, for this was unusual in my discussions in America. He firmly exclaimed to me that I had no right whatever to compare them—that is, the people of his area—with these "goddamned savages," for, he said, "We are not animals!"

That was, of course, a challenging remark, for whatever else the human being may be, he does remain an animal, par excellence, and his primarily biological reactions, whatever his color, are those of reproduction and maintenance. For my own part, I can discover no satisfactory evidence of alteration of forces or function in the reproductive equipment of *genus homo,* whether red, brown, black, white, yellow, or American.

The doctor's remark surprised me because, speaking generally, I had not heard these views expressed in public since I had been in the United States of America. This was obviously a sore point, upon which I had inadvertently trodden for the first time, but I did not feel either the person or his dogmatic assertions demanded a serious reception upon this occasion.

I replied, "You have me at a disadvantage, sir, for I would not dream of comparing my hosts and the people of this state with either 'goddamned savages' or human beings who are *not* animals, because I do not know of such specimens. I have never, in all my travels, come across any goddamned savages. In fact, I doubt if they exist, even in the most pagan tribes. I know only too well the white-damned blacks. Perhaps you refer to them? If so, I agree with you. Our lot in life is not comparable to theirs any more than mine is comparable to yours, if you are not animal."

One of the greatest joys during our long tour of America was the opportunity, on occasions like this, to gather as medical men and colleagues for discussion over a drink or at lunch, or after touring a hospital. There was no asperity in our discussions, or an absence of humor. We were earnest and thoughtful; we agreed and differed. I would not have missed one moment of that three and a half months that enabled us to exchange opinions and expose our respective ideas to analysis and dissection.

Any English doctor making a tour of the American hospitals will be struck by the luxury and magnificence of these modern buildings. I became more and more impressed with the meticulous care that had been taken to provide every possible accessory to comfort and convenience in the newer structures. The organization and equipment for the feeding of patients and staff would have left nothing to be desired in a most expensive first-class hotel. I found it difficult to decide whether I was ashamed of the English hospitals or whether I felt sympathy for the people of England that they did not have enough money to supply them with buildings adequately equipped and comfortable.

On the other hand, I often felt that they were much better off, particularly in regard to obstetrics. In one magnificent new hospital I was brought into a ward of twenty beds in the obstetric unit called the recovery room. It was here that women who had had their babies were put until they recovered consciousness or had settled down safely from the unnatural interferences to which the majority had been subjected at the deliveries of their normal, healthy babies. There was a special nursing staff for this recovery room, and it was not unnatural that I wondered what they were recovering from, and why there should be such a large place organized for that particular purpose. Did American women, having borne a baby, have to go through a stage of recovery requiring so much specialized attention? It was certainly not so in other countries, except in rare and complicated cases.

I noticed that over each of the beds there was a tap that supplied oxygen, this gas being available through tubes and pipes just as gas for a stove might be, or the electrical wiring for a building. I was directed to notice its proximity to the blood bank; every new mother was as near as possible to grouped blood, stored ready for transfusion should it be required. I was interested to hear that quite a number of patients did have blood transfusions, the number varying considerably in different hospitals, depending on the obstetric routine and the clinical opinion of the attendants.

We went on to a special ward for newborn babies, where they were immediately put into an oxygen tent for one hour, whether they were healthy or not, whether they were born with interference or without. Their first duty of life, impressed on them by the hospital authorities, was that they should spend their first hour of extrauterine existence in an oxygen tent. They were not allowed the security of mother's arms or the warmth of her body, but were placed all alone in an unnatural gas, water, and air mixture (40 percent oxygen, 75–80° Fahrenheit, approximately 70 percent humidity), as a psychological boost into a new life! I wondered why one hour in an oxygen tent, with a higher percentage of oxygen in the breathed air than they had been accustomed to in the placental blood, was more advantageous than lying in the arms of a healthy mother, experiencing from the moment of birth the security and warmth that are the natural heritages of a newborn child.

I passed on to a laboratory near to the babies' nurseries whose function, at first, I did not understand. Then I was told it was the milk bank, where the pediatricians came to write the formulas for the milk of each baby, because it was unusual for a woman to feed her baby from the breast. The organization of the milk bank was made quite clear to me—it was magnificently done, and had women not been born with breasts at all, I can't imagine anything that would have been more efficient.

I learned that when a woman was admitted to the hospital she was put into a labor room and prepared for the birth by being washed and given an enema and a shave, and was then immediately given a "shot." I asked what the "shot" was and was told it was an injection given as routine when women came into the hospital. They were usually rather anxious, and this helped to calm them down before labor progressed too far. A nurse was in attendance and, from time to time, made the rounds of the labor rooms to see how the women were getting on. The nurses were advised not to answer any questions a woman asked, but simply to tell her to be patient. She was given medicine, usually atropine by injection and 100 to 150 milligrams of Demerol, when the stresses increased, usually at about three-fifths dilatation of the cervix. Some of the staff preferred to give Demerol and hyacine, sometimes combined with a dose of nembutol. It was impressed upon me that no patient who did not wish for medication was forced to have it. It was pointed out, however, that it was highly unlikely that a woman would refuse, even though she was not having much physical pain.

The difficulty is that if she is given 100 to 150 milligrams of Demerol she will react, like so many women, in a manner that *lowers her discretion* and *intensifies,* to a large extent, *a negative emotional attitude* toward her labor activities. If she is given hyacine, there is no doubt her discretional sense will be partly or entirely destroyed.

As we passed the labor ward I heard two women cry out. How well I knew that horrifying noise. One woman was particularly uncontrolled; she was terrified, and only in pain because she was trying to overcome her discomfort by resisting it. The thought went through my mind, Can't she be told how to stop making it painful for herself? Hasn't she been told how to breathe? Similar thoughts always pass through my mind when I hear a woman distressed in early labor. But I knew these women were only semiconscious; a routine sedative had already been given, and they could not help themselves.

We moved on into the most immaculate changing room, where I was told the patients' attendants put on sterile garments before they delivered a woman. Nearby was a room where obstetricians rested while waiting for a child to be born. This was fitted with cupboards and closets for clothes, with a beautifully tiled and decorated washroom and shower.

I was then shown into an anteroom that contained a vast supply of instruments in glass cases, visible to all who might pass by, including the patients. There were hoards of drugs in capsules, vials, and bottles, in test tubes and mysterious boxes, all ready for immediate exhibition should occasion be deemed to have arisen. There were syringes and needles for all manner of analgesic and anesthetic injections; some were given to desensitize the whole woman and others for different areas and parts of the woman. Some robbed her of consciousness and others of discretion. It seemed there was no possibility of an emergency arising that could not be dealt with immediately, but there was *no provision for the absence of emergency or abnormality.* I was told it did not happen!

I felt that I was in the general atmosphere of a great nation, *so efficiently equipped for war under the pious persuasion of*

self-preservation and peace that war became almost inevitable.
In fact, the thinking seemed to be that it would be a shame to
have had so much money spent without putting the equipment
to use, even though this meant misusing it. Those of us who
have seen three wars no longer think of that. We find the mind
of man today has so reached a comprehension of the physical
world that it gives him power to destroy the human race. Man
tends to shrink from the belief that there is a force greater
than he. There is a trend in American obstetrics toward an
element of servitude to mechanization and the materialization
of childbirth and motherhood. But man, however brilliant, has
no right to assume command of the ship of human destiny
before he even knows its purpose.

I believe there is an Omnipotence that makes our presence
here purposeful. I cannot understand it, but I have only to
look at the ordered brilliance of natural phenomena to seek
some explanation of these mysteries in creative genius which
are still beyond the comprehension of man. I am never without a sense of awe, no matter how many hundreds, thousands
of babies now, I have seen into the world. I experience a sense
of awe at the magnificence of the physical and emotional
perfection of a woman when she takes her child into her arms
and knows at last she has received the gift of God for which
she has so earnestly prepared. Surely prevention is better than
cure?

Women have written me of their experiences of being tied
down to the table, their limbs fixed, their faces buried in a
mask against their wishes, their bodies cut although there was
plenty of room for the child to pass, and their infants pulled
into the world by instruments in the manner that Soranus of
Ephesus said should never be, for force should never be used
to empty the womb.

Here in this place I was seeing it for myself. I looked at
everything. By this time we had reached the delivery area. The
delivery table was an astonishing mechanical contrivance
upon which I understood women were pilloried so that, with-

out resistance, all sensations, pleasant and unpleasant, could be taken from them. Consciousness was retained in some cases, but the sensations of birth were thought to be extremely painful and thus deleted.

I found on this stainless steel and chromium-plated table a variety of pedals and handles that swung, tilted, raised, lifted, and dropped all parts and parcels of the contraption. There were rests in which a woman's legs were fixed so that she could neither move nor use them. Her body lay flat, with her head on the same level as her buttocks, reducing, almost minimizing, the mechanical advantages of the distribution and attachment of the muscles of expulsion. At the sides of the table, just about level with her hipbones, were strong metal fixtures through which saddle-leather straps and buckles passed. I asked if these were still used, having remembered that some obstetricians had discarded them, but learned that strapping down of the hands was routine practice. Every woman's hands were restrained so that she was unable to move her arms while her child was being expelled through the birth canal, or while the surgeon was removing it with instruments from the pelvic outlet, which had been operated on and had to be repaired with stitches. At the upper end of the table there were similar sockets through which straps could pass to fix not only the shoulders but, if necessary, the head of the patient, who might possibly, in her dazed condition, resist complete unconsciousness because she wished to be awake enough to see and greet her baby.

I asked my host whether a woman was conscious of the indignity of giving birth in this way, when she finds herself immobile upon the machine called a bed, fully aware of her position, her immobilization, and her exposure. My friend replied that he thought women were completely satisfied with the situation, and also commented that it made the job much easier for him. He could desensitize the whole woman or any part of her. Her position on the delivery table had nothing to do with it, so long as she escaped the agonies.

I don't wish to make my comments in any sense a satire. Rather, it is with astonishment that I wonder how such things can still be found as representing the most modern of all advances in childbearing. This vast expenditure, plan, and provision was, to me, a major condemnation of the creative genius. I had a picture of mere man, swathed in green and white masks, caps, gowns, and maybe boots, telling the Almighty it was just too bad He did not know His job. It was a good thing man was there to do it for Him. I had seen all this before, and it hurt.

I was given a gown and mask to put on and taken to observe a delivery. A young and beautiful girl was lying flat on the delivery table, her head resting on a small rubber pillow. Her legs were strapped into deeply guttered supports, and widely opened; her wrists were strapped in padded cuffs, which were attached to the table. She was still and quiet, with her eyes shut, until a contraction came. Then she opened her eyes and looked at the nurse standing beside her. It was an impersonal look received with an impersonal look. I should have preferred a faint smile or a gentle pat on the girl's arm.

The attending doctor sat on the stool between his "victim's" feet, which were on the level of his head. He looked over his shoulder and nodded to a nurse, who wheeled forward a table on which was an array of surgical and obstetric instruments covered by a sterile towel. He looked up at his professor, who was beside him, silently observing.

"She is quite normal, sir, and a pretty quick labor. She is fully dilated now, so I will get the baby. It is not big."

As he said that, he made a deep cut with a pair of scissors, about an inch and a half downwards and outwards, as if cutting into the center of the clock face down to seven o'clock on the dial. I turned to follow my host, who led the way out of the delivery room. Perhaps by some strange transference, he felt my feelings and guessed my thoughts correctly.

The day after this exhibition of kindness by incarceration, I happened to see, in a daily paper, a picture presented, along with a number of letters of remonstrance, that was intended to call attention to the dastardly cruelty of the Russians, the most unjustifiable desecration of life, human or otherwise, flaunted under the name of science. It was a picture of the passenger the Russians had the day before sent into space aboard a rocket—a small dog, depicted with a most benign, self-sacrificing expression on its face as it lay there, its hind legs tied down and its forepaws fixed in straps; it was manacled and shackled but supplied with artificial food and adequate oxygen. This, the fear-inducing illustration of ultimate cruelty, was thrust under my nose by a very good obstetrician and personal friend of mine, with the sort of look on his face that said, "Now, how about that?" .

I am, above all things, an animal lover, and sometimes would rather see chastisement administered to a naughty teen-ager than to a helpless animal, but instead of rising up in my wrath I found it very difficult to suppress the most unwelcome grin that threatened to show itself on my face. For when I heard the words "ultimate cruelty," I thought immediately of the woman I had seen the day before, her legs immobilized by straps, her hands strapped down, a band across her forehead so that she could not move her head and so that she could be given an anesthetic without being allowed to turn away. I saw by her side and all around her oxygen apparatus and food for reinforcement of nutrition, should her metabolism require support. She was helpless, placed there in order to accept the tenets of science in the name of humanity. She had become an experimental piece in the hands of a scientist, and at any moment might be shot in part or in toto into the outer space of unconsciousness.

I could not help seeing a perfectly straightforward simile. I realized the indignity, indeed the cruelty that women should be robbed of the greatest natural achievement, the reward of happiness that has been provided by the physiological law. This experience, if properly prepared and conducted by an understanding attendant, could influence not only her own life but that of her husband and newborn baby, and therefore, in time, the social circle in which we live.

We need to ask again, what is the underlying purpose? What is the biological objective of the reproductive faculty? What are we breeding for at all? Those of us who look after women bearing children must realize that every newborn child may be a potential leader of mankind. Our responsibility goes even further, for we need to be making good mothers while we make babies, in order to make a society worthy of a progressive culture. Are we going to allow our cultural desires to take us down to a level below that of our fathers and forefathers? It is our job to cultivate the stock of tomorrow.

Is the United States willing to accept the long-term results of the substitution of materialism for the metaphysical, the eternal or everlasting? The people of New York reacted strongly when the Russians put their first satellite in orbit. There was a feeling that they had suffered loss of "face," but what went through my mind was, Does this great people realize the astuteness of the Russians in adopting the use of procedures of natural childbirth?

In many of the hospitals I visited I was confused and baffled by the passion for interference with a healthy natural function. Again and again I heard of: episiotomies, 100 percent; forceps, 50 to 75 percent; induction by appointment, up to 70 percent in some places. The high rate of forceps deliveries came as a shock to me. In most countries the forceps rate is between 5 and 8 percent. When, therefore, I was told that forceps were used in up to 75 percent of deliveries in some hospitals, I at once sought justification for this high figure. Such a percentage in a hospital in England or any of the European countries I have visited would call for an inquiry. I soon learned that a school of thought that had considerable following in the United States believed that the only safe method of delivery was by forceps operation. This necessitated some form of general or local anesthetic and, of course, an episiotomy. Childbirth became a surgical performance.

I looked up statistics published by several hospitals, and found that one of the most famous ones had published tables representing the percentage of forceps deliveries of all cases in the hospital for the years stated:

Year	Clinic	Private
1954	17.5%	50.9%
1955	21.4%	46.0%
1956	18.7%	42.4%

Two questions arose in my mind. Why was the forceps rate of the white, brown, and black clinic population so much lower than for white private patients whose fees were higher? Anatomically and obstetrically, private patients do not present variations that require more help or more interference, unless their "higher intelligence" made it more difficult for them to accept the natural law. The attendant factor seemed to be an influence in this case—what was it? I made some inquiries, but received no satisfactory reply.

The operation of episiotomy is another example of routine interference, without clinical indication, without consideration of its causes or prevention. In many of the hospitals I visited I find that episiotomy is considered to be a necessary routine operation and, what has astonished me even more, that students are taught it is dangerous to deliver a child without cutting the outlet of the birth canal.

Like many other phenomena of childbirth, the cause of the tight outlet has never been carefully investigated. We are told the birth canal is tight, small, or that the head is large, in the wrong position, and so on, but when I asked, *"Why* is this?" the answer has usually been, "Well, because it is." That is all that can be said about the causation of something that is obviously abnormal or pathological.

There are recognized conditions that demand this operation. In England we generally consider there are eight indications, which I need not go into now. They are quite definite, easily diagnosable, and, for one who is not sufficiently experiericed to rely entirely upon his own judgment, make a very suitable list of the indications upon which he can base his practical application. But when it comes to results, I must say it is quite extraordinary.

In a large modern textbook I have read that episiotomy is a highly prophylactic operation because it prevents prolapse of the womb, incontinence of urine, undoubtedly prevents stillbirth of the child in some cases, and most certainly prevents the aftereffects of infantile cerebral hemorrhage.

I suggest that the operation of episiotomy could not possibly prevent all these complications and sequelae of labor! The damage causing these conditions is sustained *before* the head of the baby reaches the perineum. In 90 percent of healthy women attended by competent obstetricians the mutilation of episiotomy is unnecessary.

At this point in one of my lectures one of the senior members of the hospital staff rose quietly and said, "But have you forgotten so much that must be taken into account? Episiotomy shortens labor, which is good for the baby and the mother. It prevents tears and is a clean incision which is much easier to repair than a tear that may be jagged and roughedged. We find, too, that it relieves the pressure on the baby's head, and it obviously cannot be good for a child to be pressed down on to that rigid perineum, drawn up and pressed down again, like a battering ram." At this, there were several nods of approval.

I asked him whether he had any idea how often he had seen a truly elastic perineum which stretched easily and large enough to allow the biggest of babies to pass without any trouble or tearing. He said he didn't remember having seen one like that because he never allowed them to get to that stage. I thought this was a very good reply, and I went on.

"May I assure you that episiotomy may shorten labor by five to ten minutes if it is performed at the right moment. But it is not good for the mother, and I am not persuaded it is good for the baby in the absence of obvious tensions. I am surprised you believe tears to be unavoidable because they are not, even in a primipara. Care must be taken and patient delivery understood and performed. The battering ram analogy amuses me. Sometimes it is 'ewe.' "

Then a delightfully suave little man almost leaped to his feet. He said, "But surely, sir, we ought to know. We deliver enough, and there is no doubt about it—in this part of the United States the heads of babies are much bigger than they used to be, and there is no reason to believe that women have grown proportionately larger at the outlet."

I could not resist it, and said, "So you really feel, Doctor, that in this particular state some social factor has placed your women in a position of disadvantage in relation to the production of your children and your children's children? How do you account for that? Do you accept the law of Julius Wolfe, 'Structure is adapted to function'?"

Then he suggested, "Well, as the brain becomes more developed, I think it is possible that the head gets bigger!"

There was a good, cheerful laugh all around the room at this ambitious concept of development, and I added, "I am not sure I could possibly provide evidence to show that you are wrong, but I have no evidence to persuade me that the youth of this great country become swollen-headed before they are born!" Fortunately this little pleasantry was kindly taken.

Whereupon my friend the professor explained, "Episiotomy is not actually performed one hundred percent of the time, but only about ninety-seven percent of the time here. About three women in every hundred have their babies before the attendant has time to give the anesthetic and perform the episiotomy."

As we discussed the condition more seriously, I pointed out that the general rigidity of the birth canal has little to do with the physical condition of the woman, but varies according to her *mental* state. We went into the question of the neurology and the protective resistance and even spasm that could occur in a frightened woman. It was also realized that if a woman had a certain type of anesthesia she could be unconscious before the influence of fear was entirely absent, so that the perineum would remain tense.

Some forms of local anesthesia, such as epidural injections, undoubtedly assist in the relaxation of the perineum, and the professor of one large university hospital told me that since he had used that particular measure he found the necessity for episiotomy was not so general. In fact, using the epidural, he was now doing only 65 to 70 percent episiotomies rather than his routine of 100 percent with other forms of anesthesia.*

We discussed the position in which women were delivered, the details of the delivery of the child, and the behavior of the mother at that time. I was surprised to find that children were not received from the mother's body in the normal physiological direction, up and over the front of her body. Nature intended every mother to take her own baby and hold it up to herself as soon as it came into the world. I was able to demonstrate easily, on a blackboard, what a large number of unnecessary tears occur because of the baby being pulled straight out from the mother.

"But," I went on, "allowing for all these details of the study of the delivery of the child, there are still a number of factors which must come into it. One is the experience which enables you to know when it is necessary to do an episiotomy in order to prevent a tear."

What impressed me about this delightful conversation was how very little some of the senior men appeared to understand the detailed mechanism of this important part of labor. One oft-repeated notion was that no woman could possibly have a baby pass through the outlet of the birth canal without a terrible pain. They taught this and believed it, so much so that if a woman did have her baby without unbearable discomfort,

* With or without an episiotomy, deadening the sensations of the perineum by injection lessens or eliminates the birth climax—the pleasurable sexual orgasm accompanying many nonmedicated births, described in the forthcoming *Childbirth and the Family,* by Helen Wessel (New York: Harper & Row, 1973).

she was looked upon as a pathological or abnormal person. In fact, when it occurred, students were usually asked to go in and talk to her about it.

I pointed out once more that, from my experience and that of many other obstetricians who followed the prenatal education accurately and delivered according to the procedures of natural childbirth, more than 90 percent of women did not desire or require any cutting to enlarge the outlet. Occasionally, if the *fourchette,* the little membrane that seems to guard the back of the outlet, bursts early, one must be alert to the possible need of an episiotomy.

But it is not fully realized what a tremendous impact episiotomy has on the minds of a large number of sensitive women. It is not a thing that is discussed freely. But owing to the fact that I have not been a gynecologist only, or just an obstetrician, but have had the privilege of being a general practitioner of women's ailments of mind and behavior as well as body, I have become aware of several matters of great interest and importance.

One is that, after episiotomy, quite a definite percentage of women have developed frigidity. I have met many who were perfectly happy in married life until after their first baby was born, when they suddenly felt a deprivation of their virginal perfection. Tumescence ceased to occur and desire became much less importunate. Both husbands and young wives, happy with their babies of six or eight months old, have been to see me to ask why it is that orgasm has deserted the wife. The husband feels that she no longer loves him, and she feels horrified that such a thing could happen when they had been so happy.

If carefully examined, the condition is usually found to be primarily a mixture of physical effects and a psychological sense of deprivation and injury. These young women have suffered birth trauma. This may be a hard thing for gynecologists to understand, for the episiotomy seems so simple, so effective, so free of danger. Yet many women have told me,

"Ever since I found it was sore to sit down for a few days after my baby was born, I felt something had happened to me that could never come right again. I seemed to lose all pride in that part of my body and didn't know whether to be ashamed of myself, angry with the baby, or just apologetic to my husband."

"A dreadful state," one woman told me, "and when I went to see my doctor about it, all he said was, 'Don't be silly!'"

Even if the damage is only in the woman's mind—her self-image as a sexual being—the effect may be as irreparable. That part of her body which, deep down in her consciousness, has meant so much because of its effectiveness and perfection, is now no longer as presentable to her man-lover as it was previously. The most secret gift to her husband's love was tarnished by her baby's arrival.

I emphasize this because it is an example of the repercussions of interference with a physiological function and the normal laws of nature of which we are not always aware. We must bear in mind the possibility of emotional disturbances in a woman's mind, below the levels of rational thought, from events that are commonplace to us. I can't emphasize this enough.

When I got into the car to be driven back to the hotel at which I was staying, my mind turned to the women in the large Dutch hospitals, and in some of the Italian hospitals, and I thought how relatively unusual it is for the doctors there to interfere with a healthy, normal birth. I wondered whether there was a closer understanding of women and their thoughts and feelings in some countries than in others. Naturally I at once thought of the native tribes of the Central Congo, and of that wonderful old midwife in Buganda who came to see me with the local government medical officer. He assured me that to his knowledge she never had tears except in grossly abnormal cases. "How in the world does she do it?" I asked him, and he replied, "She is a child of nature and understands it from A to Z, and she has had fifteen babies herself!"

My visits to other hospitals seemed to be arranged as a salve to my injured obstetric conscience. In Cleveland, Cedar Rapids, Buffalo, Milwaukee, Seattle, New York, Denver, Santa Fe, and many other large towns I found groups or even whole hospitals that had turned away from the mechanistic orgy of sensate materialism. Here women were being educated and trained, made adequate in mind and body to carry out the programs required by the laws of nature. Everywhere I was told of decreased operative deliveries and a lowered rate of stillbirth and neonatal deaths. There was no maternal morbidity attributable to childbirth, very few blood transfusions were required, and childbirth was approached by women without fear or anxiety for its outcome. A father remarked how everyone at the hospital where his child was born had put him at ease. He described it as a hosptial for human, friendly, family-centered care. Another father commented by saying, "I can't say enough about the most loving, kind, and wonderful care." That atmosphere was combined with obviously first-class obstetric work. Thus as I traveled from place to place I found one or the other approach to childbirth, but with the "natural" spreading rapidly.

We learned many things about the Americans that helped us to understand some of their motives and behaviors. When people ask me, "What do you think of Americans?" I say, "Which Americans? From what point of view? Give me a more definite question and I will tell you if I have any experience upon which to give an opinion." We found so little common to all the states, but there were some things that were invariable—the kindliness and thought for its visitors.

Finally my conversations ceased, but I had no desire to leave. There was much I did not want to lose and so many I would miss. And I was conscious of an aching fear that one gets for the safety of a friend in danger! I wanted to stand up and shout, "For goodness sake, look to your production plants! The repair depots will take care of themselves."

24

In Conclusion

As this imperfect collection of observations is concluded, it may well be asked of me, "Why have you written this book?" There is no more exacting task and no occupation more thankless than the public expression of heretical views. It has been many years since I published my first series of observations and outlined the theory and practice of natural childbirth. That teaching has borne much fruit, and so I write more fully, hoping, not without justification, that more of my medical brethren may be persuaded to give this method fair and prolonged trial. I am not prompted by missionary zeal that seeks to proselytize the obstetric world, but only to invite attention to bare and irrefutable facts.

It is primarily to the youth of our profession that I appeal: to those who have just qualified and to those who are about to qualify. It is for you to join in the battle against pain. Each one of you has it within his power to observe carefully the phenomena of labor; each one of you has the birthright of investigation. Do not accept the conservative teaching of generations past without careful examination. For the most part, such teaching will stand scrutiny and will be proved correct in general principle. But from time to time you will be amazed at the inadequacy of the evidence upon which accepted principles are borne. Be critical of culture; look long and carefully before you accept its tenets; take notice of the subtle ways and means by which youth is robbed of its power and its instinctive genius. Be accurate in your deductions, and delve deeply into the details of each succeeding problem. Analyze your observations, and do not be slow to ask "why." Develop an inquiring mind; seek guidance and advice while you have around you those competent and willing to help you. There is no reason to be humble in your questioning, and certainly no justification for aggression in your differing. Learn from your mistakes, for if you seek the truth honestly, the errors that you make will be of service in your search. As you scramble from one pitfall to the next, you will gain strength and experience. The borderlands of the realm of knowledge are shrouded in a mist that is not penetrated by the earliest efforts of the beginner. As he gains a greater foothold within those realms, so the mist clears, until he finds the vista of unending possibility, the existence of which he had not previously envisaged. There is no such thing as knowing all. Cowper wrote:

> Knowledge is proud that he has learned so much,
> Wisdom is humble that he knows no more.

If, therefore, you feel humble because of your limited accomplishments, recognize that in humility alone lies the true urge and goad to further progress. Let your practice be founded upon the judgment of the intelligent, and your reputation upon the honest opinion of those who are in the best position to judge. Above all, your own personal satisfaction will raise you to a different plane; your work will be in a different cause; you will not be numbered among the "Gehazis who seek only money." Your belief is not in today, but rather in tomorrow and those distant tomorrows which will bring nearer to man his ultimate knowledge. Your faith is in the law of nature; your science is to be an adjuvant and not an impediment in its implementation.

But medicine is a science of opinion, and opinions differ, not only in diagnosis and treatment but in philosophy and ideals. In obstetrics you must form your own philosophy without fear, and observe with equanimity the ideals of those about you.

The privilege of attending women in childbirth is far greater than you are taught to realize. The public applauds the genius of skilled surgeons; famous physicians are beloved and respected for their healing power; great gynecologists are both surgeons and physicians within a limited field. Their lives are given up to the noble work of succoring the sick, curing the diseased, and mending the broken.

The casualties of living are the first call of the medical profession. But obstetricians do not work among casualties; their work is primarily among the supremely healthy members of the community. They watch over and improve original models from the great factories of human life; their responsibility is to improve the stock and render it fit to meet the new demands that modern communal existence makes upon each succeeding generation. The health of mothers and their babies should be the first consideration of an obstetrician.

You must make your choice now, and to your innermost self lay down the principles upon which your future will unfold. There are many paths leading to the rock of a physician's calling. Along the well-worn roads thousands pass, blindly following the lead of orthodoxy, pushing and jostling in a throng that steadily advances with the years to a comfortable plateau called Mediocrity. Here men gird themselves with mental and material armor, and search the descent to old age for respectable nooks and crannies where they may rest and watch the sun go down. It is possible to decorate a well-selected niche with an accolade, so that those who pass by may whisper to their friends, "Behold!"

There are also the untrodden paths that require not only youth, but freedom and fortitude. Those of you who seek a new truth must blaze a trail of your own. The jewels of our science lie off the beaten track. Press on in danger; with the risk of failure you have the urge to persevere. You will clamber among landmarks accepted by your forebears as immutable. Accept nothing, for under each established fact is the foundation of a new future. Gold is hidden in the solid vein of quartz. Climb alone up the precipice that leads to no plateau, but only to high peaks from which you can look down and see the truth you have uncovered on your way. You need no social armor in your isolation, need seek no comfortable haven of rest: sharpen your ax, respike your shoes, and struggle on, conscious always of the vision of youth, guided by the hand of experience to a greater reward than public recognition.

Pioneers pass on unheard and unlamented until the trail they blazed is followed by a few who have believed. At the end they are discovered where their life's work finished, mourned only by the wild flowers of the wilderness they loved.

Part IV

THE PHYSIOLOGY OF CHILDBIRTH

The following chapter on the physiology of childbirth was compiled primarily from material written by Grantly Dick-Read in 1933. The chapter was then submitted for comment to Dr. Berry Campbell, Ph.D., Professor of Physiology and Acting Chairman at the California College of Medicine, University of California, Irvine. The following reply was received in February 1971:

I have read the chapter of Grantly Dick-Read's book on natural childbirth with great interest and I have enjoyed the search through the literature to which it led me.

The chapter in question is remarkable. Before the discovery of the important role of estrogen and progesterone in the conditioning of the uterus to nervous regulation and even before the understanding was had of the role of acetylcholine, norepinephrine and epinephrine, not to mention oxytocin and the prostaglandins, a consideration of the clinical role of the balanced autonomic innervation of the uterus is given which still has great logical force.

Compared with other medical fields, the amount of scientific publication in obstetrics is remarkably sparse. However, there is a scattered literature on the subject in the last decade in which the same matter is reviewed in the framework of modern neuro-endocrinology. The modern work is best exemplified by Shabanah, *et al.*[1]*

The chapter from Grantly Dick-Read's book is most impressive when one realizes that the succeeding 40 years, though bringing much new and unexpected factual knowledge into the picture, have

* References for Chapter 25 begin on page 389.

born out his essential thesis completely. The reason for this, it seems to me, is that the base of his viewpoint is an astute and valid clinical observation. The physiological data are presented to show that they are compatible, but I doubt if it was from the physiological data that he drew his conclusions. It is most impressive that Dr. Read has been borne out so well by recent scientific advances.

25

The Physiology of Childbirth

There is a tendency these days, when publication in the press familiarizes the man in the street with the most dramatic exploits in the laboratory, to accept each new discovery as "the last word." So wonderful do the revelations of science appear that the idea of introducing simplicity as a means of unearthing the even greater revelations of nature is not well reveived. But it is essential to good obstetrics to begin with a clear understanding of the knowledge we have of the structure and mechanics of the uterus and birth canal when it is time to expel the fetus.

STRUCTURE OF THE UTERUS AND BIRTH CANAL

The Uterus

There are three definite muscular layers. Externally, longitudinal fibers sweep up from the lower uterine segment posteriorly over the fundus uteri, and down to the lower uterine segment anteriorly. These fibers have become enormously enlarged with the growth of the fetus, and many new fibers, or muscle cells as they are sometimes called, have made their appearance. They may be increased to fully ten times their length and five times their breadth during pregnancy. The middle layer has fibers interlaced in all directions, among which are the large and relatively dilated uterine blood vessels; the contraction of these fibers obliterates the passageway of the blood vessels. The inner layer are the circular fibers that surround the body of the uterus.

Longitudinally, the uterus may be divided into upper uterine segment, which comprises the greater part of the organ—its muscle wall is thick and powerful—and lower uterine segment, which is a thin part of the uterine body, comprising approximately three inches of uterine wall above the internal os. These two merge into each other imperceptibly, but the musculature of the lower uterine segment is weak compared to that of the upper.

It must be recognized that these divisions of the uterus are not defined by any anatomical limits. Uteri vary, and there is no fixed law where the upper and the lower uterine segment shall join.

In the same way it must be fully recognized that although the presence of (1) outer longitudinal, (2) the middle mixed, and (3) the inner circular muscle fibers are described as if they were anatomically separable and structurally apart from each other, this is not really so. The most careful dissectors have found it difficult to demonstrate clearly the muscle layers of the uterus in any given case, but the general structure and the whole organ does show that there is some such division, and although fibers in all directions may be intermixed, there is little question that they each play their part with an individuality essential to the perfection of the process.

The Cervix Uteri

The cervix uteri, like the body of the uterus, hypertrophies during pregnancy, although relatively to a small extent. Increased vascularity alters its hard, almost cartilaginous consistency to a loose and spongy elasticity. Some physiologists have observed a lengthening of the circular muscle fibers in the cervix, but its most definite property during pregnancy is elasticity. It does not have a sufficient supply of longitudinal muscle fibers to give it any power of expulsive contraction, and the internal os begins to dilate at the earliest stage of parturition. Some authorities consider that the internal os disappears and the upper part of the cervix uteri merges into the lower segment some weeks before the termination of pregnancy. The cervix uteri is attached around its whole surface to the vagina, higher posteriorly than anteriorly, so that its protrusion into the vagina makes it appear that the posterior wall is longer than the anterior. This explains the disappearance of the posterior lip before the anterior lip when the cervix is fully dilated. As the longitudinal muscles of the body of the uterus draw up the lower uterine segment, the cervix uteri is not so much stretched by the wedgelike mechanism of the descending structures, but is absorbed and pulled up by its continuity with the lower uterine segment, until the power of retraction of the uterine muscle fibers has flattened the cervix in continuity with the lower uterine segment and the upper limits of the cervical vaginal attachments. The whole birth canal thus becomes uniformly smooth, and without any constricting bands of protruding or thickened tissue, and the fetus will rotate within a well-lubricated and homogenous surface in its passage down to the vulval orifice.

The influences that may adversely affect this apparently simple mechanical procedure are largely dependent upon the ease with which the cervix uteri is pulled over the advancing presenting part, and the elasticity with which it merges into the wall of the birth canal.

The Vaginal Canal

The vaginal canal also has circular and longitudinal muscle fibers. They are weak and relatively ineffective during labor, and, unless some gross abnormality in either the fetal or maternal structure occasions undue pressure upon its walls, the dilatation of the vagina seldom gives rise to any complication. Its mucous lining pours out a copious secretion of lubricant.

The Vulva

The vulva, like other parts of the birth canal that have to dilate in order to allow free passage of the fetus, is endued with enormous elasticity. Unless some influence mars the natural process of labor, the vulva—and most important—the skin of the perineum itself will stretch without damage. The muscles of the pelvic floor will normally relax, as will the sphincter muscles of the vagina. The anterior triangle is relaxed and pulled upwards by the attachment of its apex to the anterior surface of the cervix uteri. The posterior triangle goes downward, its apex being attached to the perineum. Thus, as every student is quick to appreciate, the descending fetus passes through a pair of swinging doors—one that has opened inward and upward, and the other downward and outward.

When the integrity of this mechanism is maintained and the forces applied without aggravating stimuli, such operations as episiotomy or artificial stretching of the vulval orifice should never be necessary. In the absence of unnatural resistance to the normal forces of parturition, there should be no laceration or injury to any muscle of the pelvic floor or at the outlet. And unless subjected to sudden force or quick distension from below before the tissues are physiologically prepared, the perineum should rarely suffer injury.

These remarks upon the structure of the uterus and the birth canal must be very clearly in the mind in order to appreciate how easily complications of labor may arise from direct or reflex activities consequent upon abnormal influences invading a normal labor. Injury to the birth canal and pelvic floor is probably one of the great causes of permanent defective health among the women of cultured races. Injury arises in the very majority of cases from the imposition of resistance, either from the birth canal itself, opposing forces from the uterus above, or within a normal birth canal that is called upon to accommodate itself to applied forces from below.

AUTOMATIC CONTRACTION OF THE UTERUS

Having briefly outlined the anatomy of the uterus, and illustrated how its structure relates to its peculiar function, we must endeavor to make clear the peculiarities of the nervous mechanism of the uterus during parturition.

The uterine muscle is known to have the power of rhythmic contraction, irrespective of nerve supply. Kurdinowski,[2] in 1904, showed that the contractions were not dependent for their origin upon impulses from the central nervous system. Franz,[3] also in 1904, published further experimental work in which he demonstrated the capability of the uterus to contract when separated from the body, and also showed that impulses from the central nervous system are not essential to contraction, adding that although there were variations in the activity of the virgin uterus, these observations applied without exception to the pregnant uterus.

Holste,[4] in 1923, demonstrated powerful uterine contractions in a definite rhythm outside the body, and apparently working entirely on its own initiative. Rein,[5] in 1902, separated the uterus of a rabbit from all its extrinsic nerves, but the young arrived by spontaneous birth.

Although it can be clearly demonstrated that the various nerves supplied to the uterus appear to have branches that are inhibitory as well as branches that are motor, one faculty of uterine muscle that is extremely important in the unravelling of the mysteries of difficult labor is the ability of the circular muscle fibers to contract independently of the longitudinal. The importance of this power of individual contraction will easily be understood when we come to discuss the activity of the cervix uteri under impulses peculiar to culture.

The work of Whitehouse and Featherstone,[6] which is mentioned later, shows that as well as having the power of automatic contraction of itself, irrespective of nerve supply, there are also nerves to the uterus that govern and control its contractions either to assist or impede that automatic action. There is also evidence of some form of inhibitory center for uterine contraction that exists in the medulla oblongata, and Jacob[7] provided some substantial evidence of this fact. Thirty-six years after Jacob's work, Marshall,[8] commenting upon it, concludes that this is borne out to some extent by the fact that the "pains" of labor can often be inhibited by the emotions and other contemporary actions of the central nervous system.

Many cases have been observed and reported of automatic birth, where the lower half of the spinal cord has not functioned and the lower half of the body, therefore, has been completely paralyzed. Edward Parker Davis[9] recorded the painless character of labor in patients suffering from *tabes dorsalis* (spinal cord disease), and in his observations notes the powerful character of the muscular contractions of the uterus in these circumstances.

Physiologists have also recorded that the muscular contractions of the uterus appear to be *definitely stronger when separated from their nerve supply than in the natural state*. Zimmerman,[10] in 1914, and Schmidt,[11] in 1915, were drawn by these conclusions to submit that the normal nerve supply to the uterus conveys an inhibitory influence.

Routh[12] recorded several cases of normal parturition in women who were suffering from paraplegia caused by lesions in the spinal cord in the mid-dorsal region. In these women no impulses from nerve centers were received above that point, but they all had normal labors without sensation. It is therefore suggested that if there is a special center for the impulses necessary to parturition it is situated below the mid-dorsal region of the spine. The existence of efferent nerve fibers from the lumbar region of the spinal cord has been shown by Frankenhauser[13] and Korner,[14] and they make their way to the uterus via the inferior mesenteric ganglia and aortic plexus.

We can therefore see three apparently definite and separate controlling influences in uterine contraction during parturition, and this is clearly set out by Marshall in his general conclusions regarding the mechanism of parturition:

(1) The act of parturition is partly automatic and partly reflex, these actions corresponding in the main to the first and second stages of labor respectively, the spinal reflexes usually commencing immediately the membranes have ruptured.

(2) Direct communication with the brain is not essential for the proper coordination of uterine action, but the brain appears to exercise a controlling influence of some kind. Thus emotions often become a hindrance to the progress of parturition. It would seem possible that this inhibition of uterine contractions is brought about by an inhibition center in the brain.

(3) Direct communication between the uterus and the lumbar region of the cord is generally essential for the occurrence of those rhythmical contractions which take place in the progress of normal labor. There is experimental evidence upon animals, however, that the uterus is sometimes able automatically to expel its contents at least as far as the relaxed portion of the genital cord, even when entirely deprived of all spinal influences.[15]

More recently we have similar conclusions based upon different methods of examination. Kuntz, in *The Autonomic Nervous System* states:

In view of the experimental data available at present it may be assumed that the uterine musculature, *like other smooth muscle,* possesses the inherent capacity to undergo rhythmic contractions, but under conditions of normal innervation the activity of this musculature is subject to both motor and inhibitory nervous influences, which may be of reflex or central nervous origin.[16]

These important conclusions have a very definite bearing upon the mechanism of labor, and in particular we must note the influences that give rise to the inhibition of muscular activity, and the means by which that inhibition of rhythmic contraction is brought about.

The conclusions of Beckwith Whitehouse and Henry Featherstone, in the *British Medical Journal* of 1923, are of

If we turn back and review the structure of the uterus, we find that the proportion of circular fibers in the cervix uteri is much higher than anywhere else in the organ, and conversely the strength of the longitudinal fibers is much less. Although the lumbosacral autonomic system is motor to the longitudinal fibers, the uterus does not depend upon it for its power of contraction. Should these stimuli be entirely nullified, the uterus will continue to contract of its own automaticity, even though the sympathetic nervous system is acting directly contrary to the normal mechanism.

We may summarize the effects of the various nerve supplies under four headings:

1. The local innervation, which is responsible for expulsive contractions.

2. The parasympathetic nerve supply, which stimulates the muscles of expulsion.

3. The sympathetic nerves, which inhibit expulsion.

4. The sympathetic nerves, which cause the muscle fibers around the large vessels of the middle layer to contract.

Factors Relevant to Nerve Supply

Now, it is clear that one of the primary and essential factors of a relatively easy labor lies in the elimination of this sympathetic stimulus. The sacral autonomic supply is a comparatively small and localized area of distribution from definite and separate upper-ganglionic fibers. On the other hand, the sympathetic division of the autonomic system is of widespread distribution and allows the reception of stimuli by one means or another through a variety of causes from practically the whole body. Cannon's metaphor facilitates the understanding of this. He states: "The sympathetic is like the soft and loud pedals, modulating all the notes together, but the cranial and sacral autonomic are like the separate keys."[20] The contracting cervix resisting dilatation and increasing uterine tension is but a single symptom of the general intensification of sympathetic activity. That it may of itself become a secondary or contributing cause of further sympathetic stimulation is highly probable, for the fact that it inhibits a normal function invites psychical as well as physical reinforcements to the already adverse influences proceeding from the higher centers through the sympathetic back to the uterus.

From the point of view of the clinician, it has long been difficult to understand why a cervix that, between contractions, appears to be patulous, soft, and elastic, resists dilatation, even though the mechanism of labor is otherwise perfect. No obstetrician has failed to notice how frequently the nervous patient is the slow dilator; so much so that the slow labor has been attributed to the resistance occasioned by the fetal head to the birth canal, or by the relative weakness of the uterine contractions, and to the slowness of the labor has been assigned the mental and physical anguish of the patient.

Surely cause and effect have been transposed! The mental anguish of the patient has added general sympathetic intensification, for the physical signs of her emotion are in reality the physical signs of an intensification of sympathetic stimuli. As surely as she vomits, has a rapid pulse, large pupils, and a cold, pallid, perspiring face, so surely in harmony with these manifestations is the presence of the resistant contraction of the circular fibers of her uterus—in particular those of the cervix uteri, which series of events calls for a further excitation through the whole vicious circle. When the longitudinal fibers press down the fetal head, it causes intense discomfort which increases as retraction as well as contraction takes place. Probably the discomfort itself adds force to the sphincterlike constriction of the cervix.

Pain

The phenomenon of pain has been evolved with a definite purpose. It is so general among all the higher forms of animal life that it is probably beneficial and not of itself harmful. It is an important device employed by nature to protect the individual from injury or the results of injury. The reaction to irritation is movement, which is demonstrated by the amoeba, the simplest unicellular form of animal life; if we place minute granules of methylene blue in contact with its surface, the response is movement in order to escape from or rid itself of the irritating particle. As we ascend the scale to the higher mammals, awareness to stimulation increases. Whether reaction is associated with volition is open to discussion, and we must presume that in the absence of consciousness, defense movements are purely tissue reflexes. We can learn very little about pain from experiments upon animals. Our knowledge must accrue from observation upon conscious human beings; they alone are able to describe their feelings. If we remove the consciousness, by any means, there is no pain appreciation and therefore vital resistance to pain is absent.

Over the surface of the body and upon various internal organs and structures, there are minute nerve endings that we know as pain-receivers, or nociceptors. In the pristine eras of human development we were exposed to attack by tooth and claw; therefore the greatest profusion of nociceptors are found over the vulnerable areas of the body where injury would have most serious consequences. The sides of the neck, under the arms, the abdomen and the chest are all extremely sensitive places, for, if engaged in combat, it would be here that tooth and claw would inflict damage and cause the physical shock that places a fighter at the mercy of his foe. If we watch kittens, puppies, or young bears at play, we can see where nociceptors are liberally distributed. There are definite areas which each endeavors to claw or bite—they roll, feint, and jump to shield these places. They are playing, but unwittingly practicing the more serious art of attack and defense.

But we need not discuss the pain-receivers of the body surface, for we are interested in those within the abdominal cavity. The uterus is poorly supplied with the organs that register pain (nociceptors), for it conforms much more to the distribution and behavior of nerves that supply the internal organs of the abdomen. The intestines and the internal organs, in particular the uterus, are not affected by external cold or heat and the abdominal wall has to be severely injured or ripped open before they can be damaged, but they are well supplied with pain receptors that record *excessive tension* or *laceration of the tissues*. No other nociceptors have been demonstrated within the abdomen—the intestines and the uterus can be burned, cauterized, handled, and moved without any sensation of discomfort to the patient, but if either of these structures is stretched or torn, considerable pain and shock result.

All nociceptors are specific, that is to say, they react to only one form of pain stimulation. It follows thus that the only pain stimulus that the uterus can record is excessive tension or actual tearing of tissues. I have been persuaded from experiment and experience that specificity is a constant phenomenon in both conditioned reflexes and sensory receptors, as Pavlov[21] and Sherrington[22] conclude. The pain of labor, whether referred or otherwise, must result from one, or both, of these specific stimuli. So we must ask ourselves: Does nature intend that childbirth should be accompanied by laceration and injurious tension? If it does, why has not this important structure adapted itself to its function, according to the law of Professor Julius Wolfe, which was, in short: "Structure is adapted to Function"? If nature does not intend this laceration and injury, then those pain-receivers are there to respond only to stimuli other than normal. We must inquire: Against what is the uterus protecting itself by giving pain sensations in carrying out a perfectly natural function? The physiological perfection of the human body knows no greater paradox than pain in normal parturition.

The biological purpose of pain interpretation is protective, and it results in muscular activity to the end that the individual may either defend himself or escape from impending danger. For instance, if a finger is accidentally put on a hot stove, almost before there is any conscious mental interpretation of what has happened it has been removed; the muscular activity of protection has been immediately employed by lifting the finger from the injurious stimulus. Pain also instructs us, lest its horrors be repeated through our carelessness. The creation of such association and experience is exemplified by the small boy who withdraws his hand as the master's cane descends.

There are, however, pains from which we cannot escape so easily, arising from the internal organs and known as visceral pains. The uterus and the pelvic organs are visceral, and therefore in this discussion we are primarily concerned with visceral pain. It must be borne in mind, also, that we are not concerned with disease but with healthy women carrying out a normal and natural function.

There is no physiological function in the body that gives rise to pain in the normal course of health. When the natural urges to perform are uncomfortable, it usually indicates that the physiological balance is being strained.

All over the body there are groups of muscles whose actions are opposed to each other. A simple example is the action of the biceps and the triceps. If we wish to bend the arm at the elbow, the biceps contract and the triceps, which normally oppose it, relax. If, on the other hand, we wish to straighten our arm, the triceps contract and the biceps at the same time relax. If both these muscles function at the same time, the arm goes into a state of rigidity. If the contractions are strong enough the whole arm quivers, and in a very short time there is considerable pain in the limb.

This arrangement also holds good for all organs of the body that fill and empty. In normal physiological action one muscle group by contraction prevents emptying of the organ, but is completely relaxed and loose when the opposing muscle groups contract to empty the organ. This convenient harmony of muscle action is seen, for example, in the bowel and urinary bladder. When the bowel is emptied, the muscles that are brought into play in order to expel its contents are not opposed by the ring of muscles, or the sphincter, at the outlet, which normally holds the bowel tightly closed. When an expulsive effort is made the outlet is relaxed. The same also applies to the urinary apparatus. Both these mechanisms may give rise to acute pain if spasmodic contraction at the outlet occurs and resists the efforts of the expulsive muscles. The condition called fissure of the anus, which is extremely painful, may cause a spasm of the sphincter muscle so that it will not relax. The two opposing muscles, acting at the same time, combine to produce acute pain from abnormal pressure. The same is true in the spasmodic tension of a baby's anus when it becomes constipated. The reflex relaxation of the sphincter ani is overcome by the unconscious influence of the sympathetic, stimulated by the anticipation of increasing pain when the tension of a hard motion causes discomfort with each expulsive effort. We see it again in the retention of urine in cases of acute urethritis, for pain inhibits the reflex relaxation of the sphincter. How often emotional excitement is the underlying cause of dyspareunia, particularly when laceration of a rigid hymen conserves memory not only of surprise but of physical pain. The spasm of vaginismus has unquestionably a strong relationship to the sympathetic stimuli emanating from the pathological emotional reactions of a psychoneurotic.

The same harmony of muscle action is seen in the uterus during childbirth. The longitudinal muscle fibers, whose action is expulsive, contract. In normal conditions the circular muscle fibers are relaxed and flaccid, allowing dilatation of the outlet to the womb and free passage of the child.

From the general principles of the construction of the uterus we deduce that labor without the pain of tension or injury depends upon:

1. Expulsive muscle activity *without resistance* from constricting muscles.

2. Expulsive nerve impulses being active and constrictor nerve impulses inactive.

3. Elasticity of structures around arteries and veins between expulsive contractions so that a full supply of fresh blood may be maintained and the waste product of muscle action freely removed.

INFLUENCES OF EMOTION UPON LABOR

In order to appreciate the influences of the emotions upon any function, it should be clearly understood that emotion is probably the cause of physiological activity, and not physiological activity the cause of emotion. The perfection of the human body as a working machine is beyond criticism. If its imperfections are to be considered, then first let the applied misuses to which it is subjected be given their full significance.

The emotions do not arise from physical stimulus; but from emotional stimulus physical changes occur that, given normal and natural circumstances, are to the end that the body itself shall be more efficient to meet the physical or mental responsibility that time and circumstance may place upon it.

It is impossible to give even an outline, in such a work as this, of the discoveries that have been made that point to the increased efficiency of the body to meet emergencies under the influence of emotional stress. The secretion of the adrenal glands is said by some physiologists to play a large part in the quality of our emotional reactions. Under certain circumstances blood corpuscles are poured out into the circulatory system to meet an emergency. Under others, the blood sugar is suddenly increased, thereby augmenting the fuel value within the circulatory system. Certain mental and emotional states have been shown to call for such reaction as will increase the coagulation power of the blood. The reserves of the body, in hiding and apparently nonexistent, are suddenly called into the fray like strong reinforcements that have been lying in readiness until such time as emergency shall demand their help.

Let us consider what occurs in natural labor. Some biochemical or mechanical change—concerning which many theories are at present not yet proved—sets up rhythmical expulsive contractions of the uterus, and the lumbosacral autonomic system, under normal circumstances, proceeds to carry out its primary function, which is the emptying of viscera. It stimulates the longitudinal fibers of the uterus to contract, or it may be more accurate to say that the local and inherent stimulus derived from the uterus itself to produce rhythmical contractions is augmented by the lumbosacral autonomic system. The lumbosacral autonomic system antagonizes the sympathetic stimuli which are motor to the circular muscle fibers and inhibitory to the longitudinal bundles, with the obvious consequence that the contracting neck of the uterus and the cervix uteri, which are chiefly composed of circular muscle fibers, adopt a state of complete relaxation. This relaxation enables the cervix quickly to be taken up; it enables the uterine muscle cells by the faculty of retraction to draw up the cervix around the well lubricated presenting part.

It is open to very serious consideration whether or not the teaching of dilatation of the cervix has, in the past, been entirely accurate. Few obstetricians can be satisfied that the presenting part forces open the cervix uteri. Unquestionably, a well-formed bag of waters or a pronounced caput succedaneum are of great assistance to the retracting longitudinal muscle fibers in their efforts to pull the cervix upward over a presenting part. How many who have been called upon to do a podalic version have found that the cervix will admit the whole hand with practically no resistance, when it has been subjected to none of the so-called dilating structures from above. I suggest that the greatest factor in the dilatation of the cervix is the inhibitory effect of the lumbosacral autonomic system upon its circular muscle fibers, and the absence of any overpowering stimulus that would retain its muscle fibers in a state of contraction.

Normally, therefore, the integrity of the process of parturition depends upon the antagonistic action of those nerves which supply the longitudinal fibers on the one hand, and the circular fibers on the other. *This applies throughout the birth canal, even to the perineum itself, for the muscles of the pelvic floor and the sphincter muscles of the vagina, and the elasticity of the perineum, are each in their turn dependent for complete relaxation upon the harmony with which the integral parts of the machinery carry out their work.*

Look upon labor, therefore, in its simple form, as being carried out primarily by the lumbosacral autonomic stimuli, in conjunction with the automatic rhythmical stimuli from the uterus, antagonizing to a very large extent any interference from the sympathetic nervous system. Although it may be that there are higher centers in the medulla and in the cortex, which can, under certain circumstances, influence the course of parturition, there are sufficient cases on record to demonstrate that no activity is required on the part of these higher centers, and if they have any control over the lumbosacral autonomic or the sympathetic nerve distribution, it plays no part that is essential to uncomplicated labor. The same applies to a corticothalamic interaction, and whatever part the optic thalamus may play when deprived by anesthesia of its subservience to cortical influence, it does not appear to affect the main principle of nerve control of parturition.

If in outline this describes the muscular activity dependent upon the nerve supply throughout the birth canal, it also enables us to see that birth itself should occasion no pressure sufficiently great to give rise to objective peripheral pain. Where there is no gross abnormality of structure in the female pelvis, the elasticity of the fetal part is such that, during the processes described above, pressure is not increased to an extent that can cause injury to the surrounding tissues.

These principles of interaction of the longitudinal and circular muscle fibers are applicable right through the pelvic canal. The pelvic floor is extremely elastic; the levator ani offers no resistance where there is no spasm. The sphincters of the vagina are not only extremely elastic, but when in a state of relaxation offer no resistance whatever to the descending fetus. The skin of the perineum, if it is not subjected to any unnatural force, will dilate without rupture in a very large number of cases—in fact it may be said that any tear in the perineum in normal labor is an injury for which the obstetrician is probably more responsible than the woman herself. Thus we see that where there is complete harmony in the action and interaction of the muscles of the birth canal, and where that harmony depends upon normal stimuli to the nerves concerned in parturition, there is no anatomical feature that creates difficulty, undue strain, or pressure too great for the surrounding tissues.

When the baby is born in the natural state, the mother is not only conscious, but she hears, as a reward for the hard work that has been hers for the previous few hours, the cry of her child. The powerful emotion known as "mother love" sweeps throughout her whole body; she receives stimuli from sight, from hearing; the joy of accomplishment adds to the intensification of her sympathetic activity. The first cry of a baby after a normal labor, if clearly heard by a fully conscious mother, has, in my experience, an action upon the uterine musculature as immediate and as powerful as pituitrin extract. Not infrequently have I called the attention of nurses and attendants who have been assisting me in maternity work to this phenomenon. I have rarely seen a postpartum hemorrhage when a fully conscious mother has heard the first cry of her child; I can remember no case of healthy retained placenta under those circumstances. But more frequently I have noticed that the placenta has been expelled from the uterus into the vaginal end of the birth canal painlessly and without any hemorrhage, before the twenty minutes have passed that I adopt as my arbitrary minimum for the time of the third stage of labor.

Such cases as these demonstrate that loss of maternal blood is pathological; that a certain amount of placental hemorrhage should occur is probably not only natural, but physiologically necessary, for, as the placenta separates from the surface of the uterus, there must be a certain amount of blood retained within its meshes distal to the point of closure, and separation of those vessels which interchange supplies upon the placental site of the uterus.

The importance of this emotion to the success of parturition cannot be exaggerated. I am persuaded quite definitely in the fundamental truth of this observation that the conscious knowledge of accomplishment of which the mother becomes aware at the end of the second stage gives rise to those emotions which nature intended as agents to the perfection of the third stage of labor.

Now let us consider what occurs throughout this process when fear creeps into the mind of the woman—when that part of her autonomic nervous system which is stimulated most strongly by this emotion takes precedence, and wields its influence to antagonize the natural stimuli of the lumbosacral distribution.

The Mechanism of Fear

Fear is alertness to the presence of danger. In other words, the reception of impulses making us aware of the actual or possible presence of phenomena associated in our minds with pain or injury. Crile has pointed out that "the phylogenetic origin of fear is injury; hence, injury and fear cause the same phenomena."[23] Fear gives rise to action—in other words, produces motor responses. In order to do this, the sympathetic nervous system is activated by impulses that are inhibitory to all visceral action, for, in order to utilize all possible physical strength for the purpose of defense, those parts of the body which are of no service in defensive action are deprived of motor activity. At the same time the adrenalin excretion is increased. In short, the influence of fear, being conveyed through the sympathetic nervous system, inhibits the pelvic autonomic. As a result of this, the neuromuscular harmony of labor in the presence of fear is disturbed in a manner exactly similar to that produced by pain.

In all cases where there is injury or pain, action is demanded by the body's protective motor responses; and where there is fear, fight or flight is its only outlet. But in labor neither fight nor flight is possible. Injury without action rapidly exhausts nervous energy, but an acute emotional state that must be suffered without escape has been shown by Crile to exhaust the cytoplasm of the Purkinje cells of the cerebellum even more rapidly. Thus acute or persistent pain, whether caused by either injury or fear, actually destroys certain elements of the nerve cells of the brain that are concerned with the integration and interpretation of pain stimuli. Therefore one of the first duties of a good doctor is to see that his patient does not suffer any unnecessary pain.

The effect of pain on the human body has been observed in all the variations of its manifestation by every physician, but in particular we must consider its effect upon women in labor. We must know to what extent the nerves supplying the muscles that take part in this act can be affected by emotional stress. The experimental evidence for this can be found in the works of such investigators as Langley,[24] Cannon,[25] Sherrington,[26] Anderson,[27] etc., in regard to the other internal organs of the body.

The essential protective emotion, fear, brings about the strongest and most efficiently reinforced of all motor responses. Its influence is diffused throughout the entire receptor mechanism and the urgency of the inborn sense of self-protection amplifies or distorts the interpretation of both facts or fantasies of the emotions. The exaggerated messages prompt the cortex to precipitate a state of emergency in preparation for offense or defense. In this way somatic or physical changes may occur as a direct result of psychological states. Sir Henry Head, one of the great pioneer neurologists, said, "The mental state of the patient has a notoriously profound influence over the pains originating in the pelvic viscera."[28] In other words, the interpretation of sensations arising from the uterus may be influenced in most astonishing ways by the mental condition of the woman concerned.

Outer impulses arrive within our consciousness through the special senses; we may see danger, or hear sounds we associate with danger. But we are also capable of imagination. In civilized life the majority of those who suffer from fear or anxiety states are not threatened by reality of danger, but by the elaboration of possibilities that, being exaggerated by mental processes, produce a condition of tense alertness to the presence of danger, when in reality no danger exists. That, unfortunately, does not prevent the physical manifestations of this emotional state. Cannon[29] and others believe that the neural arrangements that are the ultimate receptors and integrators of emotional expression are situated in the optic thalamus.

This is particularly interesting when studying childbirth, for, as we have already pointed out, this is that part of the brain which is responsible for the integration of visceral pain stimuli.

Thus, we have the two great protective mechanisms, pain and fear, with a common center—the optic thalamus, for the perception of sensory stimuli and the discharge of motor impulses. In short, the influence of fear, being conveyed through the sympathetic nervous system, inhibits the pelvic autonomic. As a result of this, the neuromuscular harmony of labor in the presence of fear is disturbed in a manner exactly similar to that produced by pain.

When labor begins there is a danger that fear may sweep aside any sense of elation the woman may have experienced initially. But fear activates the sympathetic nervous system, which overrides, by its powerful influences, all other nerve stimuli throughout the body. It activates the machinery for either fight or flight; it creates a state of tension throughout the individual that provides for an increase of muscular power. But the sympathetic nerve supply to the uterus unfortunately supplies the circular fibers that inhibit the opening of the uterine outlet and resist the expulsive efforts of the longitudinal fibers of the uterus. As soon, therefore, as this protective apparatus is brought into play in order to overcome or fly from the painful recording of uterine sensations, so much more is the cause of pain introduced.

Since fear causes resistance by interfering with the normal harmony of muscle action, two powerful muscles are set against each other. This quickly increases enormously the tension of the uterine muscle. Tension above a normal amount is registered by special nerves and interpreted as pain in the higher brain centers. This creates a very serious complication of labor arising through fear, and that concerns the blood supply to the uterus through the placenta to the baby. This is sometimes overlooked.

Through this fear system or sympathetic system, the body reacts primarily not in a separate focus but *all over at the same time,* in order to protect itself against danger. The first principle of protection is to see that all possible fuel is conveyed to those muscles which will be used either in order to fly or to fight. At the same time, all the organs of the body that do not need the maximum blood supply are deprived of their blood to a large extent simply by contraction of the arteries supplying the organs that are useless in the act of defense. One of the organs useless in defense is the uterus. Under the influence of fear the blood vessels and the muscles supplied by the sympathetic or fear nervous system, actually limit the amount of blood going to and coming from the uterus. For a short time this can be done without disturbing the well-being of the infant, for it requires a very much lower oxygen pressure in the blood with which it is supplied than the adult musculature. But if this persists for any length of time without remission, it is quite likely fear itself is enough to deprive the baby within the womb of oxygen, and therefore to cause injury to some of its intricate organs, particularly the brain, and sometimes even cause intrauterine death.

Fear stimulates strongly the circular muscle fibers of the birth canal. As these circular fibers contract, their tone is increased while their elasticity is impaired, and the relaxation of the fibers is incomplete. The automatic action of the longitudinal muscle fibers of the uterus and pelvic canal not only presses down the presenting part, but the lower uterine segment adds tension in its endeavor to pull up the cervix and slide it gently over the fetal head.

So we find that where unpleasant emotions rule, the first unnatural factor becomes physically manifested in the mechanism of labor itself by a definitely resistant cervix—resistant not only to the down-coming presenting part, but resistant to the efforts of the longitudinal muscle fibers to draw it up by their faculty of retraction. For it must be remembered that there is also a local nerve supply for the uterus that enables the longitudinal fibers to continue to contract even though the autonomic supply has been cut out by sympathetic overstimulation.* So the uterus goes on contracting just the same, in

* In a recent paper by Shabanah and others ("The Role of the Autonomic Nervous System . . .") reporting from McGill University the following statements (reprinted by permission) are made as the result of some impressive experiments:

"Impressions creating anxiety and fear or, on the other hand, excitement or painful sensation, awakening the primitive defense reaction, produce a form of stress which brings about sympathetic hyperactivity. Spontaneous pain sensation due to a pelvic lesion or pain triggered from the parametria as in dyspareunia may precipitate a vicious circle. Sensory impulses travel through the two reflex arcs, the spinal and the cortical, referred to above. Since both the sympathetic and the parasympathetic contain sensory fibers, both systems are stimulated equally and, therefore, remain in balance as long as pain is not registered at the cortical level. When it is, as is normally the case, *sympathetic hyperactivity* [italics ed.] is thus created, affecting the uterus partly through its nervous connections and partly through the adrenal glands. This results in an elevation of the tissue and blood catecholamines, which in turn impair myometrial activity and induce vasospasm" (pp. 855–856).

"The preceding experimental findings in addition to other experimental and clinical observations raise the possibility that most if not all the previously mentioned, unexplained obstetrical and gynecological clinical conditions may well be etiologically related to abnormal neuro-

spite of the sympathetic nervous system being activated. We have then a condition of the expulsive fibers pushing against the circular fibers; we have two opposing groups of muscles working one against the other. The normal and natural result of this is that there is excessive tension, and soon a painless natural function is made into an extremely painful and therefore abnormal condition.

Tension is thus introduced from above, tension from within, and from the fact that the presenting part is pushed down into the pelvis, the lower part of the cervical canal, long after it should be completely drawn up and contiguous with the lower uterine segment. Instead, it is pressed low down into the pelvic cavity, maybe to the coccyx posteriorly, or even to the upper surface of the pubic bone anteriorly before full dilatation is achieved.

This is the painful first stage. It is pathological because it is opposed to normal physiological activity. Fear and apprehension mean real physical pain, not only subjective but objective, organic pain, intrinsic and extrinsic in the periphery that is active during labor. With what torment the cervix becomes fully dilated—the fact of pain is established in the mind of the woman—the dilatation of the outlet begins, and a similar series of events follows. The pelvic floor has been damaged, the levator ani injured because its anterior attachment has not been drawn up before pressure is occasioned by the presenting part. The vaginal sphincter can be seen, by anyone who has ever observed it, as two strong muscle bundles, tense and inelastic. This hypersensitiveness and tension is carried backward to the sphincters of the anus, and it may be noticed that

---

humoral causative factors reflected in a final picture of *autonomic imbalance—sympathetic hyperactivity*" (p. 856).

"These experiments in addition to certain clinical observations raise the possibility that most if not all of the above-mentioned unexplained obstetrical and gynecological conditions noted clinically may well be etiologically related to abnormal neurohumoral causative factors reflected in a final picture of *autonomic imbalance—sympathetic hyperactivity*" (p. 858).

when fear is present the pains of the second stage are frequently heralded by spasmodic contractions of the sphincters of the anus and vagina. Instead of relaxation and elasticity, therefore, tension is encountered, pain is experienced, protective spasm again augments the tension, and so again the forces join in battle on unequal ground, for sooner or later the great muscles of expulsion will either break down the resisting tissues or injure the fetus in their efforts.

In order to combat this situation, fear must be prevented. Physical relaxation is essential, and the learning of correct breathing patterns during pregnancy in order to employ them in labor. Education, correct relaxation, and breathing will prevent, so far as is possible, the harmful effects of fear, which are pain, tension, and the deprivation of oxygen in the tissues of a healthy woman.

The Mechanics of Dilatation

If we examine the action and reaction of the forces about the fetal head during the first stage of labor from the point of view of pure mechanics, the importance of cervical tension in relation to the expulsive and dilating force of the uterine musculature may be clearly demonstrated.

In consideration of the normal case, resistance occasioned by molding of the bones of the fetal head upon the bones of the pelvis during the first stage cannot be taken into account. It is, in fact, extremely unlikely that the bony structure of the pelvis during the first stage of normal labor exerts any force upon the fetal head that is relatively important in the dilatation of the pelvic canal. Cases of abnormalities of bony structure of pelvis or fetus do not come under this heading.

Let the fetal head be likened to a ball passing through an expanding ring, the cervix uteri. More accurately, the cervix may be described as a series of expanding rings. If the tension of the cervix uteri is increased, then the expulsive force must be proportionately increased. Retraction and automatic expulsive contractions continue, irrespective of the inhibition of the pelvic autonomic stimuli, until gradually they overcome the resistance either by dilatation or by rupture of the ring muscle. Rupture occurs in the majority of cases when the tension remains abnormally great.

It is obvious also that parturition under these circumstances necessitates a muscular strain upon the mechanism out of all proportion to that which nature intended. It is not difficult to appreciate why modern woman may suffer from lacerations, displacements, bruisings, and internal injuries. It is also clear that such tension cannot exist without pain.

It is my belief that subinvolution of the uterus is not infrequently due to an excessive strain placed upon the fibers of expulsion in their efforts to overcome the inelastic and tense circular fibers of the cervix uteri. This is augmented by the tension that is placed upon the thin and relatively meager musculature of the lower uterine segment. When the cervix is torn by the oncoming fetal head, large vessels are frequently ruptured, for the blood supply of the cervix at that time is enormously increased. Many serious postpartum hemorrhages have occurred from the split lateral walls of the cervix uteri.

Cases have been noted in which the fetal head has started to come down in the occipito posterior position, when the pelvis presents no abnormalities, and when no reasonable cause has appeared for so serious a complication.

It can be shown that rotation into the posterior position is much more easily accomplished when the cervix uteri has resisted full dilatation and has been pushed down only partially dilated before the fetal head. By presenting a thickened, almost obstructive band upon the wall of the birth canal, it deflects the occiput from the simple course, and by its presence influences the occiput to swing through the greater segment to the posterior position.

The ease with which these cases of persistant occipito posterior presentation, without any skeletal abnormality, can be rectified after full dilatation of the cervix, must be considered from this point of view, that in the absence of full dilatation the cervix uteri played some part in the presentation of the fetal head. A state of complete relaxation is necessary before rotation can be performed, but how frequently with the attainment of the occipito anterior position the child will almost fall through the pelvic canal.

At the outlet, *tension* is the greatest of all predisposing causes of rupture of ther perineum. The fourchette may go, but too frequently the sphincter of the vagina is either partially or totally torn at the posterior end. An effort may be made by the insertion of a few stitches to obviate this trouble, but how rarely does a torn sphincter regain its full power of contractility.

To the casual observer these points may be of small importance, but above all things an obstetrician must be a humanitarian. To produce a child and injure the mother is the same thing as producing the mother and ruining the wife, and many physicians will readily acquiesce to the suggestion that this is synonymous with domestic strain, if not ultimately with personal estrangement.

It is almost superfluous to add what must be obvious to the least critical, that these observations are not intended to explain the origin of all complications of labor, but rather that in intensified emotions, we have a factor that not only makes labor painful when it should be painless, but introduces difficulties and complications that need never arise.

One of the most astounding results of the application of the principles outlined above is the almost entire elimination of such complications to labor as have been mentioned. Given anatomical efficiency, physiological integrity can then be acquired by the elimination of negative emotions, substituting the peacefulness of muscular relaxation.

BIBLIOGRAPHICAL REFERENCES FOR CHAPTER 25

1. E. H. Shabanah, A. Toth, and George B. Maughan, "The Role of the Autonomic Nervous System in Uterine Con-

tractility and Blood Flow. I. The Interaction Between Neuro-hormones and Sex Steroids in the Intact Isolated Uterus," *American Journal of Obstetrics and Gynecology* 89, no. 7 (August 1, 1964): 841–880.

2. Kurdinowski, "Physiologische und pharmakologische Versuche an der isolirten Gebarmutter," *Arch, f. Anat. u. Phys., Phys. Abth.,* 1904.

3. Franz, "Studien Zur Physiologie des Uterus," *Zeitsch. f. Geburtsh. u. Gynak.* 53 (1904).

4. Holste, "Untersuchungen am uberlebenden Uterus," *Arch, f. exp. Path. u. Pharmakol.* 96, no. 1:25.

5. Hermann Friedrich Rein, *Physiology* (Collected Works), Part 3, "Animal Physiology and Physiology of Perception" (Office of Military Government for Germany, Field Information Agencies Technical, British, French, 1948).

6. Beckwith Whitehouse and Henry Featherstone, *British Medical Journal,* 1923.

7. Jacob, *Ueber die Rythmischen Bewegungen des Kaninchen Uterus.*

8. Francis Hugh Adam Marshall, *Physiology of Reproduction,* 3rd ed. (London, New York: Longmans, Green, London, 1910; 3rd ed. 1952).

9. In *Complications of Pregnancy* (New York: Appleton, 1923).

10. Zimmerman, 1916. See also "Soluble Extract of Corpus Luteum in the Vomiting of Pregnancy," *Louisville Mont. Journal Medicine and Surgery* 23 (1929).

11. Schmidt, "Spontane Geburt bei Poliomyelitis ant. acuta. Dissertation," 1915.

12. Charles Henry Felix Routh, *The Causes and Prevention of Infant Mortality* (London: J. Churchill, 1860).

13. Fritz Frankenhauser, "Die Bewegungsnerven der Gebarmutter," *Jenaische Zeitsch. f. Med.* 1 (1864).

14. Korner, *Studien d. Phys. Instituts zu Breslau,* 1865.

15. Marshall, *Physiology of Reproduction.*

16. Albert Kuntz, *The Autonomic Nervous System* (Philadelphia: Lea & Febiger, 1929, 4th ed. 1953).

17. Whitehouse and Featherstone, *British Medical Journal,* 1923, p. 406.

18. Ibid.

19. Walter B. Cannon, *Bodily Changes in Pain, Hunger, Fear and Rage* (1st ed., New York: Harper & Row, 1929. 2nd ed., New York: Harper & Row, 1963).
20. Ibid.
21. Ivan Petrovich Pavlov, *Conditioned Reflexes; an Investigation of the Physiological Activity of the Cerebral Cortex* (London: Oxford, 1928; New York: Dover, 1960).
22. Sir Charles Scott Sherrington, *The Integrative Action of the Nervous System,* 1906 (New Haven: Yale University Press, 2nd ed. 1948); *Reflex Activity of the Spinal Cord* (Oxford: Clarendon Press, 1932). See also Judith P. Swazey, *Reflexes and Motor Integration: Sherrington's Concept of Integrative Action* (Cambridge, Mass.: Harvard University Press, 1969).
23. George Washington Crile, *Man—An Adaptive Mechanism* (New York: Macmillan, 1916); *The Origin and Nature of the Emotions* (Philadelphia and London: W. B. Saunders, 1915); *A Physical Interpretation of Shock, Exhaustion, and Restoration, an Extension of the Kinetic Theory* (London: Frowde, 1921).
24. John Baxter Langley, *Via Medica* (London: Hardwicke, 1867); *Brain,* 1903; *Journal of Physiology, 1908.*
25. In *Bodily Changes in Pain, Hunger, Fear and Rage.*
26. In *The Integrative Action of the Nervous System.*
27. Sir Thomas McCall Anderson, *Lectures on Clinical Medicine* (London: Macmillan, 1877); Langley and Anderson, *Journal of Physiology* 19 (1893–94, 1895–96): 71–131, 327.
28. Sir Henry Head, *Studies in Neurology* (London: Hodder & Stoughton, 1920); "Certain Aspects of Pain"; *British Medical Journal,* 1923; see also Kenneth W. Cross, and others, *Henry Head Centenary* (London: Macmillan; New York: St. Martin's Press, 1961).
29. In *Bodily Changes in Pain, Hunger, Fear and Rage.*

Epilogue

Pioneers Pass On
Jessica Dick-Read

Childbirth Without Fear has had an indelible impact upon the world as far back as 1932, when the subject first appeared in England under the title *Natural Childbirth*. In 1942 *The Revelation of Childbirth* brought a "gleam" of sanity to a country locked in the deadly combat of World War II. With so many dying in warfare, Dick's work brought promise of a happier rebirth.

In 1944, born of "The House of Harper," *Childbirth Without Fear* was offered to the women of America, still in a period when our very future as a human race was so sadly blurred by man's inhumanity to man. Dick's poignant message gave courage to those women who believed they were being denied their right—the right to fulfill their proudly cherished heritage of giving birth in surroundings of kindness, dignity, and peace.

The war ended, and with its passing women the world over heard that "call from out of the wilderness," and responded. Now, mainly through Dick's freeing childbirth from ugly and ignorant concepts, once again women everywhere can give birth more wisely, with their personal dignity restored.

To all potential mothers I can but simply say, he was *great*. I am proud not only to have been a beloved wife but also to have been at his side as, in the face of many conflicts, he introduced many through his teaching and guidance to the loveliness and truth that is childbirth.

To me, *Childbirth Without Fear* still remains Dick's "living" work. Some have asked whether he died a disappointed man. No, he certainly did not, though he was very tired due to the strain imposed by many tours and his determination, in writings and lectures, to exert all efforts in behalf of safer, kinder obstetrics. But he strongly believed that a light was beginning to glimmer among many of his profession who were at least attempting to put into practice the efficacy of natural childbirth. From my heart I say that I know that, though he never lived to see the full flowering of his great work, he died content in the knowledge of having tendered and nourished a "late" budding.

During mid-1955 Dick suffered his first fairly serious heart attack, and another during a tour in Europe the following year. But he continued his work, and came ahead to the United States and Canada in late 1957 for a lecture tour. A third heart attack occurred on this tour, while he was lecturing in Toronto in 1958.

Ironically, it was not a heart attack, as we feared might happen, that took his life. In January of 1959 a different kind of attack, a cerebral hemorrhage, occurred. After a few days' rest Dick again made one of his vital recoveries, and, quite truly, one could not believe that he had suffered in any way. But the second attack of that kind came soon after Easter. Dick was hospitalized for observation, in his old hospital, the London, in Whitechapel. Fortunately, his illness was short lived. When the end was considered by his doctor to be but a matter of hours, Dick looked up at me and said, "Home, Lovey."

With all speed I made arrangements to get him back to our home in Norfolk, and he lived for another nine days, happy, conscious, and content in the knowledge of being among those who loved him so. Toward the end his speech was gone, but through his eyes he continued to register and express that wonderful humanity and intelligence which I am unable to find words to define. His passing was peaceful, and as in 1942 when he held his beloved mother's hand as she crossed the threshold, I held his, and so the link remains unbroken.

APPENDIX

Glossary of Terms for Lay Readers

Abruptio placenta. A premature tearing away of the placenta from the wall of the uterus, before the baby is born.

Afterbirth. The placenta and membranes in which the baby developed, expelled after the birth of the baby.

Amniotic fluid. The colorless fluid in which the baby floats in the womb before birth, enclosed in the membranes.

Analgesia. Insensibility to pain without loss of consciousness.

Anesthesia. Partial or complete loss of sensation, with or without loss of consciousness, depending on type used.

Anterior. Before, in front of, toward the front.

Birth canal. The passageway through which the baby is born, the uterine opening and vagina.

Caput. Usually referred to as the soft swelling of the presenting part of the baby's scalp.

Centimeter. A unit of linear measure. One finger width equals about two centimeters.

Cervix. The lower, narrower end of the uterus, often called the "neck" of the uterus, through which the baby leaves the uterus and enters the vagina during birth.

Coccyx. The end of the vertebral column, beyond the sacrum; the tailbone.

Contraction. The tightening of a muscle.

Cyanosis. The slightly bluish discoloration of the skin caused by lowered oxygen and increased carbon dioxide in the blood.

Dilatation. The gradual opening of the cervix.

Dorsal. Pertaining to the back.

Dyspareunia. Painful coitus.

Dyspnea. Difficult breathing usually accompanied by pain.

Ejaculation. The ejection of semen from the penis.

Episiotomy. A small, straight cut made in the tissues (perineum) at the opening of the vagina, to enlarge the passageway.

Expulsion. The second stage of labor, pushing the baby out.

Fetus. The developing baby from twelve weeks pregnancy until birth.

Flaccid. Describing completely relaxed, absent muscular tone.

Fourchette. A fold of mucous membrane at the lower end of the vaginal opening.

Fundus. The top of the uterus, furthest from the opening.

Hemorrhage. Excessive bleeding.

Hypertrophy. Increase in the size of an organ due to growth or normal functioning.

Hyperventilation. Too rapid breathing, causing a loss of carbon dioxide from the lungs, numbness of hands and fingers, trembling, racing of heart, muscle cramps, and fainting.

Imprinting. In humans, usualy referred to as "human socialization."

Internal os. The opening of the cervix inside the uterus.

Ischemia. The obstruction of circulation of blood to a part of the body.

Labor. The rhythmical contractions of the uterine muscles that open the cervix and expel the baby, membranes, and placenta.

Laceration. Tearing of the skin or muscles.

Lactation. The secretion of milk.

Lightening. The settling of the baby lower into the abdomen in late pregnancy.

Lochia. The discharge from the birth canal during the first few weeks after giving birth.

Lumbar. Describing the area of the lower back.

Meconium. The dark bowel movement of all newborns.

Membranes. The "bag of waters," a sac of thin membranes in which the baby floats within the uterus during pregnancy.

Multipara. A woman giving birth to her second or subsequent babies.

Neurasthenia. Complaints of weakness, exhaustion, depression.

Nociceptors. The nerve endings that receive pain sensations.

Occipito anterior. Describing the condition in which the back of the baby's head faces the front of the mother's body during birth, his face downward.

Occipito Posterior. Describing the condition in which the back of the baby's head faces the back of the mother's body during birth, his face upward.

Occiput. The back of the head.

Ovary (pl. ovaries). One of two almond-shaped female glands situated on each side of the uterus at the end of ligaments, close to the Fallopian tubes.

Ovum. The cell or "egg" discharged from an ovary and carried to the uterus through the Fallopian tube.

Parturient. Describing a woman in labor.

Parturition. The process of giving birth.

Pelvic cavity. The space within the pelvis.

Pelvic floor. The muscles and outer tissues supporting the contents of the pelvic cavity.

Pelvis. The basin-shaped ring of bones at the bottom of the trunk of the body, which support the spine and rest on the legs.

Perineum. The tissues between the anus and the vagina.

Placenta. The spongelike organ attached to the uterine wall of the mother, and to the baby by the umbilical cord. The baby receives his nourishment and expels his wastes by means of the placenta.

Podalic version. The turning of the fetus so that the feet are born first.

Posterior. Behind, in back of, toward the back.

Postmature. Describing a baby born after the normal length of pregnancy.

Postnatal. After the baby is born.

Postpartum. After the baby is born.

Precipitate. Describing a rapid birth, occurring unexpectedly.

Premature. Describing a baby born before the normal length of pregnancy, and usually weighing under 5 pounds 8 ounces.

Prenatal. Before birth.

Primigravida. A woman giving birth to her first baby.

Puerperium. The period of time following birth until the pelvic organs return to the nonpregnant condition, usually about six weeks.

Sacrum. The triangular bone at the base of the spine, attached to the bones of the pelvis and formed of five united vertebra, directly below which is the coccyx, or tailbone.

Sperm, spermatozoa. The mature male sexual cell, which fertilizes the egg of the female.

Thoracic. Pertaining to the chest area.

Tumescence. Condition of swelling, or being distended.

Umbilical cord. A tubelike structure connecting the baby to the placenta, 12 to 36 inches in length.

Uterus. The organ in the female pelvis in which a fetus can develop; the womb.

Vagina. The passage from the cervix to the vulva, about five inches in length.

Vascularization. The process in which new blood vessels develop in a structure, to increase the supply of blood.

Vernix caseosa. The whitish cheesy deposit covering the baby's skin at birth. If left undisturbed it gradually is absorbed into the baby's skin.

Vulva. The external female genitals, composed of the inner and outer folds of tissue (*labia minora, labia majora*), clitoris, and vaginal opening.

Sources of Information

International Childbirth Education Association, Inc. (P.O. Box 5852, Milwaukee, Wis. 53220).

The ICEA is a federation of individuals and of community childbirth education groups throughout the United States and other countries. Because of its wide contacts, it is a valuable resource agency for all those who want information concerning childbirth education opportunities in various areas, or current trends in childbirth literature and practice.

ICEA Supplies Center (208 Ditty Building, Bellevue, Wash. 98004).

The Supplies Center makes available a wide range of books, pamphlets, films and teaching aids on every aspect of family life for both lay and professional people.

Maternity Center Association (48 East 92nd Street, New York, N.Y. 10028).

The MCA is a progressive training center for good obstetrics, dispersing timely information on methods and research, and frequently sponsoring cross-disciplinary workshops and seminars for improving the quality of maternity care.

American Society for Psychoprophylaxis in Obstetrics (36 West 96 Street, New York, N.Y. 10025).

This organization is dedicated to furthering the teaching of the Lamaze-Pavlov approach as it has been adapted to this country, training couples for childbirth in education classes throughout the country. It also accredits teachers in this method of childbirth preparation.

La Leche League International (9616 Minneapolis Avenue, Franklin Park, Ill. 60131 [telephone 312 455-7730]).

The LLL offers help to women who want to breastfeed their babies, through literature, member groups in many communities, and a medical board of consultants for counsel in unusual breastfeeding problems.

American Institute of Family Relations (5287 Sunset Boulevard, Los Angeles, Calif., 90277).

The AIFR has been a responsible resource center for all aspects of family life for many years, including materials on sex education and education for childbirth. A wide range of publications are available on request.

Sources of Supplies

Cal Fitzhugh Obstetrical Backrest
  American Sterilizer Company
  Erie, Pa.

Natural Childbirth Backrest,
Catalog No. 012-80166
  IPCO Hospital Supply Cor-
  poration
  161 Sixth Ave.
  New York, New York 10013

Universal Backrest, Catalog
No. 46, S-2639A
  Will Ross Incorporated
  Health Products Division
  4285 N. Pt. Washington Road
  Milwaukee, Wisconsin

Newborn Warmer
  IMI
  4321 Birch Street
  Newport Beach, Calif. 92660

Bibliography

BOOKS

Pregnancy and Childbirth

A Baby Is Born. New York: Maternity Center Association, 1964.

Bing, Elizabeth. *Six Practical Lessons for an Easier Childbirth.* New York: Grosset & Dunlap, Inc., 1967.

————. ed. *The Adventure of Birth: Experiences in the Lamaze Method of Prepared Childbirth.* New York: Simon and Schuster, Inc., 1970.

Bowes, *et al. The Effects of Obstetrical Medication on Fetus and Infant.* Monograph of the Society for Research in Child Development, vol. 25, no. 4. Chicago: University of Chicago Press, 1970.

Bradley, Robert, M.D. *Husband-Coached Childbirth.* New York: Harper & Row, Publishers, 1965.

Chertok, Leon. *Psychosomatic Methods in Painless Childbirth.* Philadelphia: J. B. Lippincott Company, 1959.

Eastman, Nicholson J. *Expectant Motherhood.* 4th ed. Boston: Little, Brown, and Company, 1963.

Eastman, Nicholson, J., and Hellman, Louis M., eds. *Williams' Obstetrics.* 13th ed. New York: Appleton-Century-Crofts, 1966.

Flanagan, Geraldine Lux. *The First Nine Months of Life.* New York: Simon and Schuster, Inc., 1962.

Goodrich, Frederick. *Preparing for Childbirth.* Englewood Cliffs, N.J.: Prentice-Hall, Inc., 1966.

Hazell, Lester. *Commonsense Childbirth.* New York: Putnam, 1969.

Jacobson, Edmund. *How to Relax and Have Your Baby*. New York: McGraw-Hill, Inc., 1959.

Kitzinger, Sheila. *The Experience of Childbirth*. Baltimore: Penguin Books, Inc., 1967.

Miller, John S. *Childbirth, A Manual for Pregnancy and Delivery*. New York: Atheneum Publishers, 1963.

Montagu, Ashley. *Life Before Birth*. New York: New American Library, 1964.

Prelude to Action. New York: Maternity Center Association, 1969.

Richardson, Stephen A., and Guttmacher, Alan F., eds. *Childbearing: Its Social and Psychological Aspects*. Baltimore: The Williams & Wilkins Company, 1967.

Standards for Obstetric-Gynecologic Hospital Services. Chicago: The American College of Obstetricians and Gynecologists, 1969.

Standards and Recommendations for Hospital Care of Newborn Infants. Evanston, Ill.: American Academy of Pediatrics, 1966.

Thoms, Herbert. *Childbirth with Understanding*. New York: McGraw-Hill, Inc., 1962.

Wessel, Helen. *Childbirth and the Family*. New York: Harper & Row, Publishers, 1973.

White, Gregory. *Emergency Childbirth*. Franklin Park, Ill.: Police Training Foundation, 1958.

Related Subjects

Bowlby, John. *Child Care and the Growth of Love*. New York: World Health Organization, 1953.

Brazelton, T. Berry. *Infants and Mothers: Differences in Development*. New York: Delacorte Press, 1969.

Cannon, Walter B. *Bodily Changes in Pain, Hunger, Fear and Rage*. Rev. ed. New York: Harper & Row, Publishers, 1963.

Chertok, Leon. *Motherhood and Personality*. Philadelphia: J. B. Lippincott Company, 1969.

Deutsch, Ronald. *The Key to Feminine Response in Marriage*. New York: Random House, and Ballantine, 1968.

Fitzpatrick, Elise, Eastman, Nicholson, J., and Reeder, Sharon R. *Maternity Nursing*. 11th ed. Philadelphia, Lippincott, 1966.

Fromm, Erich. *The Art of Loving.* New York: Harper & Row, 1956.

Haire, Doris. *Implementing Family-Centered Maternity Care with a Central Nursery.* ICEA of New Jersey, 1968. Available from ICEA Supplies Center.

Montagu, Ashley. *The American Way of Life.* New York: Putnam, 1967.

Montagu, Ashley. *Touching: The Human Significance of the Skin.* New York: Columbia University Press, 1971.

Nesbitt, Robert. *Perinatal Loss in Modern Obstetrics.* Philadelphia: F. A. Davis, 1957.

Newton, G., and Levine, S., eds. *Early Experience and Behavior.* Springfield, Ill.: Charles C Thomas, 1968.

Newton, Niles. *Family Book of Child Care.* New York: Harper & Bros., 1957.

————. *Maternal Emotions.* New York: Hoeber Medical Division, Harper & Row. 1955.

Pryor, Karen. *Nursing Your Baby.* New York: Harper & Row, Publishers, 1963.

Shapiro, Sam, and Nesbitt, Robert. *Infant Perinatal and Maternal and Childhood Mortality in the United States.* London: Cambridge University Press, 1968.

Stender, Fay. *Husbands in the Delivery Room.* 2nd ed. Milwaukee: International Childbirth Educational Association, 1968.

Trobisch, Walter. *I Loved a Girl.* New York: Harper & Row, Publishers, 1965.

————. *I Married You.* New York: Harper & Row, Publishers, 1971.

The Womanly Art of Breastfeeding. Chicago: La Leche League, 1963.

Waller, H. K. *The Breasts and Breast Feeding.* London: William Heinemann Ltd., 1957.

Wiedenbach, Ernestine. *Family-Centered Maternity Nursing.* 2nd Ed. New York: J. P. Putnam's Sons, 1967.

FILMS

A Story About Childbirth (1966). Black/white, sound, 30 min. A young couple experience childbirth together, John S. Miller,

M.D., attending. No perineal views. Education for Childbirth Association, Box 154, San Anselmo, Calif. 94960.

Birthright (1968). Color, sound, 15 min. A prepared couple shares their experience. Brief perineal views. CEA of Greater Philadelphia, Box 8741, Philadelphia, 19101.

Childbirth for the Joy of It (1968). Color, sound, 20 min. Several normal, nonmedicated births reveal how different couples react differently to childbirth. No perineal views. Jay Hathaway Production Services, 4846 Katherine Avenue, Sherman Oaks, Calif., 91403.

Childbirth, the Great Adventure (1963). Color, sound, 20 min. A young couple prepare and experience their first child's birth, Morris Gold, M.D., attending. No perineal views. Childbirth Education League, Box 231, Lynnwood, Wash. 98036.

Childbirth Without Fear (1956). Color, sound, 20 min., 1956. Four births attended by Grantly Dick-Read, M.D., in South Africa. Several perineal views. Universal Education and Visual Arts, 221 Park Avenue South, New York, N.Y. 10003.

Human Reproduction (code #647550) McGraw-Hill Text Films, 330 West 42nd Street, New York, N.Y. 10036.

Husband-Coached Childbirth—A Modern Preparation for Parenthood (1968). Color, sound, 30 min. Emphasis on good communication between doctor and couple, Jack Hoage, M.D., attending. Two perineal views. Mr. Arthur Emr, 11740 Sunset Boulevard, Los Angeles, Calif. 90049.

Natural Childbirth (1966). Black/white, sound, 30 min. A shared experience, emphasizing the father's role, Robert A. Bradley, M.D., attending. Jay Hathaway Production Services, 4846 Katherine Avenue, Sherman Oaks, Calif. 91403.

Index

Abraham, Johnston, 289, 291–92
abruptio placenta, 32, 107, 397
Academy of Medicine (New York), 302
Academy of Psychosomatic Medicine (Chicago), 333
Addington Hospital (Durban, South Africa), 306
adrenal glands, 377, 381
Africa
  South Africa, 306, 308–16
  tribal societies, 20–21, 317–23, 336–37, 352
afterbirth, 78–79, 228–30, 248
  African tribal attitudes toward, 321
  emergency procedures, 239
afterpains, 252
American Society of Psychoprophylaxis, 105*n*.
amnesia, *see* Second stage of labor
Anderson, Sir Thomas McCall, 31, 268, 382
anemia
  iron-deficiency, 44–46
  physiological, 45
anesthesia, analgesia, 25, 46–47, 64–67, 104, 108–9, 206, 218–19, 292, 315, 340–41, 350
  abnormality and, 219

  deaths due to, 109
  deep anesthesia, 65
  education in, 48–49, 65
  neuromuscular tension, 61
  prevention vs., 66–67
  psychological hazards, 65
  suggestion and, 67
Angelergues, 330
Antenatal and Postnatal Care (Browne), 291
anus, fissure of, 376
Aristotle, 19, 47
asepsis, 26–27
Atlee, H. B., 118
attitudes (*see also* Attitudes, maternal; Emotions; specific emotions)
  Christianity, 21–25
  culture vs. natural law, 28–30
  of doctors, 5–6, 282ff., 303ff.
  Greece, ancient, 17–19
  of husband, 5–6
  Judeo-Christian, 21
  mental imagery, 13–36
  of nurses, 5–6
  primitive societies, 17, 20–21, 28–30, 318ff.
  religion and, 20–25, 285–86
attitudes, maternal (*see also* Attitudes; Emotions; specific emotions), 37, 266–67, 271–72, 277–79, 380–81

attitudes (*cont'd*)
  education, prenatal, and, 4–5,
    15–17, 34–35
  iron-deficiency anemia of
    mother and, 44–46
  types, 49–50
autonomic nervous system
  fear and, 381ff.
  uterine contractions and,
    366ff., 378ff.

backache, 35
  in labor, 62–64, 107–8, 207
bacteriology, 27
bag of waters, 53, 58, 154, 197,
  218, 235
Beck, Joan, 132
Bible (*see also Christianity*), 23–
  24
Bieniarz, J., 202*n.*
Birth of a Child, The (Grantly
  Dick-Read), 306
birth canal
  nervous system and, 378–79,
    385–87
  structure of (*see also* specific
    subjects), 364–65
blood
  adrenal secretions and, 377
  circulation, emotions and, 31–
    32
  loss, maternal, 380–81
bottle-feeding, 255
Bourrel, A., 329–30
bowels, 35, 151
  reflex relaxation of muscles,
    375–76
Bowes, 206*n.*
breastfeeding (*see also* Breasts),
  92–98, 241
  advantages of, 245–46, 253–4
  afterpains, 252
  colostrum, 240–44
  on demand, 244–45
  diet, mother's, 256
  emergency procedures, 238–39

immediate, of newborn, 123,
  226, 238–39
impossibility of, 255
nipples, care of, 253
position, 254–5
rejection of, 304
relaxation and milk flow, 254
supplementary feeding and,
  244
breasts (*see also* Breastfeeding),
  97
exercise for firming, 187–91,
  258
nipples, 150–51, 253
sensitivity and enlargement,
  157
supporting, 149
breathing, *see* Respiration
Brindeau, Professor, 305
British Medical Association, 284
British Medical Journal, 301,
  368–69
Browne, Francis James, 291, 292
Browne, Sir Thomas, 267
Buganda, 352
Bwalya Kalunda, 318

Caesarian section, 22, 47, 129
Campbell, Berry, 360–1
Canada, 334, 393
Cannon, Walter B., 86*n.*, 370,
  371, 382, 383
Carey, Harvey, 247
Catholic Church (*see also*
  Christianity), 325
cervix, cervical canal, 363–64
  fear reaction, 34, 161
  first stage of labor, 6–7, 58, 61,
    200
  hemorrhage, postpartum, 388
  mechanics of dilation, 387–89
  nervous system and dilatation
    of, 378–79
  sympathetic stimuli and
    contractions of, 371–72
childbed fever, 25–26

childbirth (*see also* Labor; specific stages, subjects)
Caesarean, 22, 47, 125
in continuum of child development, 124–25
emergency procedures, 234–39
family and, 81–102
history, 17–28
ideal, example of, 139–41
instrument deliveries, 282, 304, 346–47
materialistic, mechanistic approach to, 325–32, 338ff.
mental imagery concerning, 13–36
natural, *see* specific subjects
preventive medicine and, 126
primitive societies, 17, 20–21, 28–30, 105, 112, 317ff., 336–37
principles of natural, in perspective, 103–42
problems of, 125–26
spirituality of, 11–12, 35–36
Childbirth Without Fear (Grantly Dick-Read), 301–2, 326, 327, 392–93
Christianity, 21–25, 35, 285–86
Claye, Andrew C., 66n.
clinics, prenatal, 37, 38
Clinique Tarnier (Paris), 305, 326
clothing, maternal, 48, 148–49
Coda, Martin W., 132
coitus
during pregnancy, 42–43
dyspareunia, 376
episiotomy and, 351
vaginal control, 195
Communism, 324–32
conception, 152–54
conditioning
color-music association, 269–70
conditioned reflexes, 13–14, 41, 328

mental imagery and, 13ff.
positive, in labor, 46–47, 67
Congo, 20–21, 336–38, 338–39, 352
constipation, 35, 151
Crile, George W., 381
crowning, 73–74, 220–21
emergency birth, 237, 238

Davis, Edward P., 367
de Kruif, Paul, 291
De Lee, Joseph, 67, 291, 292
depression, 35
diet, *see* Nutrition
Dick-Read, Grantly
Africa, 308–23, 336–37
Birth of a Child, The, 306
acceptance of theories of, 286ff., 300–1, 305
childbirth, observations of, 266–67, 277–79, 281, 284ff., 299, 315, 317ff., 339ff.
Childbirth Without Fear, 301–2, 326, 327, 392–93
childhood and youth, 263ff.
clinic, obstetrical, 284ff., 290
color association, 269–70
death, 393
education for childbirth, 286ff.
general practice, 283
internship, 270–72
Introduction to Motherhood, 306, 324, 327
Isleworth hospital project, 306–8
lectures and lecture tours, 290–91, 292, 302–5, 393, 333–53
London Hospital, 270–72, 280, 282–83
marriage, 283–84
military service, World War I, 279–80
Motherhood in the Post-War World, 300

Dick-Read, Grantly (cont'd)
   Natural Childbirth, 289–92,
     302, 327, 392
   notoriety, 309–12
   principles of, in perspective,
     103ff.
   rejection of theories of, 282ff.,
     303–5, 309–12
   relaxation, 279, 287
   Revelation of Childbirth, The,
     300–2, 309, 392
   Russian approach to painless
     childbirth and, 324–32
   South Africa, 306, 308–16,
     324
   training, medical, 267ff.
   translations of books by, 301,
     324, 326
   war injuries, 274–75, 290, 308
   World War II, 297–99
Dick-Read, Jessica, 300, 313,
   392–93
dyspepsia, 35

Eastman, Nicholson J., 103, 112
education in pregnancy (*see also*
   Pregnancy; specific subjects),
   37–51, 105, 152–61, 286ff.
   anesthesia or analgesia, 48–49
   attitudes and, 4–5, 34–35
   clothing, 48
   diet, 41–42, 48
   doctor–patient relationship,
     43–44
   fertilization process, 152–54
   fetus, development of, 154–56,
     157
   husband, 47, 81–82, 87–89,
     113–14, 137–38, 287
   hygiene, 48
   illegitimacy and, 126–27
   inadequate, hazards of, 38–39
   labor, 38ff., 48ff.
   media and, 16–17
   mental imagery and, 15–17
   negative, 15–17

newborn, potential of, 130–34
nutrition, 137
physical fitness, 40, 136–37,
   184–95
postpartum, 138–39, 141
program, ideal, 134–39
in relaxation, 40, 50–51, 137,
   169–83
in respiration, 40, 164–67
sex, 100, 293
South Africa, 313–14
teamwork, 47–48
training classes in late
   pregnancy, 138
women as teachers, 313
Egypt, ancient, 17
Ehrlich, Paul, 131
elation, maternal, 4–6, 52–55
Elizabeth, Princess, 309–10
Ellis, Harlan, 103–42
emergency, natural childbirth in,
   234–39
   afterbirth, 238, 239
   bearing down, 236–38
   breastfeeding, 239
   fear and, 235–36
   head, emergence of, 237, 238
   newborn, holding, 238–39
   onset of labor, 234–35
   pain, 236
   position, 236, 237, 238
   relaxation, 237
   umbilical cord, 238–39
   urination, 236
emotions (*see also* Fear; Love)
   adrenal glands and, 377
   Aristotle, 19
   birth and, 9–12
   crises of, in labor, 58–59, 62,
     71–72, 73–74, 200, 219–20,
     237
   development of, 3–4
   in labor, influences upon, 377–
     89
   mental imagery and, 13–14
   Soranus of Ephesus on, 19

episiotomy, 346–52
exaltation, maternal, 52–53, 78–80
exercise, 184–85
    for abdominal muscles, 257–58
    for breasts, 187–91, 258
    breathing, 257
    labor "work" position, 194
    for pelvic floor muscles, 194–95, 257
    pelvic rock, 186, 258
    postnatal, 256–59
    prenatal, 184–95
    squatting, 186–87

Fairbairn, John, 289
family (see also Husband), 81–102
    maternity care centered on, 124–25, 136–39
fear, 14–15, 103, 380–87
    emergency childbirth and, 235–36
    imagination and, 383
    information sources and, 15–17
    language and, 54
    naturalness of, 27
    nervous system and, 380ff.
    pain and, 19–21, 30–35, 160–61, 235–36, 281, 284–85, 291, 381–87
    physical complaints and, 35
    relaxation and, 50–51
    religion and, 20–21, 285–86
    tension-pain syndrome, 31–35, 235, 381–87
    uterine circulation, 31–32
Featherstone, Henry, 366–67, 368–69, 370
fetus, development of, 154–56
fingernails, care of, 150
first stage of labor, 4, 55–67, 209–10
    attendance, 60–61, 200, 201
    backache, 61–64, 207
    bag of waters, 58, 197

bearing-down, 7, 208, 236–37
cervix, cervical canal, 6–7, 58, 61, 200
    doctor–patient relationship, 55–57, 59
    early, 197–202
    emergency procedures, 234–37
    emotional crisis, 58–59, 200
    examination and preparation, 117–18, 199
    late, 202–6
    neuromuscular tension, 61
    nourishment, 58, 200
    onset, 4–6, 53–55, 196–97, 234–35
    pain, relievers, see Anesthesia, analgesia
    position, 108, 202–3
    relaxation (see also Relaxation), 6–7, 199, 205–6
    respiration, 67, 204–5
    show, 197
    sleep, 199–200
    transferral to birth room, 118
    transition, 61–64, 206–8
    uterus, 6
Flanders, 277–78
Fourth International Congress of Catholic Doctors, 325
France, 305, 326, 328, 329–30, 334
Frankenhauser, Fritz, 367
Franz, 366
Fuller, John I., 133

Galton, Francis, 13
Gardiner, Charles Fox, 268
Germany, 334
Gilliatt, Sir William, 306–7, 309–10
Goodrich, F. W., Jr., 324
Great Britain, 263–74, 280–301, 306–8

Greece, ancient, 17–19
Guttmacher, Alan F., 134

hair, care of, 149–50
Haire, Doris, 248n.
Hardin, Garrett, 131
Harlow, Harry, 114, 133
Hay, Jack, 317
Head, Sir Henry, 45, 282, 382–83
headache, 35
Heardman, Helen, 166n.
Hellman, Louis M., 103, 112
hemorrhage, postpartum
    cervical, 388
    placental, 380–81
hemorrhoids, 195
Hersilie, 330
Hess, Eckhard H., 133
Hippocrates, 17–18
Holland, 352
Holste, 366
hospitals, 114–24
    acceptance of natural child-
        birth, 334
    American, 338–42
    checking into, 47, 54, 197–99
    early, 25–27
    equipment, 118, 123n., 140
    furnishings and facilities, 139–
        40
    maternity care, ideal program,
        135–39
    nurseries, 246–47
    nursery care, 248–49
    nursing care, see Nurses, nurs-
        ing care
    prenatal classes, 37, 38
    rooming-in, 141, 246–47, 249–
        50, 255–56
    teamwork, 47, 60, 116–24
husband, 81–92
    anxiety, 16
    attitudes, 5–6, 81ff.
    educating, 47, 81–82, 87–89,
        113–14, 137–38, 287
    family and child relationships,
        96–102
    labor and birth, 90–91, 113–14,
        116–24, 140–41, 200ff.,
        212–14
    neuropsychiatric, 125–26
    primitive cultures, 112
hygiene, personal
    bowels, 151
    breasts and nipples, 150–51
    fingernails, 150
    hair, 149–50
    skin, 149
    hypnotism, 296, 325

illegitimacy, 126–27
imagination, fear and, 383
imprinting
    color-music association, 269–
        70
    mother-child, 127–29, 133–34,
        270
International Childbirth Educa-
    tion Association, 105n.
Introduction to Motherhood
    (Grantly Dick-Read), 306,
    324, 327
iron deficiency, anemia due to,
    44–46
Isleworth (Great Britain), 307–8
Israel, A. J., 311–12
Italy, 334, 352

Jacob, 367
Jacobson, Edmund, 50, 314
Jeffereys, M. D. W., 269
Johannesburg (South Africa)
    Sunday Times, 310
Jones, George W., 301–2n.
Journal of the American Medical
    Association, 301

Kegel, Arnold, 194n.
Koch, Robert, 27
Korner, 367

Kroger, William, 333
Kuntz, Albert, 368
Kurdinowski, 366

labor (*see also* specific stages, subjects), 52–80, 234–39
    African tribal usages, 320–21
    anesthesia or analgesia (*see also* Anesthesia, analgesia), 25, 46–47, 48–49, 64–67
    atmosphere and physical surroundings, 57–58
    conditioning and suggestion in, 46–47, 67
    dilatation, mechanics of, 387–89
    doctor–patient relationship, 55–57, 59, 68
    education in (*see also* Education in pregnancy), 38ff., 48ff.
    elation, 4–6, 52–55
    emergency procedures, 234–39
    emotional crises of, 58–59, 62, 71–72, 201, 219–20, 237
    emotions, influence of, 235–36, 377–89
    exultation, 52–53
    first stage, 4, 52–53, 55–67, 196–210
    husbands and, 90–91, 113–14, 116–24, 140–41, 200ff., 212–14
    induced, 297
    injuries, 365
    obstetrical principles, 52
    onset, 4–6, 53–55, 196–97, 234–35
    physiology of (*see also* specific subjects), 362–89
    precipitate, 235
    premature, 126, 138
    psychological responses to, 4–12
    restraints, use of, 48, 342–43, 345
    second stage (amnesia), 7–9, 52–53, 67–78
    third stage, 78–80, 226–30
    urination during, 236
lactation, *see* Breastfeeding
Lamaze, Ferdinand, 305, 326, 328, 330
Lancet, The, 300
Langley, John Baxter, 31, 268, 270, 382
Lanteujoul, Professor, 305
Lewis, Sir Thomas, 32
lightening, 157–58
Lister, Joseph, 26
lochia, 230, 252
London *Daily Mirror*, 309
London *Evening News*, 310–11
London Hospital, 271–72, 280, 282–83
Lorenz, Konrad, 114, 133
love
    birth and, 9–12, 78–80, 380
    emotional development and, 3–4
    mental imagery and, 13
Lurye, Dr., 327

Maloney, James Clark, 133
Manson, Dr., 317
Marshall, Francis H. A., 367, 368
"Maternal Happiness" (address; Grantly Dick-Read), 291
maternity care, *see* Postnatal care and health; Prenatal health and care; specific subjects
Maternity Center Association, 302–3
Mead, Margaret, 113, 133–34
Melbourne (Australia) *Sun*, 309
mental imagery, 13–36
    Christianity, 21–25
    history and, 17–28
    imprinting, 127–29, 133–34, 270
    information sources, 15–17
    love and, 13

mental imagery (cont'd)
  paganism, 20–21
  science and, 25–28
Metallurgic Hospital (Paris), 328
Middle Ages, 21–22
midwives, 18, 22–23, 135
Moffatt Mission (South Africa), 317
Montagu, Ashley, 132
Montessori, Maria, 132
morning sickness, 41–42
Morris, Norman, 134
Motherhood in the Post-War-World (Grantly Dick-Read), 300
muscles
  analgesics, 61
  blood circulation and pain, 32
  nervous system and responses of, 366ff., 384ff.
  pain, and inhibition of reflex relaxation, 375–77
  tension and pain (see also Relaxation), 6, 31–35, 160–61, 286, 291
  uterus, 158–60, 362–63, 366ff.

Natal (South Africa) Daily News, 310
National Health Service (Great Britain), 306
Natural Childbirth (Grantly Dick-Read), 289–92, 302, 327, 392
nausea, 41–42
nervous system
  fear and, 381ff.
  uterine contractions and, 366ff., 378ff.
newborn and their care, 123, 240
  body contact with mother, 226, 240–41
  bottle-feeding, 255
  breastfeeding, see Breastfeeding
  cleaning, 123
  emergency procedures, 238–39
  holding, 123, 238–39
  imprinting and separation, 127–30, 133–34
  immediate routine, 232–33
  potential, developing, 131–34
  presentation to parents, 9, 123–24, 225–26
  rooming-in, 246–47, 249–50, 255–56
  vernix caseosa, 123
  warmth, 123
Nicolayev, A. P., 326, 332
Nightingale, Florence, 25
Ninth British Congress of Obstetrics and Gynecology, 290–91
nurses, nursing care, 37
  attitudes, 5–6
  doctor relationship, 55
  emotional crisis in labor, 200
  labor coaching, 140
  -patient relationship, 54–55
  postpartum education of mother, 141
  prenatal care, 135
  standards, 25
nutrition, 48, 147–48
  breastfeeding and, 256
  education, 137
  first stage of labor, 58, 200
  infant (see also Breastfeeding), 255
  minerals and vitamins, 148
  in nausea, 41–42

obstetricians, 25, 37, 157
  attitudes, 5–6
  education of pregnant women, 40ff.
  examinations in pregnancy, 37–38, 40, 42
  examinations of parturient, 117–18, 199
  -nurse relationship, 55
  objectives of care in pregnancy, 39–40

obstetricians (*cont'd*)
  orthodoxy, need to question,
    354–57
  -patient relationship, 43–44,
    55–57, 59, 68, 296–97
  postnatal visit to, 252
  prenatal care, ideal, 135
  principles of natural childbirth
    in perspective (*see also* spe-
    cific subjects), 103–42
  relaxation, 183
occipito posterior position, 388–
  89

pain, 104–5, 106–12
  absence of in normal course of
    health, 375
  acceptance of necessity of, and
    belief in, 17ff., 27, 284–86
  anesthesia, *see* Anesthesia,
    analgesics
  backache in labor, 62–64, 107–
    8, 236–37
  blood circulation, restricted, 32
  cervical dilation, 7
  "curse of Eve," 23–24, 25
  fear and, 19–21, 30–35, 160–
    61, 235–36, 281, 284–85,
    291, 381–87
  first stage of labor, 6–7
  mental imagery and, 14–15
  moans and, 8–9
  muscular tension, 6, 31–35,
    160–62, 286, 291
  nervous system and, 373ff.
  pathology, 107
  pelvic floor, 71–73, 108
  pubic area, 108
  purpose of, 372–73, 374–75
  receivers (nociceptors), 61,
    373–74
  reflex relaxation of muscles,
    inhibition of, 375–77
  relaxation and, 51
  respiration and, 107
  scars, psychological, 15, 47, 97

  second stage of labor, 8–9
  as term for contraction, 54,
    117
  uterine contractions and, 107,
    373–77
  vulva, 9, 73–74
Paris (France), 305, 326, 328
parasympathetic nervous system,
    and uterine contractions,
    371ff.
Pasteur, Louis, 27
Pavlov, Ivan P., 13–14, 325,
    326–31, 374
pelvis, pelvic muscles
  firming muscles, 194–95, 257
  labor ("work") position exer-
    cise, 194
  nervous system and, 379–80
  pain, 71–73, 108
  pelvic rock exercise, 186, 258
  squatting exercise, 186–87
perineum
  episiotomy, 346–52
  insensitivity, 9
  nervous system and, 379
  repair, 79–80, 225–6
Pfaffenberger, Clarence, 133
physical fitness, 40, 184–85
  exercises, postnatal, 256–59
  exercises, prenatal, 186–95
  fear and, 35
  posture, 185–86, 251, 258–59
physiology of childbirth (*see also*
    stages of labor; specific sub-
    jects)
  contraction, automatic, of
    uterus, 366–69
  emotions, influences of on
    labor, 377–89
  sympathetic stimuli, effects of,
    369–77
  uterus and birth canal, struc-
    ture of, 362–65
placenta, 154–55
  afterbirth, 78–79, 228–30, 248

placenta (*cont'd*)
  afterbirth, African tribal atti-
    tudes toward, 321
  hemorrhage, postpartum, 380–
    81
Platonov, 326
Polynesia, 113
population explosion, 131
Portugal, 334
postnatal care and health, 251–52
  afterpains, 252
  breastfeeding, *see* Breastfeed-
    ing
  diet, 256
  exercise, 256–59
  household chores, 251–52
  lochia, 252
  obstetrician, visit to, 252
  rooming-in, 246–47, 249–50,
    255–56
posture, 185–86, 251, 258–59
pregnancy, 37ff., 84
  anemias, 44–46
  clothing, 148–49
  coitus during, 42–43
  culture vs. natural law, 28–30
  discomforts of, 35, 41–42
  education in, *see* Education in
    pregnancy; specific subjects
  exercises, 184–95
  family relationships in, 81ff.
  fertilization process, 152–54
  fetus, development of, 154–56,
    157
  full term, 196
  health of mother and child, 86
  high-risk, 127, 135
  hygiene, personal, 149–51
  lightening, 157–58
  nutrition, 41–42, 48, 147–48
  obstetrician (*see also* Obstetri-
    cians), 157
  physical examinations, 37–38,
    40, 42
  prenatal care, 130–31, 134–38
  prudery concerning, 81, 88

  psychological manifestations
    of, 84ff.
  quickening, 42
  superstitions, 85
  uterus in, 156–58
prematurity, 126, 138
prenatal health and care (*see also*
    Education in pregnancy;
    Pregnancy; specific sub-
    jects), 146–47
  clothing, 148–49
  hygiene, 149–51
  nutrition, 41–42, 48, 147–48
  program, ideal, 134–38
  updating, 130–31
primitive societies, 17, 20–21,
    28–30, 105, 112, 317–23,
    336–37, 352
"Prophylaxis of Fear" (address;
    Grantly Dick-Read), 290
"Psychological Aspects of Ma-
    ternal Welfare" (address;
    Grantly Dick-Read), 291
psychoprophylaxis, 326–32
psychosomatics, 30

quickening, 42

racism, 337–38
Rein, Hermann F., 366
relaxation (*see also* First stage of
    labor), 6–7, 56–58, 112–13,
    168–69, 205–6
  breathing, 177–78
  crowning, 220–21
  education in, 50–51, 137, 169–
    83
  facial, 171–72, 205
  fear and, 50–51
  milk flow, 254
  of obstetrician, 183
  positions for, 178–79
  practicing, 173–77
  preparation for, 169–70
  recognition of tension, 170–73,
    179–83

relaxation (*cont'd*)
  residual tension, 179–83
  second stage, 211, 216–18
religion
  Christianity, 21–25, 35, 285–
    86
  fear and, 20–21, 285–86
  pagan, 20–21
  spirituality of childbirth, 11–
    12, 35–36
respiration, 107, 108, 162–63
  breath-holding, 166–67
  education, 40, 164–67
  first stage of labor, 67, 204–5
  full deep, 164, 257
  hyperventilation, 125
  rapid, 167
  relaxation, 177–78
  second stage of labor, 67–68,
    69, 74, 216, 220
  "sleep" breathing, 164–66
  "work" breathing, 164
Revelation of Childbirth, The
    (Grantly Dick-Read), 300–
    2, 309, 392
Revue Nouvelle Médécine, 329–
    30
Ribble, Margaret A., 94*n*., 132,
    133, 245*n*.
Richardson, Stephen A., 134
Rivers, William H. R., 269
Roesslin, Eucharius, 22
Roman Empire, 21
Roth, Lawrence, D., 324
Routh, Charles H. F., 367
Russia, 324–32

Sawyer, Blackwell, 306
Scandinavia, 334
science
  advances in, 25–28
  religion and, 35–36
Schmidt, 367
Scientific Council of the U.S.S.R.
    Ministry of Public Health,
    325–26

Scott, John Paul, 133
second stage of labor, 211, 224
  amnesia and alienation, 7–9,
    52–53, 68–71, 74, 212
  bearing down, 7, 68–69, 72, 73,
    74, 118–22, 221, 237–38
  birth, 74, 122–24, 221–22
  crowning, 73–74, 122, 220–21,
    237, 238
  early, 211–16
  emergency procedures, 237–39
  emotional crises, 71–72, 73–
    74, 219–20
  moans, 8–9
  pain relief, *see* Anesthesia and
    analgesia
  perineum, 9, 221
  position, 118, 214, 350
  relaxation, 211, 216–18, 220–
    21
  respiration, 67–68, 69, 74, 216,
    220
  sleep, 7, 68, 212
  umbilical cord, 74, 123
  vulva, 9, 73–74
  well-established, 216–20
Semmelweis, Ignaz Philip, 26
Seventh-Day Adventist Mission
    Hospital (South Africa),
    317
sex education, 100
Shabanah, E. H., 385–86*n*.
Sherrington, Sir Charles Scott,
    374, 382
Shipley, Arthur Everett, 268
Simpson, James Young, 25
show, 197, 235
skin, care of, 149
Soranus of Ephesus, 19, 21, 22,
    23
South Africa, 306, 308–16, 324
South African Medical and Den-
    tal Council, 310–12
South America, 334
Soviet Union, 324–32
Spain, 334

spirituality of childbirth, 11–12, 35–36
Sunday Pictorial, 310
sympathetic nervous system
  emotions and, 372
  fear, influence of, 31–33, 381ff.
  uterine contractions, 366ff., 378ff.
sympathy, 6

tension, muscular
  pain and, 6, 31–35, 160–61, 286, 291, 370ff.
  recognition of, 170–73, 179–83
  relaxation, *see* Relaxation
teeth, care of, 150
third stage of labor (exaltation) (*see also* Newborn), 78–80
  afterbirth, 78–79, 228–30
  emergency procedures, 238–39
  lochia, 230
  maternal love, 78
  perineum, repair of, 79–80, 225–26
  return to room after birth, 124
  shivering attacks, 226–28
  uterus, 78, 79, 226
Thoms, Herbert, 324
Time magazine, 85n.

umbilical cord, 74, 123, 154–55
  emergency procedures, 238–39
United States, 301–5, 306, 324, 333–53, 393
urethritis, 376
urination
  during labor, 236
  frequency in pregnancy, 42
U.S.S.R., 324–32
U.S.S.R. Academy of Medical Science, 325
uterus
  abdominal supports, 149
  afterbirth, 78–79
  afterpains, 252

bearing down, and prolapse of, 321
blood circulation, 31
breastfeeding and, 94–95
cervix, *see* Cervix, cervical canal
contractions, nervous system and, 366ff., 378ff.
contractions, pain and, 107
fear reactions, 31–33, 235
fetus, 154–56
first stage of labor, 6
inhibition of contractions, 367, 370
in pregnancy, 156–58
involution, 95
ischemic, 32
muscle structure of, 158–60, 362–63
nerve supply of, 369–71
onset of labor, 53–54
pain receptors (nociceptors), 373–74
third stage of labor, 78, 79, 226

vagina, 96, 195, 364
  nerve supply, 370
  vaginismus, 376
varicose veins, 195
Vellay, Pierre, 326, 330
Velvosky, Dr., 325, 326
vernix caseosa, 123
vulva, 9, 73–74, 365

waters, bag of, 53, 58, 154, 197, 218, 235
Weiss, Dr., of Hamburg, 22
Wessel, Helen, 24n., 350n.
Whitehouse, Beckwith, 366–67, 368–69, 370
witchcraft, 17
Wolfe, Julius, 374

Zimmerman, 367